Pediatric Considerations in Disaster Settings

Lisa Umphrey • Joseph Wathen
Conrad W. Wanyama • Dan Alaro
Celia Wanda Kariuki • Caren Ito Emadau
Rosemarie Gachie-Lopokoiyit
Editors

Pediatric Considerations in Disaster Settings

A Concise Guide to Advocating
for Children's Needs

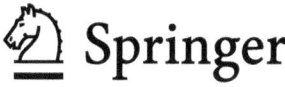

Springer

Editors
Lisa Umphrey
Center for Global Health
Children's Hospital Colorado
Aurora, CO, USA

Joseph Wathen
Emergency Medicine
University of Colorado Anschutz Medical
Aurora, CO, USA

Conrad W. Wanyama
KEMRI-Wellcome Trust
Kilifi and Nairobi, Kenya

Dan Alaro
Kenya Pediatric Association
Nairobi, Kenya

Celia Wanda Kariuki
Mama Lucy Kibaki Hospital
Nairobi, Kenya

Caren Ito Emadau
Pumwani Maternity and Referral Hospital
Nairobi, Kenya

Rosemarie Gachie-Lopokoiyit
The Pediatric Clinic Karen
Nairobi, Kenya

ISBN 978-3-031-85500-9   ISBN 978-3-031-85501-6   (eBook)
https://doi.org/10.1007/978-3-031-85501-6

This Springer imprint is published by the registered company Springer Nature Switzerland AG
The registered company address is: Gewerbestrasse 11, 6330 Cham, Switzerland

If disposing of this product, please recycle the paper.

Contents

Chapter 1
Understanding Disasters: Exploring Core Definitions and Concepts

Israa Khan, Geoffrey Winstanley, Jessica Landry, Stephen Berman, and Lisa Umphrey

Definition of Disasters

Objectives

- Identify events that have the potential to cause disasters
- Describe the individual and social factors that contribute to vulnerability, coping mechanisms, and risk

Definitions

What defines an event as a disaster? Why is one hurricane or tornado considered a disaster, while another with even stronger winds is merely labeled a bad storm? The key lies in how the population is affected, both directly and indirectly, including damage to infrastructure. According to the United Nations International Strategy for Disaster Reduction (UNISDR), a disaster is a serious disruption in the functioning of a community or society due to hazardous events interacting with exposure,

I. Khan (✉) · J. Landry · L. Umphrey
Department of Pediatrics, Section of Hospital Medicine, University of Colorado School of Medicine Anschutz Medical Campus, Aurora, CO, USA
e-mail: Israa.khan@childrenscolorado.org

G. Winstanley
Center for Global Health, Aurora, CO, USA

S. Berman
University of Colorado School of Medicine, Aurora, CO, USA

Department of Epidemiology, Colorado School of Public Health, Aurora, CO, USA

© The Author(s), under exclusive license to Springer Nature Switzerland AG 2025
L. Umphrey et al. (eds.), *Pediatric Considerations in Disaster Settings*,
https://doi.org/10.1007/978-3-031-85501-6_1

vulnerability, and capacity, leading to human, material, economic, and environmental losses (UNISDR 2009). In 2019, the acronym was officially changed to UNDRR (United Nations Office for Disaster Risk Reduction) from UNISDR to better reflect its name but the definition remains the same.

Disasters are often seen as a combination of three factors: (1) exposure to a hazard, (2) the presence of vulnerability, and (3) insufficient capacity or measures to manage or mitigate the consequences. The impacts of a disaster may include loss of life, injury, disease, and harm to the physical, mental, and social well-being of affected individuals. Additionally, there can be significant damage to property, destruction of assets, loss of services, social and economic disruption, and environmental degradation. Disasters interrupt normal life, causing physical and emotional distress, an overwhelming sense of helplessness, and, frequently, a need for external assistance due to the magnitude of the damage.

Although there are many ways to define disasters, they generally have three defining elements. First, an event or phenomenon significantly impacts a population or environment. Second, certain vulnerabilities or conditions exacerbate the impact. For example, a hurricane causes far more damage in areas with poorly constructed infrastructure compared to regions with well-built structures. Identifying these vulnerabilities is crucial for preparedness and disaster prevention. Third, local resources are often insufficient to address the problems caused by the event. Disasters frequently overwhelm healthcare systems, not only causing unexpected deaths but also creating large numbers of wounded and sick who exceed the community's healthcare capacity. Clinics and hospitals may be damaged or destroyed, and medical personnel directly affected, which hampers recovery efforts and increases morbidity and mortality.

A clear example of this dynamic is the 2023 earthquake in Turkey and Syria [27]. The 7.8 magnitude quake caused over 56,000 deaths in both countries. Even before the earthquake, 4.1 million people in affected areas of Syria required humanitarian assistance, a situation worsened by ongoing conflict, economic instability, and inflation. The earthquake damaged 55 health facilities in northwest Syria, suspending services in 15 of them, severely restricting access to healthcare. With aftershocks continuing, some areas resorted to using tent hospitals as safer alternatives to unstable buildings. This disaster demonstrates how preexisting burdens on the medical system, combined with external assistance challenges, can intensify the chaos and fragmentation of the response (United Nations Office for the Coordination of Humanitarian Affairs [UNOCHA] 2023). See Table 1.1 for other examples of recent disasters.

An important illustration of these dynamics is shown in Fig. 1.1, which highlights the relationships among hazards, vulnerabilities, and capacities in the context of disaster impact.

Similarly, pandemics, such as the COVID-19 pandemic (2020) and epidemics such as the Ebola epidemic in West Africa (2014–2016), can overwhelm even well-functioning healthcare systems by sharply increasing the demand for medical care. These disasters, initially local, can expand to become global crises. During the COVID-19 pandemic, despite displays of resilience and adaptation, many people

Table 1.1 Examples of Natural Disasters

Type of disaster	Location	Date	People affected	Death toll
Heatwaves	South Asia (India and Pakistan)	March–May 2022[a]	Millions	90
Earthquakes	Morocco	September 2023	500,000	2946
Floods	Libya	September 2023	884,000	11,300
	China	July 2023	Four million	51
	Pakistan	June–November 2022	33 million	1739
	East Africa (Kenya, Ethiopia, Uganda, Tanzania, Burundi, and Somalia)	May 2024	1.6 million	473
	Brazil	April–May 2024	Two million	172
Wildfires	California	June–November 2023	500,433	4
Volcanic eruptions	Mount Nyiragongo, Democratic Republic of Congo	May 2021	400,000	32
	Hunga Ha'apai, Tonga, South Pacific Ocean	January 2022	84,176	4
Tornadoes	Northeastern Texas, southeastern Oklahoma, Southwestern Arkansas, and Northwestern Louisiana (30 tornadoes were recorded)	November 2022	28 million	2
Pandemic	Worldwide	December 2019—ongoing	771 million cases	Approximately seven million

Sources:
https://www.fema.gov/disaster/current
https://www.climate.gov/news-features/blogs/beyond-data/2022-us-billion-dollar-weather-and-climate-disasters-historical
https://reliefweb.int/disasters
[a]There have been ongoing annual heatwaves in South and Southeast Asia (India, Pakistan, Bangladesh, Thailand, Lao PDR, Myanmar, and Cambodia)

suffered from fatigue, cognitive impairments, anxiety, and a sense of hopelessness. This led to a phenomenon known as a "foreshortened future," where individuals could no longer envision their future or plan for it, such as by pursuing education, employment, or marriage [28]. Disasters, therefore, can significantly increase vulnerability and have lasting psychological, social, and economic impacts (World Health Organization [WHO] 2021; Centers for Disease Control and Prevention [CDC] 2022).

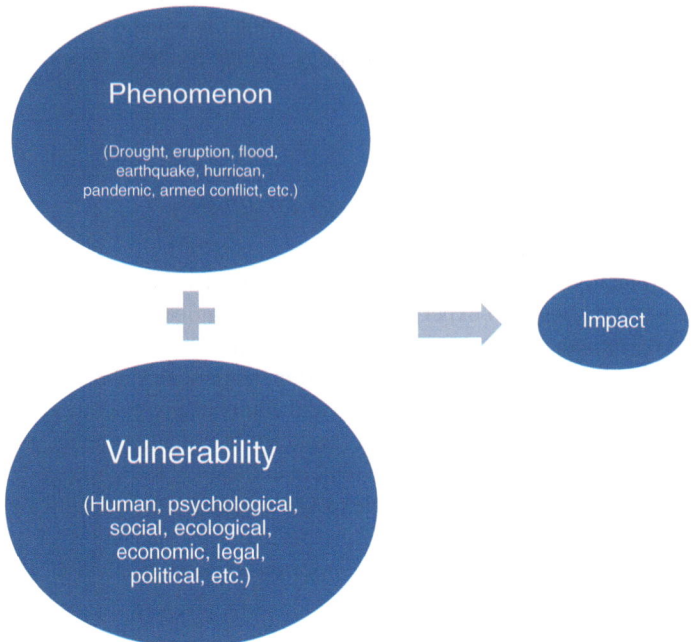

Fig. 1.1 Framework of disaster components

Classification of Disasters

Disasters can be categorized into two broad groups: those caused by natural forces and those resulting from human activities.

1. Natural Disasters

   Natural disasters arise from natural phenomena, including earthquakes, volcanic eruptions, hurricanes, wildfires, tornadoes, and extreme weather conditions. They can be classified into rapid onset disasters, such as earthquakes and tsunamis, and those with a more gradual onset, like droughts that lead to food insecurity, malnutrition, or famine. For instance, in February 2023, a devastating earthquake struck Turkey and Syria, with a magnitude of 7.8, resulting in over 56,000 deaths and displacing millions [27]. Similarly, Hurricane Ian impacted Florida in September 2022, causing significant flooding and destruction, with damages estimated at $50 billion. Despite advancements in technology, accurately predicting the climatic and geological changes that can trigger disasters remains a significant challenge. Consequently, preparing for natural disasters continues to pose difficulties.

The unpredictability of these events highlights the necessity for countries to develop effective disaster-response plans and mobilize resources swiftly and efficiently. Establishing a well-defined organizational structure is also crucial for coordinating national and international assistance. While certain regions of the world have made significant strides in sanitation and disaster response, developing countries remain highly vulnerable due to their fragile economies, healthcare systems, and transportation infrastructure. In recent years, the occurrence of disasters, the human toll in terms of those affected and fatalities, and the economic losses attributed to these events have risen steadily on a global scale, as illustrated in Figs. 1.2 and 1.3.

2. Human-Made Disasters

Human-made disasters result from human actions, whether intentional or unintentional. They can be subdivided into three main categories:

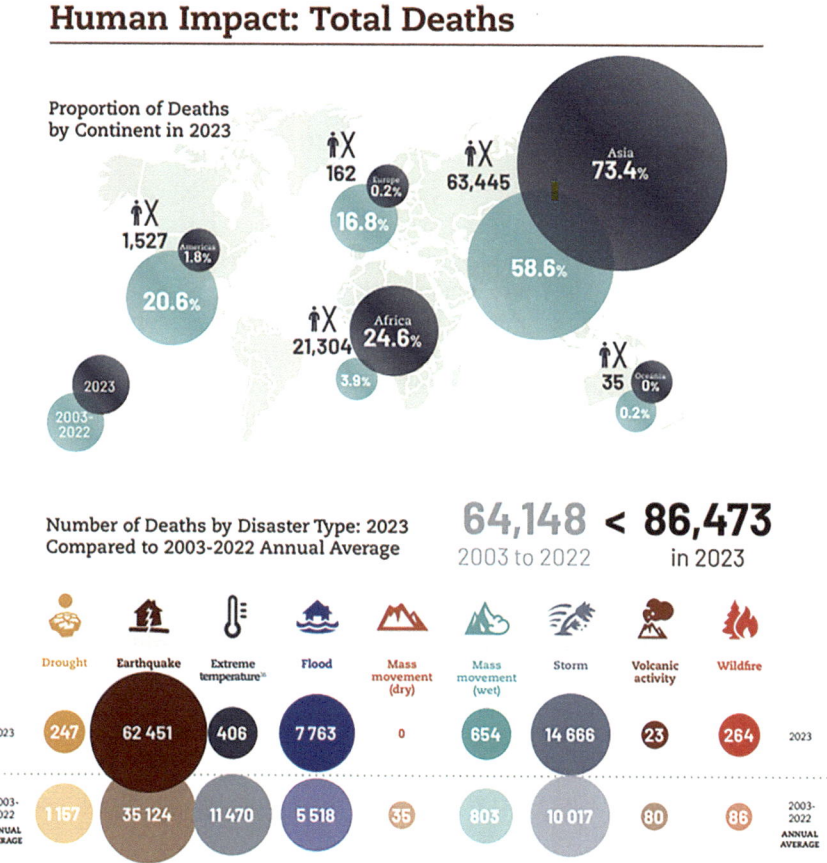

Fig. 1.2 Human impacts of disasters in 2023—total deaths. (*Source: OCHA—CRED. 2023: Disasters in numbers. Brussels: CRED, 2024. This document is available at* https://files.emdat.be/reports/2023_EMDAT_report.pdf)

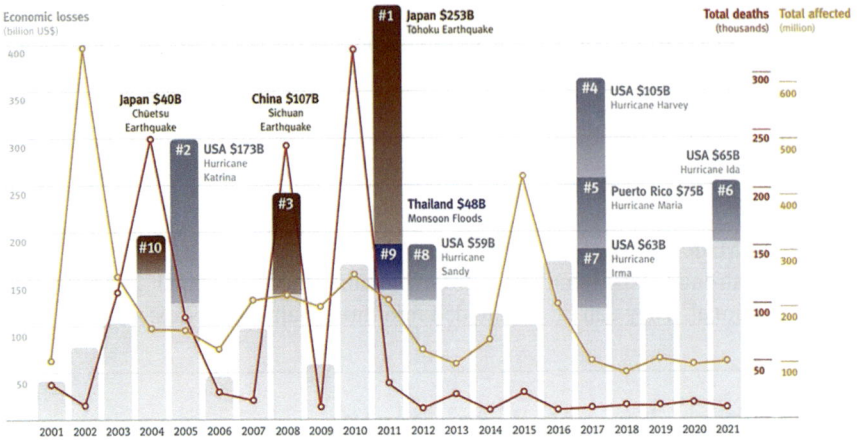

Fig. 1.3 Top 10 economic losses and disaster trends (2001–2021). (*Source: 2021 Disasters in numbers: extreme events defining our lives:* https://www.cred.be/sites/default/files/2021_EMDAT_report.pdf)

1. *Technological Disasters*

    Unregulated industrialization and inadequate safety standards have increased the risk of technological or industrial disasters, which may include infrastructure failures, power outages, or hazardous material leaks [7]. Recent examples include the train derailment in East Palestine, Ohio, in February 2023, which resulted in the release of toxic chemicals, and the chemical spill in Palestine in July 2023, which led to widespread environmental contamination. Although these disasters occurred recently, their impacts may last for years and continue to affect the health of the local populations.

2. *Armed Conflict and Violence*

    Human-made disasters can also include events such as mass shootings, intentional fires, mutinies, and suicide bombings. Armed conflicts lead to broader societal breakdowns, impacting governance, social protection, economies, pediatric healthcare and essential services while causing prolonged population displacement [4–6]. Recent armed conflicts in Ukraine, starting in February 2022, have resulted in widespread violence and the displacement of millions, particularly affecting children who may become victims of violence or be forced to participate in hostilities. The number of children affected by armed conflict has increased steadily in recent years due to population growth, urbanization of war, and a rising number of global conflicts [8, 10, 14, 24, 26].

3. *Complex Humanitarian Emergencies*

    The term "complex humanitarian emergency" refers to crises stemming from international or civil wars. These situations typically result in the mass displacement of people from their homes due to safety concerns. Ongoing conflicts in Syria, which began in 2011, have led to the displacement of millions and disrupted essential services, including food distribution, water supply, electricity, and sanitation . Communities may find themselves stranded and isolated, unable to access necessary assistance. Such emergencies are frequently marked by a breakdown in social and physical infrastructure, including healthcare systems. Furthermore, implementing any emergency response in these contexts can be challenging due to political instability and unsafe environments.

Displaced Populations

Natural disasters and complex emergencies can compel individuals to leave their homes in search of safety elsewhere. The United Nations High Commissioner for Refugees (UNHCR) has a primary mission to protect the rights and well-being of people who have been forced to flee, including their right to seek asylum and find refuge in another country. Among the groups that UNHCR supports are refugees and internally displaced persons (IDPs). Figure 1.4 illustrates trends concerning refugees, asylum-seekers, and IDPs who require protection; Fig. 1.5 illustrates the number of people in need of international protection.

Refugees often escape their home countries due to war, violence, famine, or a well-founded fear of persecution based on political, ethnic, religious, or national grounds. Individuals recognized as refugees are entitled to specific protections under international humanitarian law. In contrast, IDPs leave their homes for similar reasons but do not cross international borders, which complicates their legal protection and assistance. As of 2023, UNHCR estimates indicate there are 36.4 million refugees and 62.5 million IDPs globally. Furthermore, approximately 110 million people were forcibly displaced worldwide by mid-2023 due to persecution, conflict,

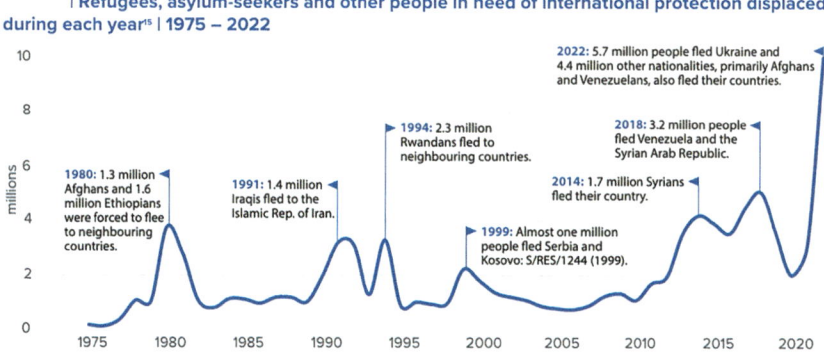

Fig. 1.4 Refugees, asylum-seekers, and other people in need of international protection displaced each year (1975–2022). (*Source: UNHCR Global Trends Report 2022:* https://www.unhcr.org/global-trends-report-2022)

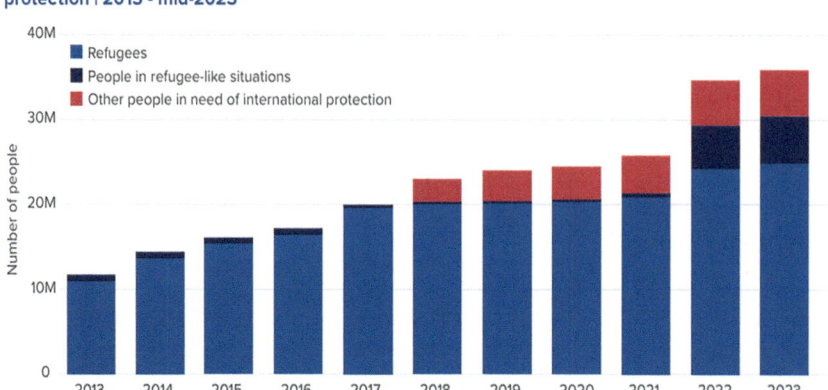

Fig. 1.5 Refugees, people in refugee-like situations, and other people in need of international protection (2013–2023). (*Source: UNHCR Global Trends Report 2023:* https://www.unhcr.org/sites/default/files/2023-10/Mid-year-trends-2023.pdf)

violence, human rights violations, or disruptions to public order. Notably, 52% of all refugees and individuals seeking international protection originate from just three countries: the Syrian Arab Republic (6.5 million), Afghanistan (6.1 million), and Ukraine (5.9 million).

Refugee and migrant women and children face unique challenges and protection risks while in transit. These challenges include family separation, psychosocial stress and trauma, health complications—especially for pregnant women—physical harm, and increased risks of exploitation, and gender-based violence. Women often serve as primary caregivers for children and elderly family members, which heightens their need for protection and support [9, 11]. Figure 1.6 depicts the age distribution of displaced persons in 2020.

The ethical, rapid, and culturally sensitive resettlement of refugees and other forcibly displaced populations requires global solidarity and a shared responsibility among the international community. This entails efforts to alleviate the burden on host countries, enhance refugee self-reliance, advocate for governments to accept fleeing families, and establish supportive conditions in countries of origin to facilitate safe and dignified voluntary returns.

Phases of Disasters

Since interventions in emergencies develop along a continuum Disastersphases, it is beneficial to categorize Pediatric disasters into four phases. This approach helps establish priorities and response activities, as well as systematize previous experiences [13] (see Fig. 1.7).

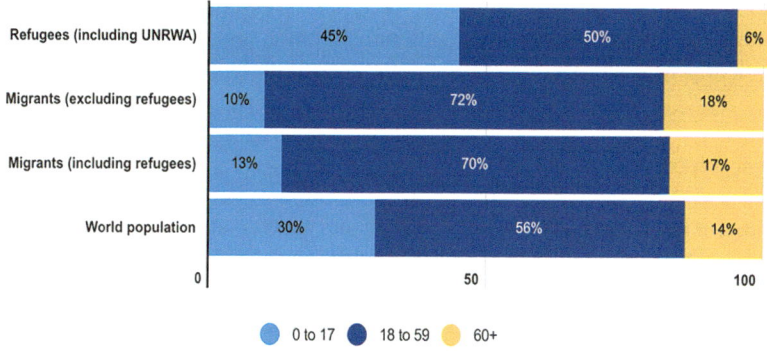

Fig. 1.6 Age distribution of refugees, international migrants, and total population (2020) as a percentage

Fig. 1.7 Phases of disaster management

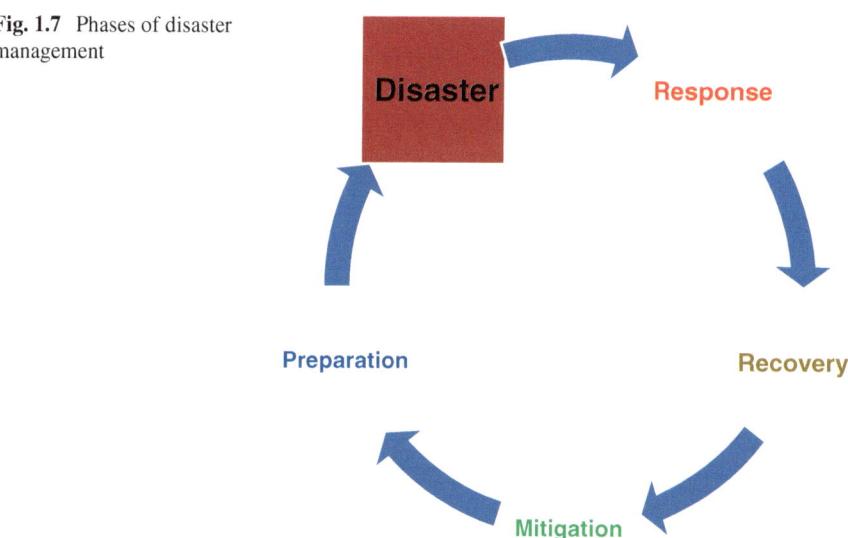

Preparedness Phase

This phase includes all planning, activities, and actions undertaken before or in anticipation of a disaster. Effective planning should be informed by an analysis of the community or organization's risk of exposure to specific disaster types. Preparedness plans must consider the frequency of each disaster, the expected magnitude of its effects, and the degree of advanced warning or suddenness of its onset and conclusion. Additionally, it is essential to assess the characteristics of populations most likely to be impacted, the types and amounts of resources available within the community or organizational structure, and the capacity to operate independently without external support for extended periods.

Response Phase

The response phase encompasses all activities and actions taken during and immediately after a disaster. This includes notifying the organizations involved in disaster response, establishing initial communication networks, conducting search and rescue operations, assessing damage, evacuating individuals, providing shelter, and carrying out various other activities. The response phase continues until initial casualties have been either rescued or officially acknowledged as lost, and sufficient resources are available to address the immediate humanitarian needs of the affected population.

This phase should persist until a comprehensive damage assessment has been completed, while simultaneously initiating plans for restoration and recovery. In conflict situations, displacement may be prolonged until safety and security are restored in the affected individuals' place of origin. For those impacted, response services may need to be offered in camps or short-term shelters, which are designed to accommodate them for limited durations. While normalcy typically returns within days to weeks following most natural disasters, in the case of conflict, it may take several years before individuals are able to return to their homes.

Recovery Phase

The recovery phase is the period during which the affected organization or community strives to reestablish self-sufficiency. This phase involves new community planning, rebuilding efforts, and the restoration of government functionality and public service infrastructure. As recovery progresses, the health status of the affected population begins to return to pre-disaster conditions, and external support services are gradually phased out.

Mitigation and Prevention Phase

This phase typically occurs when conditions are beginning to revert to their pre-disaster state. Mitigation involves a thorough examination of all aspects of emergency management to identify "lessons learned." These insights are then applied to prevent the recurrence of the disaster or to minimize the impact of future events. Mitigation encompasses preventive and precautionary measures, such as revising building codes, redesigning public utilities and services, evaluating mandatory evacuation procedures and warning policies, and educating community members. Both mitigation and preparedness are ongoing processes, as insights gained from previous disasters inform planning for future ones.

Effects of Disasters

Disasters impact communities in numerous ways, presenting significant public health hazards for various reasons. They can result in an unexpected number of deaths and injuries that surpass the local resources' capacity to respond, necessitating external assistance. Additionally, disasters can devastate health infrastructure, hindering immediate response efforts and disrupting preventive activities, which can lead to long-term increases in morbidity and mortality. They may also have detrimental effects on the environment, raising the risk of infectious and transmissible diseases, thereby affecting overall health, causing premature deaths, and diminishing future quality of life. Furthermore, disasters can influence the psychological and social behaviors of communities, create food shortages with severe nutritional implications, and trigger large-scale population movements—both spontaneous and organized—to areas where health services may be overwhelmed by the increased demand.

Mortality Considerations in Disasters

Objectives

- Recognize crude mortality and under-5 mortality rates as indicators of disaster severity
- Identify the environmental factors linked to increased morbidity and mortality rates
- Describe the five leading causes of death in humanitarian emergencies in developing countries

Severity of a Disaster

The 2023 earthquakes that struck Turkey and Syria illustrated how various factors can independently escalate the severity of a disaster. These factors include the population's health and socioeconomic conditions, inadequate preexisting infrastructure, and the magnitude of the event itself. Consequently, the severity of a disaster fluctuates based on its intensity and the vulnerability of the affected population.

For instance, earthquakes of similar magnitude can have markedly different outcomes depending on the region. The earthquakes in China (2008), Haiti (2010), and Turkey (2023) led to numerous collapsed structures, including schools and hospitals, resulting in a higher casualty rate. In contrast, earthquakes of comparable magnitude in Tokyo (2009) and Chile (2010), along with the Turkish earthquake in 2023, caused significantly fewer fatalities, largely due to the implementation of earthquake-resistant building techniques and stringent construction codes.

Public health officials often utilize the Crude Death Rate (CDR), also known as the Crude Mortality Rate (CMR), as a key metric for assessing the severity of a disaster based on the number of lives lost. The CMR serves as a vital statistics summary rate that reflects the number of deaths occurring within a population during a specified time frame, typically a calendar year. It is defined as the number of deaths in a specific geographical area within a year per 1000 individuals in that area at mid-year. To calculate the CMR, the total number of deaths is divided by the total population, and this figure is then multiplied by 10,000. The CMR can be expressed in various units, such as deaths per 10,000 per day, deaths per 1000 per month, or deaths per 1000 per year.

As a rough indicator of mortality rates within a country, the CMR is significantly influenced by the age distribution of the population. Many countries will eventually experience an overall rise in the death rate, despite ongoing reductions in mortality across all age groups. This trend is primarily driven by declining fertility rates and increased life expectancy, leading to an aging population. In developing nations, the typical CMR ranges from 0.4 to 0.7 deaths per day per 10,000 people. A CMR exceeding 1 death per 10,000 people per day or an under-5 mortality rate (U5MR) of more than 2 deaths per 10,000 per day was once regarded as the standard threshold for indicating a humanitarian emergency. However, as baseline mortality rates have significantly decreased since this standard was established, it is no longer adequate for evaluating the need for humanitarian interventions. For example, the global U5MR fell by 60%, from 93 deaths per 1000 live births in 1990 to 37 in 2022. Despite this progress, enhancing child survival rates continues to be an urgent priority.

Today, we focus on assessing the increase in CMR compared to a baseline, the duration of this increase, and the number of people affected. To evaluate the progression of a disaster and the effectiveness of relief efforts, it is essential to monitor the CMR over several relevant time intervals. For example, following the mass movement of Rwandan refugees into Eastern Zaire (now the Democratic Republic of the Congo) after the Rwandan genocide, the CMR in that region surged to 40 to 60 times above the corresponding reference value. Typically, the CMR peaks during the initial phase of a disaster.

Vulnerable Victims

Most diseases linked to disaster events can be effectively prevented through adequate interventions, particularly by addressing the basic lifesaving needs of the affected population. These essential needs encompass shelter, food, clean water, sanitation, healthcare services, and security measures. While immediate mortality rates during any disaster do not disproportionately affect a specific age group, the overall population tends to bear the brunt of these fatalities. However, in the aftermath of such events, the mortality rate often rises significantly among the most vulnerable populations.

The groups at greatest risk include children—especially those separated from their families—pregnant and breastfeeding women, individuals without a spouse or support system, single-headed households led by women, disabled persons, and the elderly. Children who are separated from their families face not only an elevated mortality rate but also an increased likelihood of experiencing various adverse outcomes, such as rape, torture, robbery, exploitation through child labor, child trafficking, and recruitment as child soldiers [4, 15]. Furthermore, due to specific physical and physiological characteristics, infants and children are particularly susceptible to exposure to toxic substances [7] and the challenges posed by overcrowding during the displacement of large populations (see Table 1.2).

During the 1991 northern Iraq refugee crisis, which followed Iraq's invasion of Kuwait, children aged 0 to 5 made up only 18% of the total refugee population, yet they accounted for a staggering 64% of the overall refugee mortality rate (see Fig. 1.8). More recently, conflicts in Gaza resulted in the deaths or injuries of 26,000 children, representing just over 2% of Gaza's child population, further devastating the already fragile health system and disrupting access to education [17, 19]. Box 1.1 outlines several mitigating factors that can help reduce the vulnerability of children during times of disaster or conflict.

Table 1.2 Characteristics contributing to the vulnerability of children

Pediatric body system affected	Risks during a disaster
Respiratory	Higher minute volume increases the risk of exposure to inhaled agents. Nuclear fallout and heavier gases settle lower to the ground and may affect children more severely
Gastrointestinal	Higher risk for dehydration from vomiting and diarrhea after exposure to contamination
Skin	Higher body surface area increases risk for skin exposure. Skin is thinner and more susceptible to injury from burns, chemicals, and absorbable toxins. Evaporation loss is higher when skin is wet or cold, so hypothermia is more likely
Endocrine	Increased risk for thyroid cancer from radiation exposure
Thermoregulation	Less able to cope with temperature problems, with higher risk for hypothermia
Developmental	Lower ability to escape environmental dangers or anticipate hazards
Psychological	Prolonged stress from critical events. Susceptible to separation anxiety

Adapted from AAP [2]

Fig. 1.8 Mortality rate among per age group refugee crisis in Northern Iraq—1991. *(Source: Mahar, Patrick & Lynch, Julia & Wathen, Joe & Tham, Eric & Berman, Stephen. Module 1 Disasters and their Effects on Children: Key Concepts)*

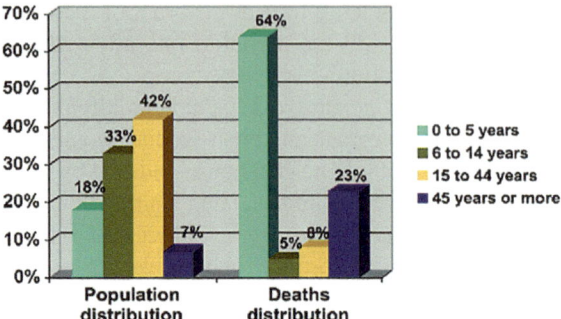

Box 1.1 Immediate Measures to Reduce Children's Vulnerability During a Disaster
- List children in the community.
- Provide visible identification tags to all children.
- Identify community leaders capable of taking care of individuals or groups of children.
- Guarantee the care and safety of refugees to provide the safest possible environment for children.
- Consider vulnerable children when planning the distribution systems.
- Assign priority to the search for parents or families of unaccompanied children.
- Post in a central place the photographs of children separated from their families to enhance their identification.
- Make sure that camps or shelters, if needed, are located as near the affected areas as possible.
- Place families and groups of neighbors together.

Causes of Mortality

The primary objective of any intervention during humanitarian emergencies is to minimize the number of deaths. While both conflict and natural disasters can lead to immediate fatalities, many preventable deaths occur in the later phases of a disaster over an extended period.

Research has consistently identified five leading medical issues as the main causes of mortality among vulnerable populations in post-war or post-natural disaster contexts [21]. Figure 1.9 illustrates the leading causes of death in children under the age of five.

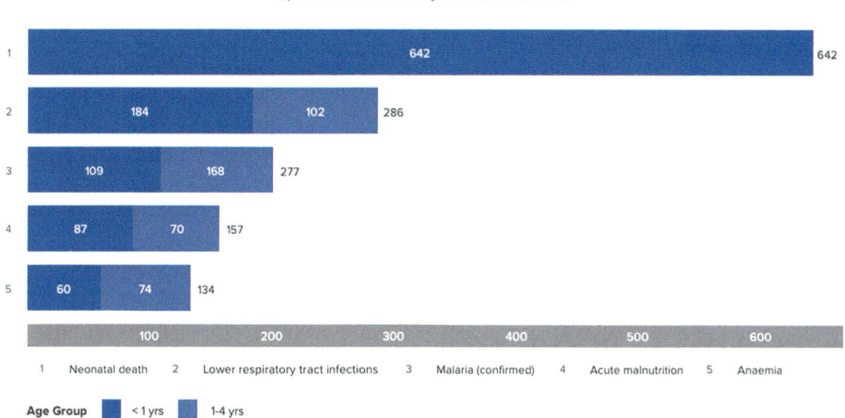

Fig. 1.9 Top Five Causes of Mortality in Children Under 5 Years. (*Source:* Liu et al. [21])

Strategies for Emergency Relief in Disaster Situations

Objectives

- Describe the ten essential emergency relief measures as defined by the World Health Organization
- Describe how these measures should be applied within the community

Every disaster or humanitarian emergency presents a distinct scenario shaped by the triggering event, climate, geography, culture, social structure, and the preexisting conditions of the affected population. Consequently, national and international organizations should prioritize conducting a rapid assessment before rushing to respond, as it is essential to gather critical information first. Interventions based on speculation rather than accurate data risk wasting time and valuable resources, ultimately exacerbating the suffering of those impacted [23]. Although similar disasters tend to follow predictable patterns of disruption, as illustrated in Table 1.2, the severity of the event and the corresponding response can vary significantly based on local characteristics.

An effective response must align with the specific needs of the local community, region, and nation, adapting continuously through ongoing reassessment. Historical data from previous disasters may not accurately predict the most pressing needs in future situations. For instance, while safe water supply is typically unaffected by mudslides, if the regional water pumping or purification system is directly compromised, addressing the ensuing shortage of safe water becomes critical to preventing disease outbreaks and excessive mortality.

The timing of resource deployment is another crucial factor to consider. Trauma is a leading cause of death in the immediate aftermath of earthquakes. If trauma surgery teams and field hospitals are deployed a week after the event, the majority of trauma-related fatalities will likely have already occurred, diminishing the effectiveness of these costly and resource-intensive interventions [3].

The World Health Organization (WHO) and the Pan-American Health Organization (PAHO) have established guidelines for the appropriate use of field hospitals in sudden-impact disasters (for further details, visit www.paho.org/disasters).

Essential Emergency Relief Measures

1. *Conduct a Rapid Assessment of the Emergency Situation and Affected Population*: A swift and accurate assessment is crucial for identifying available resources, unmet needs, and imminent risks facing the affected population. This information enables optimal use of available resources.

   (a) *National Level*: Assessments are generally performed by expert teams tasked with quickly defining the magnitude of the emergency, evaluating environmental conditions, assessing infrastructure damage, identifying health and nutrition needs, and gauging local response capacity.

   (b) *Community Level*: In the immediate aftermath of a disaster, local resources will primarily drive the initial response. Communities must be equipped to conduct local assessments of the disaster's impact. Healthcare professionals should be prepared to evaluate health issues within their communities and develop mechanisms for disseminating this information to contribute to regional or national assessments. Ongoing assessments should inform both rescue and recovery efforts, and re-evaluations should occur whenever significant changes arise. The quality and specificity of collected data should be maximized to the extent possible. Resource managers utilize this information to determine how to allocate resources during large-scale disasters.

2. *Provide Adequate Shelter and Clothing*: Inadequate shelter can lead to exposure to extreme weather conditions, resulting in preventable deaths after disasters. Proper shelter can also help lower the caloric needs of affected populations and reduce disease transmission.

   (a) *Community Level*: Ensure that all individuals have access to sufficient shelter that provides adequate personal space and climate-appropriate protection. Short-term shelters should prioritize vulnerable populations while keeping individuals close to their communities and family networks. Resources should generally focus on rebuilding within the community instead of creating large camps or temporary settlements outside the disaster area.

3. *Ensure Adequate Nutrition*: Food requirements are typically estimated at a minimum of 2100 Kcal per person per day, but it is essential to consider the preexisting nutritional status of individuals and the overall population.

   (a) *Community Level*: Develop a plan for equitable food distribution, monitor food stores, and ensure safe food storage, handling, and preparation. Special attention should be given to meeting the nutritional needs of vulnerable groups. As resources permit, establish targeted supplemental and therapeutic feeding programs for malnourished individuals.

4. *Provide Effective Sanitation and Clean Water*: The estimated minimum requirement for drinking water is 3–5 liters per person per day, but it is recommended that each person has access to 15–20 liters per day to cover all needs, including washing and cooking.

   (a) *Community Level*: Re-establish supplies of clean water, sanitation, and waste disposal services as quickly as possible. For immediate needs, there should be at least one latrine per 20 individuals, and in the long term, each family of five should have access to one latrine.

5. *Establish a Diarrhea Control Program*: An increase in diarrheal diseases is a common consequence of disasters due to disruptions in sanitation infrastructure and healthcare services.

   (a) *Community Level*: Implement community-based education on household sanitation measures, diarrhea prevention, and symptom management, especially for young children. Healthcare centers should prepare to treat dehydration cases and optimize the use of low-cost strategies like oral rehydration solution (ORS) and zinc supplementation. It is also crucial to recognize potential cases of cholera and dysentery.

6. *Consider Mass Immunizations*: The COVID-19 pandemic highlighted the challenges of managing transmissible diseases among large populations, and mass immunization can be an effective strategy for reducing mortality in the aftermath of disasters. Measles has historically been a significant cause of death in crowded and displaced populations. Immunization against measles, along with vitamin A supplementation, should be routinely considered as a preventive measure after disasters affecting vulnerable groups. Additionally, *Streptococcus pneumoniae*, rotavirus, and *Haemophilus influenzae* type b frequently lead to outbreaks post-disaster, making mass immunization vital for under-immunized populations. Tetanus immunization and tetanus immunoglobulin may also be necessary for large numbers of patients injured during disasters. Other vaccines, such as those for influenza, varicella, hepatitis A, typhoid, and COVID-19, should be considered if there is a risk of outbreaks in crowded settings. The cold chain required to maintain vaccine potency poses the greatest challenge in areas with unstable infrastructure.

   (a) *National Level*: National and international agencies collaborate to determine the necessity of mass immunization following specific events. If deemed essential for part or all of the population, national authorities will manage logistics for the mass immunization and distribution campaign, including cold chain requirements, personnel, and materials.

(b) *Community Level*: Health officers must promptly assess the availability of vaccines and the cold chain as part of the healthcare evaluation. Healthcare professionals should monitor cases of transmissible diseases and develop a plan for mass immunization targeting vulnerable groups within the community. Establishing trusted lines of communication with the community early on is crucial for reducing misinformation regarding prevention, treatment, and vaccination strategies.

7. *Establish Minimum Reproductive Health and HIV Services, and Enhance Primary Medical Care*: In fragile communities, preventable causes of mortality will lead to the majority of disaster-related deaths in the weeks and months following the event. These casualties can be mitigated through community health education and improved access to primary care. Critical services should include emergency obstetric and neonatal care, management of sexually transmitted infections, addressing the health impacts of sexual and physical violence, ensuring safe blood transfusions, and adhering to universal precautions in health facilities, including field hospitals. Initial efforts should focus on identifying individuals who were receiving treatment for chronic diseases before the disaster to restart their care and identify potential complications from missed treatments.

(a) *Community Level*: Health professionals should coordinate with emergency transport and response systems within their communities. Healthcare interventions during the rescue phase should aim to minimize fatalities caused by the event (e.g., trauma, drowning). Following the rescue phase, healthcare resources should concentrate on re-establishing and enhancing access to quality primary care, especially for the most vulnerable groups.

8. *Implement Disease Surveillance and Health Information Systems*: Effective health information and disease surveillance systems are essential for identifying priorities and monitoring the effectiveness of health interventions.

(a) *National Level*: Health authorities will utilize available information to define initial priorities for resource allocation. They should establish specific surveillance guidelines for each disaster to track relevant disease and mortality trends.

(b) *Community Level*: Each healthcare delivery setting should immediately implement a disease surveillance and health information collection system based on established WHO, PAHO, or governmental guidelines. Healthcare professionals should regularly share this information with higher-level health authorities.

9. *Organize Human Resources*: The shock and disruption caused by an event can hinder a disaster-affected population's ability to respond effectively and in an organized manner. Having a predefined emergency plan with clearly identified leaders can assist the local community in coping until external resources arrive.

(a) *Community Level*: Develop an emergency plan and designate community leaders responsible for:

  (i) Conducting rescue operations
  (ii) Carrying out assessments (e.g., health services, transportation, food, sanitation/water systems)
  (iii) Organizing food and water distribution
  (iv) Maintaining waste management and sanitation programs
  (v) Managing health services
  (vi) Handling corpses and gravesite management
  (vii) Identifying unaccompanied minors and other highly vulnerable individuals (e.g., elderly or persons with disabilities) and organizing a caregiver program

10. Coordinate Activities

(a) *National Level*: In large-scale disasters, numerous national and international agencies will work to assess, develop plans, contribute resources, and establish funding priorities at national and regional levels. Effective collaboration among these agencies, each bringing unique expertise and resources, is crucial. All agencies will ultimately rely on the quality of assessments conducted in affected communities to make informed decisions, gather necessary resources, and determine the capacity of each community to implement plans that will reduce mortality, alleviate suffering, and facilitate recovery.

(b) *Community Level*: Develop local emergency plans that integrate with regional and national plans and agencies. Familiarize yourself with the mechanisms for collecting and communicating information (e.g., assessments, surveillance data) during disasters. Building relationships with key individuals within and outside the community before a disaster occurs is essential.

Types of Organizations Involved in Disasters

Objectives

- Identify national and international organizations that may respond to disasters in your country
- Recognize the resources, strengths, and limitations of these organizations

In cases where local resources fall short during a disaster, support from national, international, or transnational organizations becomes crucial. Each organization has its own distinct structure, culture, response capability, technical expertise, logistical resources, and a particular focus—whether thematic or regional.

Before a disaster occurs in a country, some organizations may already be engaged in emergency relief activities. In times of crisis, certain organizations can quickly mobilize and redirect their resources to provide immediate assistance. However, ensuring effective coordination and cooperation among these organizations is essential, though often challenging, in the chaotic environment of a large-scale emergency. Two main types of organizations typically provide assistance: governmental and non-governmental organizations (NGOs).

Governmental Organizations

Governmental organizations operate under the authority of a country's current government. This category also includes intergovernmental organizations, such as the United Nations (UN), which function under the collective leadership of multiple governments.

Examples of governmental organizations include:

- National Ministries: These agencies, operating at the national level, have the authority to plan and implement disaster response efforts. For instance, in 1986, a regional conference on disasters was held to enhance disaster preparedness and response across Latin America and the Caribbean. Following this, many nations appointed health disaster coordinators within their Ministries of Health (MoH). These coordinators oversee health-related relief efforts during emergencies, regularly update emergency plans, and conduct training for healthcare professionals to ensure ongoing preparedness.
- International Relief Providers: Box 1.2 highlights governmental agencies that offer financial aid and technical support to nations affected by humanitarian crises.

  Effective collaboration between these organizations is essential to managing disaster relief efficiently and ensuring that those affected receive timely and appropriate assistance.

Box 1.2 Government Agencies Involved in International Disaster Responses
- Canadian International Development Agency (CIDA) www.acdi-cida.gc.ca
- European Commission Humanitarian Organization (ECHO) www.acdi-cida.gc.ca
- Japan International Cooperation Agency (JICA) http://www.jica.go.jp/worldmap/english.html
- United Kingdom Department for International Development (DFID) www.dfid.gov.uk
- United States Agency for International Development (USAID): https://www.usaid.gov

Non-governmental Organizations (NGOs)

Non-governmental organizations (NGOs) are nonprofit, mission-driven entities that focus on advocacy or service delivery to address social or political issues. These organizations operate independently of government support. Currently, thousands of NGOs—both international and national—are active worldwide. While many NGOs are small and concentrate on specific projects such as education, providing tools, or training in sustainable development, only a few possess the resources necessary to engage in development promotion or disaster response on a global or regional scale. Each NGO operates according to its mission statement, which guides its activities.

NGOs typically receive funding through private or institutional donations. Private funds offer more flexibility, allowing NGOs to allocate resources freely in alignment with their mission. In contrast, institutional donations often come with conditions, requiring NGOs to adhere to agreements specifying how, where, and when the funds will be used.

Some NGOs adopt a "right to interfere" policy, which enables them to operate across borders without formal approval from the host country. While NGOs generally strive for neutrality, some may take a more active role in exposing injustices they observe. They excel in emergency situations within their areas of expertise, such as providing water or distributing food. However, most NGOs cannot operate independently in disaster settings and often rely on the United Nations, the military, or other agencies for security, transportation, communication, logistical support, or medical care for their personnel.

NGOs often have a unique advantage in providing direct assistance to communities due to preexisting relationships and an understanding of local culture, public health needs, and issues. Their familiarity with the affected communities allows them to respond more effectively. Furthermore, many NGOs transition from disaster relief to long-term development, demonstrating a commitment to rebuilding and supporting community growth. Box 1.3 lists several significant NGOs, some of which are discussed in greater detail.

Box 1.3 Non-profit and Other Organizations Involved in Disaster Response

1. Action Against Hunger, https://www.actionagainsthunger.org/
2. ActionAID International, https://actionaid.org/
3. Amnesty International, https://www.amnesty.org/en/
4. CARE International, https://www.care-international.org/
5. Clinton Health Access Initiative (CHAI): https://www.clinton-healthaccess.org
6. Danish Refugee Council, https://pro.drc.ngo/

7. Direct Relief, https://www.directrelief.org/
8. International Committee of the Red Cross/Red Crescent: https://www.icrc.org/en
9. International Medical Corps, https://www.internationalmedicalcorps.org/
10. International Rescue Committee (IRC): https://www.rescue.org
11. MedGlobal: https://medglobal.org
12. Médecins du Monde (MDM): https://medical-volunteers.org/contact/#volunteer
13. Médecins sans Frontières / Doctors Without Borders (MSF): https://www.doctorswithoutborders.org/
14. Office for the Coordination of Humanitarian Affairs (OCHA), www.unocha.org
15. Oxfam International, https://www.oxfamamerica.org/
16. Partners in Health: https://www.pih.org
17. Pan American Health Organization (PAHO), www.paho.org
18. Refugee Health Alliance (RHA). https://www.refugeehealthalliance.org
19. Save the Children: https://www.savethechildren.org/
20. The Gates Foundation: https://www.gatesfoundation.org
21. United Nations including, www.un.org
22. United Nations High Commissioner for Refugees (UNHCR), www.unhcr.org
23. United Nations International Children's Emergency Fund (UNICEF), www.unicef.org
24. World Food Program (WFP), www.wfp.org
25. World Health Organization (WHO): https://www.who.int/emergencies/situations
26. World Vision, https://www.worldvision.org/

Military Groups

Both local and foreign military forces can be mobilized to assist in responding to natural disasters or complex emergencies. The military's unique capabilities make them highly effective in such situations. One of their greatest advantages is their speed; few organizations can match the military's ability to swiftly mobilize large-scale logistical operations. They also provide security, ensuring the protection of environments, populations, and supplies during relief efforts. Their extensive fleet of planes, helicopters, and land and naval equipment allows for efficient transportation of resources to affected areas. Additionally, the military excels in maintaining supply lines, even in challenging environments, thanks to their experience in logistics. With a well-defined command structure, control, and communication systems, they can quickly adapt to evolving situations. Military forces are also self-sufficient in the field, as they bring the necessary supplies to sustain their personnel.

Specialized units, such as engineering teams and preventive medicine units, can offer valuable technical assistance. These units are equipped to perform rapid epidemiological evaluations, outbreak investigations, and water purification, among other vital tasks. Furthermore, military field hospitals and medical evacuation capabilities can be helpful, especially in specific disaster scenarios. For guidance on the appropriate use of field hospitals, see the WHO-PAHO guidelines.

Despite these advantages, the use of military forces in disaster response comes with notable challenges. Military field hospitals, for instance, are typically designed to care for soldiers with combat injuries, which may not align with the primary healthcare needs in a disaster, where women and children often require preventive and primary care. Additionally, the supplies available through military channels may not always be suitable for addressing the specific health concerns or food needs of the affected population. Another limitation is that the military, as a government asset, can sometimes prioritize political or strategic objectives over humanitarian goals. Their presence can also create tension within certain communities, and relief workers, who depend on neutrality for their safety and effectiveness, may be compromised by an association with military forces. Finally, military operations are costly, and the expense of mobilizing military resources for disaster relief can be significant.

Medical Responders in Disasters

After disasters, many pediatricians and other healthcare professionals volunteer their services for short periods. During the initial phase of disaster response, the greatest pediatric needs include air transport teams, surgical teams (comprising a surgeon, operating room nurse, anesthesiologist, and critical care pediatrician), and pediatricians trained in emergency medicine and critical care. It is essential for volunteers to work through an established organization, whether governmental or nongovernmental, that understands the local context and adheres to ethical standards in relief efforts [8].

When deploying a response team in the immediate aftermath of a disaster, it is crucial to have personnel who can manage the types of injuries typically associated with that specific event. For instance, in a major disaster like the 2023 earthquake in Turkey and Syria, most injuries were likely due to collapsed buildings, resulting in crush injuries, open wounds, and various orthopedic traumas. Therefore, teams must be equipped with both the personnel and supplies necessary to treat these injuries. In the case of a disaster caused by an explosion, such as a large industrial accident or bombing, the pattern of injuries may overlap with those seen in earthquakes but will also include a significant number of burns and blast-related injuries. For these situations, teams should include specialists in burn care, along with those experienced in treating other forms of trauma.

Box 1.4 provides technical recommendations for planning disaster response teams, and Table 1.3 outlines a list of pediatric supplies and equipment that can be

Table 1.3 Suggested equipment for pediatric care provision during disasters

Vital signs and monitoring
Stethoscope
Thermometer
Sphygmomanometer/blood pressure cuffs—premature, infant, child, adult
Pulse oximeter and probes/sensors
Monitoring equipment if available
Portable monitor/defibrillator (with settings <10)
Pediatric defibrillation paddles
Device to check serum glucose and strips to check urine for glucose, blood, etc.
Airway management/breathing
Simple face masks—infant, child, adult
Pediatric and adult masks for assisted ventilation
Self-inflating bag with 250 cc, 500 cc, and 1000 cc reservoir
Oral airways
Suction catheters and machines
Tongue blades
Optional for intubation
Laryngoscope handle with batteries (extra batteries AA, laryngoscope bulbs)
Miller blades—0, 1, 2, 3 Macintosh blades 2,3
Endotracheal tubes: uncuffed—3.0, 3.5, 4.0,4.5, 5.0, 6.0, cuffed—7.0,8.0
Laryngeal mask airways
Stylets—small, large
Easycap (ETCO2) analyzer—2 sizes
Adhesive tape to secure ETT
Laryngeal mask airways
Circulation/intravascular access or fluid management
IV catheters—18-, 20-, 22-, 24-gauge
Butterfly needles—23-gauge
Intraosseous needles—15- or 18-gauge, or Eazy IO device
Boards, tape, tourniquet IV
Pediatric drip chambers and tubing
Orthopedic and wound materials
Splints and gauze padding
Plaster for casting, not fiberglass (hard to remove)
Cotton padding for Jones bandages
Ace wraps
Sling
Gauze
Bandages or wraps
Tape
Tournique
Procedures
Nasogastric tubes—8, 10, 14F

(continued)

Table 1.3 (continued)

Scissors, scalpels, hemostats, forceps
Surgical equipment for amputations, incision and drainage of wounds, laceration repairs
Chest tubes
Chest tube stylettes
Chux
Miscellaneous
Broselow tape
Warm water source and portable showers for decontamination
Personal protective equipment (PPE)
Headlamps with replacement batteries

vital when caring for children in disaster settings. It is important for response teams to understand the local supply and resource provision systems or to work within the supply chains approved by the responding agency. Issues such as unreliable supply chains, cold chain requirements, medication safety, and the improper handling of medical waste from unsolicited or inappropriate donations can create ethical, logistical, and legal challenges in disaster response settings.

Box 1.4 Examples of Technical Recommendations for Disaster Situations [1]

Frequent effects of specific disasters

- Volcanic eruptions: Respiratory issues due to ash, environmental contamination, and infrastructure damage
- Earthquakes: Traumatic injuries, structural collapses, disruption of essential services like electricity and water
- Floods: Waterborne diseases, destruction of homes, and loss of crops
- Hurricanes: Storm surges, flooding, wind damage, and widespread displacement

Vulnerable groups and special needs

- Children, elderly, and pregnant women: Increased need for medical care, protection, and appropriate shelter
- People with disabilities: Access to mobility aids, tailored medical assistance, and safety measures
- Individuals with chronic conditions: Continuity of care for diabetes, heart disease, and other chronic illnesses
- Mental health: Addressing trauma, anxiety, and depression caused by disaster-related stress

Transmissible Diseases and Vector Control

- Cholera and tuberculosis: Higher transmission risk in crowded shelters and camps.
- Vector control: Essential to prevent outbreaks of malaria, dengue, and other vector-borne diseases
- Hygiene measures: Emphasis on sanitation and clean water to stop disease spread

Immunization Needs in Disaster Contexts

- Measles: Rapid vaccination campaigns to prevent outbreaks in densely populated shelters
- Equine encephalitis: Targeted vaccinations in areas prone to the disease, especially after floods or hurricanes
- Children and vulnerable groups: Prioritized for immunization to protect against highly contagious diseases

Food safety and nutrition

- Food preparation: Guidelines to ensure safe cooking and storage in disaster environments
- Nutrition: Focus on providing balanced meals, especially for children and pregnant women
- Prevention of foodborne illnesses: Safe handling practices to avoid outbreaks caused by contaminated food supplies

Environmental sanitation and shelter health

- Rodent control: Measures to reduce the risk of disease transmission in camps and shelters
- Water supply: Ensuring access to clean drinking water in temporary settlements
- Waste management: Proper disposal systems to maintain hygiene and reduce infection risks
- Shelter design: Guidelines for safe, clean, and hygienic temporary housing solutions.

https://www.who.int/publications/i/item/a-strategic-framework-for-emergency-preparedness

Coordination of Disaster Response Teams

Coordinating the efforts of governmental and non-governmental organizations in a disaster zone is a significant challenge. After a natural disaster, the government, its agencies, and military of the host nation usually assume operational command.

Most countries have now established governmental authorities responsible for managing disaster planning and response on a global scale, along with sector-specific coordinators, such as those focused on health. External agencies or foreign governments typically provide support through technical assistance and additional resources. For instance, the Pan American Health Organization (PAHO) has developed technical manuals and training programs designed to help nations plan and coordinate disaster responses at both regional and national levels.

In complex emergencies stemming from conflict, command of operations, including the coordination of humanitarian aid, is typically under the control of the armed forces or government authorities. Coordination can become especially difficult in these scenarios when hostile groups are nearby and attempt to obstruct civilian aid. In such cases, humanitarian assistance may be manipulated as a political or strategic tool.

Communication During Disaster Responses

Effective communication between disaster relief teams, coordinating groups, and logistical teams is crucial in disaster situations. Advances in technology have provided a variety of communication devices, each with its own strengths and limitations. Communication networks and contingency plans are essential components of disaster preparedness [13].

- *Radios* are beneficial for short-range communication when a disaster relief team is dispersed. However, their limited range means they cannot connect teams or organizations that are far apart.
- *Satellite phones* are an excellent option for maintaining communication between the team and their home country. They are particularly useful when traditional telephone services are unavailable or when there is no infrastructure, as they use orbiting satellites to transmit data. Despite their reliability, satellite phones are expensive and limited in availability. Additionally, many portable satellite phones require a clear view of the sky for their antennas to function properly.
- *Cellular phones* offer a convenient method for communication, allowing for voice calls, emails, and SMS texting between team members and coordination efforts with the home country. However, cellular networks depend on infrastructure that may be damaged or destroyed in the disaster. Moreover, in the immediate aftermath of a disaster, cellular networks can become overloaded due to the high volume of users.
- The widespread availability of the *internet* through satellite links or data provided by cellular networks also allows for various communication methods, including email and social media. This diversity in communication platforms enhances the ability to share information in real time, although internet access may still be limited depending on the local infrastructure and connectivity post-disaster.

Effective coordination and communication are key to ensuring that resources are deployed efficiently and that relief efforts reach the people who need them most, despite the inherent challenges of operating in a disaster zone.

Myths and Realities of Disasters

Objectives

- Identify common myths and realities surrounding disaster response and recovery
- Describe effective disaster response strategies that prioritize local capacities and address vulnerabilities

Myths and Realities of Disasters

The Pan American Health Organization (PAHO) has identified several common myths and misconceptions surrounding the public health impact of disasters [22]. Understanding these myths and the truths that counter them is crucial for effective disaster planning and management.

One prevalent myth is that foreign medical volunteers with extensive medical training are urgently needed in disaster situations. In reality, local populations typically handle immediate lifesaving needs. They include healthcare workers and first responders who are already familiar with the community and its unique challenges. Only when there is a specific skill set unavailable in the affected country, such as advanced surgical techniques or specialized trauma care, is there a genuine need for foreign medical personnel. Otherwise, the introduction of foreign teams can create additional challenges and strain existing resources.

Another common misconception is that any form of international assistance is necessary right away. This notion can lead to hasty responses that lack proper assessment and coordination. Rushing to provide aid without understanding the actual needs can cause chaos and inefficiency. In fact, many immediate needs are met by the victims themselves, along with their local governments and agencies, who are often the first to respond. It is more effective to wait for a thorough needs assessment to identify genuine gaps in assistance, allowing for a more targeted and appropriate response.

There is also a belief that epidemics and plagues are inevitable following disasters. However, this is not the case; epidemics do not spontaneously emerge after a disaster, and the presence of dead bodies does not automatically lead to catastrophic outbreaks of exotic diseases. The key to preventing disease in the aftermath of a disaster lies in improving sanitary conditions, ensuring access to clean water, and providing education on hygiene practices to the affected population. These preventive measures can significantly reduce health risks.

Many people believe that disasters bring out the worst in human behavior, leading to looting and rioting. While it is true that isolated incidents of antisocial behavior can occur, research shows that the majority of people respond to disasters with compassion and cooperation. In times of crisis, communities often come together to support one another, demonstrating remarkable resilience and solidarity. Rather than descending into chaos, many individuals take on roles as helpers, volunteers, and caregivers.

Another myth is that the affected population is too shocked and helpless to take responsibility for its own survival. Contrary to this belief, many individuals find new strength and determination during emergencies. For example, in the aftermath of the 1985 Mexico City earthquake, thousands of volunteers organized themselves to sift through rubble in search of survivors [5]. Such actions illustrate the capacity for self-reliance and collective effort in times of crisis.

It is also a common misconception that disasters strike randomly, without regard to social or economic factors. In reality, disasters tend to disproportionately impact the most vulnerable populations, particularly the poor, women, children, and the elderly. These groups often face heightened risks due to their limited access to resources and support systems. Therefore, relief efforts must prioritize these populations to address their specific needs effectively.

Another belief is that relocating disaster victims to temporary settlements is the best solution for those displaced. However, this should be considered a last resort. Many humanitarian agencies recognize that funds typically allocated for tents can be better utilized to purchase building materials, tools, and other resources that support long-term reconstruction within the affected area. Establishing temporary settlements can sometimes hinder recovery efforts by diverting resources from more sustainable solutions.

Many people assume that food aid is always necessary following natural disasters. In reality, natural disasters rarely result in widespread crop failure, meaning that massive food aid is not always required. Local food supplies can often meet the needs of affected individuals, reducing dependency on external aid and encouraging community resilience.

There is a prevalent belief that disaster victims always need clothing donations. However, used clothing is seldom needed and may often be culturally inappropriate. Although disaster victims might accept donated clothing, it is rarely worn due to issues related to fit, style, or cultural relevance. Instead, targeted support that respects local customs and needs is far more beneficial.

Finally, it is a common misconception that life returns to normal within a few weeks after a disaster. The reality is that the effects of disasters can be long-lasting, with affected countries often losing significant financial and material resources in the immediate aftermath. Rebuilding and recovery can take years, and successful relief programs must be designed with a long-term perspective, recognizing that international interest tends to wane even as needs and shortages persist. Acknowledging these myths and their realities can lead to more effective disaster response and recovery efforts, ultimately benefiting affected communities.

Conclusion

Disasters are largely unavoidable and beyond our control, yet we can mitigate their impact through better preparation, which in turn reduces human suffering. As Vernon Law once remarked, "Experience is a hard teacher. She gives the test first and the lessons afterward." To improve disaster preparedness and planning, knowledge and understanding are essential. Pediatricians play a crucial role in this process, ensuring that the unique needs of children are appropriately addressed in disaster planning and response efforts. Pediatric volunteers must be well prepared, with proper training, access to necessary materials and resources, and consideration of mental health challenges they may face during their work.

Acknowledgments Acknowledgment of former chapter authors: Patrick Mahar, MD; Col. Julia A. Lynch, MD, FAAP; Joseph Wathen, MD; Eric Tham, MD, MS, FAAP; Sathyanarayanan Doraiswamy, MD; Allen G.K. Maina, MD.

Resources

1. A strategic framework for emergency preparedness. WHO; 2017. Accessed 10 October 2024. https://iris.who.int/bitstream/handle/10665/254883/9789241511827-eng.pdf?sequence=1.
2. AAP. Pediatric education for prehospital professionals. London: Jones & Bartlett Publishers; 2006.
3. Aguirre AS, Rojas K, Torres AR. Pediatric traumatic brain injuries in war zones: a systematic literature review. Front Neurol. 2023;14:1253515. https://doi.org/10.3389/fneur.2023.1253515.
4. Bendavid E, Boerma T, Akseer N, et al. The effects of armed conflict on the health of women and children. Lancet. 2021;397(10273):522–32. https://doi.org/10.1016/s0140-6736(21)00131-8.
5. Child Landmine Survivors: An Inclusive Approach to Policy and Practice. Save the Children. Accessed 12 September 2024. https://bettercarenetwork.org/sites/default/files/Child%20Landmine%20Survivors%20-%20An%20Inclusive%20Approach%20to%20Policy%20and%20Practice.PDF.
6. Childhood in Rubble: the humanitarian consequences of urban warfare for children. 2023:1–72. May 2023. file:///Users/lisaumphrey/Downloads/4703_002-ebook%20(1).pdf.
7. Chung S, Baum CR, Nyquist AC. Chemical-biological terrorism and its impact on children. Pediatrics. 2020;145(2). https://doi.org/10.1542/peds.2019-3749.
8. Conflict SHi. Critical condition: violence against health care in conflict. Insecurity Insight: data on people in danger. 2023. Accessed 19 June 2024. https://insecurityinsight.org/wp-content/uploads/2024/05/2023-SHCC-Critical-Conditions.pdf.
9. Council on Community Pediatrics. Providing care for immigrant, migrant, and border children. Pediatrics. 2013;131(6):e2028–34. https://doi.org/10.1542/peds.2013-1099.
10. Hageman JR, Alcocer AL. The effects of armed conflict on children. Pediatr Ann. 2021;50(10):e396–7. https://doi.org/10.3928/19382359-20210918-01.
11. Hazer L, Gredebäck G. The effects of war, displacement, and trauma on child development. Humanit Soc Sci Commun. 2023;10:1–19.
12. Health AAoPCoE. Pediatric environmental health. American Academy of Pediatrics; 2018.
13. Health emergency and disaster preparedness. PAHO. Accessed 10 October 2024. https://www.paho.org/en/topics/health-emergency-and-disaster-preparedness.

14. How is the term "armed conflict" defined in international humanitarian law? ICRC. 2024. Accessed 12 September 2024. https://www.icrc.org/sites/default/files/document_new/file_list/armed_conflict_defined_in_ihl.pdf.

15. Inter-agency Guiding Principles on Unaccompanied and Separated Children. International Committee of the Red Cross. 2004. Accessed 12 September 2024. https://www.unhcr.org/sites/default/files/legacy-pdf/4098b3172.pdf.

16. Jawad M, Hone T, Vamos EP, Cetorelli V, Millett C. Implications of armed conflict for maternal and child health: a regression analysis of data from 181 countries for 2000-2019. PLoS Med. 2021;18(9):e1003810. https://doi.org/10.1371/journal.pmed.1003810.

17. Kadir A, Shenoda S, Goldhagen J, Pitterman S. The effects of armed conflict on children: policy statement. Pediatrics. 2018;142(6). https://doi.org/10.1542/peds.2018-2586.

18. Kadir A, Shenoda S, Goldhagen J. Effects of armed conflict on child health and development: a systematic review. PLoS One. 2019;14(1):e0210071.

19. Kirollos M, Anning C, Fylkesnes GK, Denselow J. The War on Children: time to end grave violations against children in conflict. Save the Children. 2018. Accessed 19 June 2024. https://www.savethechildren.org.uk/content/dam/global/reports/education-and-child-protection/war_on_children-web.pdf.

20. Landmine and Cluster Munition Monitor. Landmine and Cluster Munition Monitor. 2024. Accessed 12 September 2024. https://www.the-monitor.org/.

21. Liu L, Oza S, Hogan D, Chu Y, Perin J, Zhu J, Lawn JE, Cousens S, Mathers C, Black RE. Global, regional, and national causes of under-5 mortality in 2000–15: an updated systematic analysis with implications for the Sustainable Development Goals. Lancet. 2016;388(10063):3027–35. https://doi.org/10.1016/S0140-6736(16)31593-8. Epub 2016 Nov 11. Erratum in: Lancet. 2017 May 13;389(10082):1884. PMID: 27839855; PMCID: PMC5161777.

22. Perspectives in Health – The magazine of the Pan American Health Organization (PAHO). 2005;10(1): https://www3.paho.org/english/dd/pin/persp21_box02.htm.

23. Political Declaration on Strengthening the Protection of Civilians from the Humanitarian Consequences arising from the use of Explosive Weapons in Populated Areas. Protecting Civilians in Urban Warfare, Department of Foreign Affairs of Ireland. 2022. Accessed 12 September 2024. https://www.gov.ie/en/publication/585c8-protecting-civilians-in-urban-warfare/#political-declaration-on-ewipa.

24. Shenoda S, Kadir A, Pitterman S, Goldhagen J. The effects of armed conflict on children: technical report. Pediatrics. 2018;142(6). https://doi.org/10.1542/peds.2018-2585.

25. Talabani JM, Ali AI, Kadir AM, et al. Long-term health effects of chemical warfare agents on children following a single heavy exposure. Hum Exp Toxicol. 2018;37(8):836–47. https://doi.org/10.1177/0960327117734620.

26. Vigne JCK. 25 Years of Children and Armed Conflict: Taking Action to Protect Children in War. UNICEF. Accessed 12 September 2024. https://www.unicef.org/media/123021/file/25%20Years%20Children%20in%20Armed%20Conflict.pdf.

27. et al. 2023 Turkey-Syria Earthquake, Center for Disaster Philanthropy, https://disasterphilanthropy.org/disasters/2023-turkeysyria-earthquake/ (2024).

28. (2023) Distortions in time perception during collective trauma: Insights from a national longitudinal study during the COVID-19 pandemic. Psychological Trauma: Theory Research Practice and Policy 15(5) 800-807 10.1037/tra0001326

Chapter 2
Preventive Medicine Strategies in Disaster Settings

Israa Khan, Geoffrey Winstanley, Jessica Landry, Dan Alaro, and Stephen Berman

The Essential Role of Population Data in Disaster Response

Objectives

- Differentiate between standard clinical practice and preventive medicine
- Identify how public health measures take precedence over individual patient care following a disaster
- Explain and utilize population evaluation tools, including rates and underlying causes of disease, in communities impacted by a disaster

In the aftermath of a disaster, health workers encounter numerous challenges. They are deeply concerned about the health and well-being of their patients, while worrying about their own families. Most possess an intrinsic desire to assist their community. Depending on the specific circumstances, pediatricians may need to apply skills that extend beyond routine practice, such as providing trauma care immediately following an earthquake. Nevertheless, in any disaster situation, preventive medicine and public health strategies are crucial for the overall recovery of the community.

I. Khan (✉) · J. Landry
Department of Pediatrics, Section of Hospital Medicine, University of Colorado School of Medicine Anschutz Medical Campus, Aurora, CO, USA
e-mail: Israa.khan@childrenscolorado.org

G. Winstanley
Center for Global Health, Aurora, CO, USA

D. Alaro
KMA Center, Nairobi, Kenya

S. Berman
Department of Epidemiology, Colorado School of Public Health, University of Colorado School of Medicine, Aurora, CO, USA

L. Umphrey et al. (eds.), *Pediatric Considerations in Disaster Settings*, https://doi.org/10.1007/978-3-031-85501-6_2

Preventive medicine emphasizes the use of population health data and public health strategies to enhance the health of entire communities. Following a disaster, the regular public health infrastructure is often severely disrupted. Much like the autonomic nervous system, which maintains bodily functions without conscious effort, this infrastructure operates continuously to support community health, behind the scenes. When public health services are suddenly interrupted, the community faces potentially catastrophic consequences stemming from a lack of knowledge about where to access preventive and treatment services. The collapse of public health systems significantly increases the risk of communicable diseases, which are linked to high morbidity and mortality rates. In these scenarios, re-establishing the public health infrastructure should take precedence over individual patient care.

Preventive Medicine as a Public Health Approach During Disasters

In clinical medicine, physicians focus on diagnosing and treating patients individually. Most healthcare is centered on the needs of individual patients. In contrast, preventive medicine addresses the underlying causes of illness in society by utilizing public health techniques to tackle these issues at the population level rather than on an individual basis [15] (Box 2.1). The "patients" in preventive medicine are groups of people, entire populations, or specific sub-groups within those communities.

The initial step in transitioning from clinical to preventive medicine is to understand the patient in this broader context. In clinical settings, physicians evaluate patients individually by assessing vital signs, completing a history and physical examination, and possibly conducting additional tests to establish a diagnosis and develop a treatment plan. However, in preventive medicine, the focus shifts from individuals to communities [15]. To accurately diagnose community health, one must assess the community's "vital signs," which are represented by mathematical data, such as rates of disease within the population.

Box 2.1 Characteristics of Preventative Medicine
- Preventive medicine is grounded in public health principles.
- It is focused on addressing health issues at a population level rather than on individual patients.
- This approach relies on mathematical data to inform decisions and strategies.
- Preventive medicine investigates the underlying causes of diseases within a community to develop effective interventions.

The Use of Rates to Measure Community Impact During a Disaster

A rate is defined as a fraction that represents the number of cases of a specific condition divided by the number of individuals within a particular population group, then multiplied by a standard number to depict the population at risk [12] (Box 2.2). Rates facilitate comparisons of data using a numerator and a denominator, such as the number of illness cases or fatalities between different communities. They also play a vital role in assessing the effectiveness of interventions within a population over time. Although many clinicians are familiar with how to calculate rates, they may not apply these calculations in their daily practice. Understanding rates is essential for grasping health issues within a community. Without this information, resources may not be allocated efficiently for the benefit of the community. This is especially crucial in post-disaster situations where resources—such as food, supplies, and time—are more limited than usual.

Box 2.2 Rates of Conditions

$$\text{Rates} = \frac{\text{person}}{\text{person at risk}} \times \text{even number}^*$$

*even number represents the size of the population (1000, 10,000, 100,000).

To calculate rates, both a numerator and a denominator are required [12]. The numerator represents the number of cases of a specific issue, while the denominator denotes the number of individuals in the community who are at risk for that issue. The resulting figure can be expressed as a fraction, a percentage (if multiplied by 100), or a rate. All these forms convey valuable information and can be converted from one format to another. Public health practitioners utilize rates to communicate important data effectively.

The reliability of a rate depends on the quality of the data used to create it. To ensure accurate numerators, cases must be clearly defined so that busy clinicians can easily categorize health problems. For instance, a standard case definition for diarrhea could be a child experiencing three or more watery stools per day. Consistency in case definitions is crucial to guarantee that rates remain comparable across different regions or can be consistently tracked over time. Additionally, precise and descriptive denominators are vital for determining accurate numerators. Basic demographic information is necessary, including the total number of affected individuals in the community and the population structure, which encompasses gender distribution and the number of individuals in specific age groups. In disaster scenarios, age groups can be categorized as (i) under 5 years, (ii) 5 to 15 years, and

(iii) over 15 years. The latter group can further be subdivided into those aged 15 to 60 years and those over 60 years.

Refer to the example in Box 2.3. If the only data available was the number of cases of pneumonia (2.3 A) District B has a higher number of cases compared to District A, suggesting that District B should be prioritized for resource allocation. However, the number of cases listed only represents the numerator of a rate. The lower half of Box 2.3 B provides information about the number of children under 5 years of age (that is the denominator) in both towns. Therefore, while Town B has more cases, it is also more populated, whereas Town A has fewer cases within a smaller population. Consequently, Town A has a higher rate per 10,000 children under 5 years old. This example highlights the importance of having both the numerator and the denominator in understanding health data.

Box 2.3 Calculation of Rates

Which district has more problems in children younger than 5 with pneumonia?
  Determine: the number of cases of pneumonia

- District A: 304 cases of pneumonia
- District B: 1054 cases of pneumonia

  (B) Determine: the number of kids younger than 5 years of age

- District A: 1597 kids <5 y/o
- District B: 12,818 kids <5 y/o

  Calculate: Rates of pneumonia per 10,000 children <5 years of age:

$$\text{District A} = \frac{304}{1597} \times 10,000 = 1904$$

$$\text{District B}: \frac{1054}{12818} \times 10,000 = 822$$

The most critical rates for assessing the severity of a disaster are mortality rates, specifically the Crude Mortality Rate (CMR) or Crude Death Rate (CDR). This summary rate is based on the number of deaths occurring within a population over a specified period, typically a calendar year. The CMR is defined as the number of deaths in a specific geographical area during a given year, divided by the mid-year total population of that area during the same year, multiplied by 1000. The CMR can be reported in various units: deaths per 10,000 per day, deaths per 1000 per month, or deaths per 1000 per year (Box 2.4). For example, in a community of 15,955 individuals experiencing 49 deaths in 7 days, the CMR would be calculated as 49 / 15,955 × 10,000 = 30.7 deaths per 10,000 people in 1 week. To obtain the daily CMR, which serves as the international standard for assessing disaster severity and response effectiveness, this figure is divided by 7 (30.7/7), resulting in a daily CMR of 4.4 deaths per 10,000 people per day.

Box 2.4 Crude Mortality Rate (CMR)

$$\frac{\text{Total number of deaths in a group}}{\text{Total number of persons in the same group}} \times 10,000$$

Expressed as deaths per 10,000 persons per day.

The under-5 mortality rate (U5MR) is another crucial measure used to assess the severity of a disaster and the community's response capacity [5, 16]. This age-specific mortality rate (ASMR) reflects the number of deaths among children younger than 5 years. The U5MR is significant because it highlights the disaster's impact on children, who are among the most vulnerable members of society. This age group is often referred to as the sentinel population, as changes in their health status become evident more quickly than in other age groups. There has been notable progress in the global U5MR, which declined by 60% from 93 deaths per 1000 live births in 1990 to 37 per 1000 live births in 2022 [16] (Fig. 2.1). Despite this significant improvement, enhancing child survival remains an urgent concern, particularly as indicated by the slower decline in neonatal mortality shown in the same figure [4]. Health-care workers become increasingly concerned about a humanitarian emergency when the mortality rate reaches 2 deaths per 10,000 children under 5 years per day. Traditionally, a CMR above 1 death per 10,000 people per day or a U5MR exceeding 2 deaths per day had been considered an emergency threshold. However, since this threshold was established, baseline mortality rates have significantly decreased. Therefore, classifying a CMR of >1 as indicative of a humanitarian emergency fails to account for the global decline in mortality rates over the last 40 years. Today, we assess the CMR's increase relative to a baseline, its duration, and how many individuals are affected. To evaluate the progression of a disaster and the effectiveness of relief efforts, it is essential to monitor the CMR over several relevant time intervals. The preferred approach is to declare an emergency when the CMR among a specific population is at least twice its "normal" value.

In addition to the CMR, attack rates are calculated during disaster situations [12]. These rates illustrate the relationship between the number of new disease cases and the total population at risk. Attack rates are classified as incidence rates, reflecting the number of new cases within a population. Conversely, prevalence rates indicate the proportion of existing disease cases within a population. Both incidence and prevalence rates articulate the specific burden of a particular disease relative to all diseases, thereby helping to establish management priorities and efficiently allocate human resources. The risk of an epidemic is represented by incidence rates, as they indicate the emergence of new cases within a population. Prevalence rates, on the other hand, measure the proportion of disease that already exists, thus illustrating endemic conditions within the population.

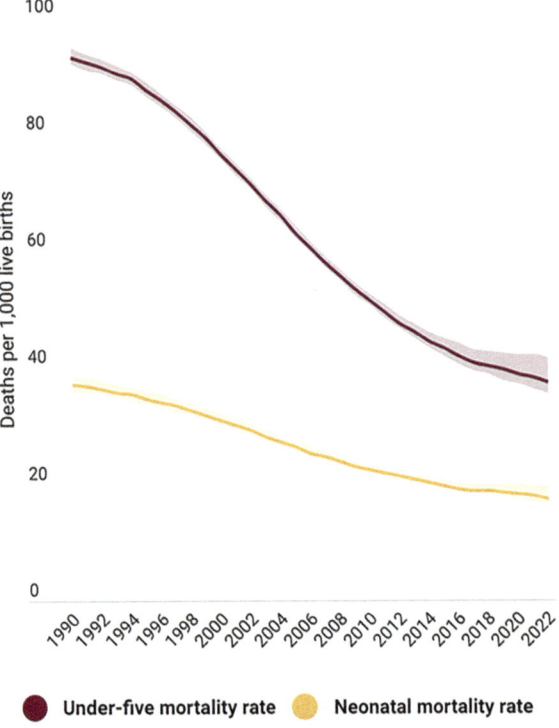

Fig. 2.1 Global mortality rates by age, 1990- 2022. (Source: UNICEF- Under-five mortality: https://data.unicef.org/topic/child-survival/under-five-mortality/#:~:text=Globally%2C%20infectious%20diseases%2C%20including%20pneumonia,View%20project%20in%20full%20screen)

Conducting Essential Needs Assessments in Disaster Responses for Targeted Relief

Objectives

- Identify the major components of a population evaluation, including demographics, pre-disaster health conditions, emergency needs assessment, health-care system evaluation, and surveillance program establishment.
- Describe the key components of an emergency needs assessment.
- Develop disaster response plans utilizing community resources such as transportation, communication, and security.

Population Evaluation

Pediatricians play a vital role in facilitating post-disaster recovery within their communities by assisting in the assessment of local population conditions. It is crucial to gather accurate data rather than relying on speculation. Frequently, disaster relief efforts are undermined, and resources are wasted by well-meaning individuals who act without the support of robust epidemiological data [17]. Box 2.5 outlines the essential components of a population evaluation.

Box 2.5 Population Evaluation

(A)   Collecting demographic data is essential for understanding the population affected by the disaster.

(B)   Assessing measures of health status prior to the disaster provides valuable context for evaluating community needs.

(C)   Health-care systems evaluation.

(D)   Conducting an evaluation of emergency needs helps identify the most urgent requirements for effective response.

(E)   Establishing a morbidity and mortality surveillance system is crucial for monitoring health trends and outcomes following the disaster.

(A)   *Demographic Data*

In the aftermath of a disaster, it is essential to collect data on the population characteristics of those affected, including numbers, age groups, ethnicity, and gender. The simplest method of counting individuals is through aerial observation, which is the least accurate way to assess the scope of a disaster, yet it may be the only option in certain situations. Visual estimates from the ground can also provide a quick approximation of the affected population.

A more precise approach involves using standard sampling techniques, such as systematic household sampling. The most effective way to gather demographic information is by counting every individual and categorizing them by age and sex. Special attention must be given to vulnerable groups, which include children under 5 years, unaccompanied minors, pregnant and breastfeeding women, the elderly, and the injured [5]. Identifying these populations is crucial, even though the counting process can be tedious, making it a top priority (Box 2.6). Humanitarian organizations like United Nations High Commissioner for Refugees (UNHCR), World Food Program (WFP), and United Nations Office for the Coordination of Humanitarian Affairs (OCHA) often register beneficiaries, so it is advisable to obtain population denominators from these agencies. Without accurate demographic data, understanding the true nature of the community's needs becomes challenging, leading to inefficient use of scarce resources.

Box 2.6 Important Demographic Data to Collect in Disasters
- Male/female ratio: Assess the gender distribution within the affected population.
- Age distribution: Categorize individuals by age groups: under 5 years, 5–15 years, and over 15 years.
- Vulnerable groups: Identify at-risk populations, including young or unaccompanied children, pregnant and lactating women, and the elderly.
- Population of the wounded and sick: Determine the number of individuals who are injured or suffering from illness.

(B) *Pre-disaster Health Conditions*

Baseline health data can be obtained from local health authorities, with immunization records serving as a valuable resource [5]. Health workers can provide insights into the prevalence and types of health issues present in the community prior to the disaster, as well as identify the areas most likely to be affected, particularly the most vulnerable households.

Pediatricians can enhance their disaster preparedness by actively participating in the development of community health plans and leading disaster drills. Ideally, public and private health-care providers should convene periodically to discuss community health challenges and practice disaster response exercises. This collaboration would enhance their understanding of the community's health issues and strengthen relationships between the public and private sectors before a disaster occurs.

(C) *Emergency Needs Assessment*

A needs assessment evaluates both the deficiencies within a community and the available resources and capacities that can be mobilized to address these issues. The primary goal of a needs assessment is to identify the gaps between existing community resources and the needs of the population [7, 8, 9, 14, 17].

Whenever feasible, it is preferable to close these gaps by mobilizing local resources immediately rather than awaiting external assistance. Emergency needs assessments, also known as rapid needs assessments, concentrate on identifying needs that can alleviate the highest levels of morbidity within the community [8]. These assessments are described in detail below and in Box 2.7. Additionally, security, transportation, and communication are critical components of an emergency community needs assessment, even though they may extend beyond the traditional health-care domain. These aspects will be discussed further at the end of this section.

> **Box 2.7 Critical Considerations for Evaluating Emergency Needs**
> - Drinking water: Ensure access to safe and sufficient drinking water.
> - Nutritional status: Assess the nutritional needs and existing conditions of the population.
> - Shelter: Evaluate the availability and adequacy of shelter options for affected individuals.
> - Basic sanitation: Address sanitation needs to prevent disease spread and maintain hygiene.
> - Local environmental conditions: Analyze environmental factors that may impact health and safety.
> - Public health needs: Identify key health issues, including morbidity and mortality rates, to guide interventions.

Water

Water is essential for survival and should always be prioritized. In the immediate aftermath of a disaster, the quantity of water is often more crucial than its quality. Providing clean water is the most effective preventive medicine intervention to curb the spread of disease. The estimated requirement for drinking water ranges from 3 to 4 liters per person per day. However, when cooking, cleaning, laundry, and personal hygiene needs are considered, the total water requirement increases to approximately 15–20 liters per person per day. Identifying immediate water sources, protecting these resources, and implementing methods to maintain and improve water quality are critical tasks. Relief agencies may eventually supply water purification systems. If there are urgent concerns regarding water contamination, chlorination can be done by adding 2 drops of bleach (sodium hypochlorite solution) per liter of water [19].

Nutritional Status

Nutritional assessments evaluate community needs alongside available local resources. The recommended caloric intake for a displaced population is 2100 Kcal per person per day [19]. Other elements of a nutritional needs assessment include the preexisting nutritional status of individuals, food availability, nutritional quality (including the presence of adequate micronutrients), food security, preparation, distribution throughout the community, and cultural factors affecting nutrition.

Common sampling techniques for assessing children's nutritional status or other health conditions include random selection (either simple or systematic) and cluster sampling.

Shelter

Regarding shelter, the World Health Organization (WHO) recommends a minimum of 3.5 square meters (m^2) of floor space per person for a displaced population in warm climates [18]. This requirement increases to 4.5 m^2 in colder climates due to the necessity of spending more time indoors for activities such as food preparation and meals. The shelter should be suitable for the local climate and culture.

Additionally, structural stability and material integrity are essential considerations. A rapid assessment of available space will help identify any discrepancies between needs and capacity. While individual family shelters are preferable to communal shelters, pre-disaster planning should identify potential local community spaces such as schools, churches, and assembly halls that can serve as emergency shelters.

Basic Sanitation

Basic sanitation measures aim to prevent the spread of communicable diseases resulting from indiscriminate defecation [18, 19]. Feces are a concentrated source of pathogens and can trigger outbreaks of diarrheal diseases. In the post-disaster context, effectively managing human waste is a top priority. One person can contaminate water sources that thousands rely on, and flies can transfer fecal matter to food supplies, leading to rapid outbreaks of food and waterborne illnesses.

Local Environmental Conditions

It is crucial to assess conditions that may impact community health, such as smoke, chemical spills, floods, landslides, collapsed structures, terrain slopes, drainage issues, and insect vectors during disaster situations.

Public Health Needs

The emergency assessment of health needs focuses on mortality rates and the primary causes of morbidity [13]. Tracking death, as the most severe negative health outcome, is essential for understanding the health landscape of a community. For the most accurate analysis, mortality data should be reported by age, sex, and cause of death. It is also important to consider any subpopulation characteristics within the community that may be relevant for tracking health equity concerns e.g., socio-economic status, religion, race, and culture.

Morbidity data is equally vital for comprehending both immediate and long-term health needs within the community. This information can be captured through patient logbooks or records that document demographics and primary diagnoses. Such data can be analyzed quickly to identify the main health threats facing the community and guide resource allocation.

(D) *Health-Care System Evaluation*

Although evaluating community health-care resources is not typically included in traditional emergency needs assessments, it plays a crucial role in the aftermath of a disaster [14, 17]. This evaluation encompasses various aspects, including human resources, medical supplies, equipment, surgical capabilities, emergency department, and primary care capacity, as well as the condition of health-care facilities.

Assessing the health-care system effectively requires a thorough understanding of community resources prior to a disaster. By collaborating with public health officials and disaster planning committees, pediatricians and other local physicians can be incorporated into community health-care worker rosters and can gain insights into where emergency medical supplies are stored. Establishing organized plans for signaling an emergency and designating a specific location for health-care workers to convene can facilitate the rapid mobilization of personnel during an emergency.

Additionally, it is vital to identify extra areas for triage and manage surge capacity, along with developing a staffing plan for these supplementary treatment spaces. The COVID-19 pandemic highlighted the challenges many health-care facilities faced due to insufficient plans for expanding treatment areas and staffing. Therefore, recognizing alternate care facilities within each community and across regions may be necessary to meet increased demands.

Pre-disaster planning, which includes assigning responsibilities for evaluating the condition of local hospitals and clinics as well as determining available medical supplies, can help prevent confusion and minimize redundant efforts during a crisis.

(E) *Building an Effective System for Morbidity and Mortality Surveillance*

Following a disaster, it is crucial for both private and public health-care workers to collaborate in establishing an integrated and coordinated system for recording and reporting diseases [10, 12]. This collaboration is one of the most vital responsibilities of health workers engaged in traditional clinical treatment. Although clinicians working long hours may perceive data collection as a distraction, it is essential for effective disaster response planning.

In an ideal situation, each health-care worker would systematically record at least the age, sex, and diagnosis of every patient. This information should be collected and provided promptly to public health authorities for analysis, allowing for rapid responses to emerging health threats. In a well-organized health-care system, electronic medical records can significantly streamline this data acquisition process.

Additional Considerations During Disaster Needs Assessments

(A) *Transportation and Communication Resources*

Effective transportation and communication systems are essential components of any disaster response strategy [8]. Reliable two-way communication methods, including radios, telephones, and internet access, are crucial for disseminating vital information, coordinating efforts among disaster responders, and facilitating external assistance. Utilizing mass media to convey emergency instructions and public health education can significantly enhance community awareness during crises. Additionally, the state of roads, waterways, and landing strips is critical for the timely evacuation of injured individuals and the delivery of emergency supplies. Ensuring access to motor vehicles, fuel, and boats is vital for rapidly reaching disaster-affected areas, thereby improving the overall response effort.

(B) *Security*

In disaster scenarios, security considerations are often underestimated by health workers. Adequate security is essential for conducting initial rapid emergency needs assessments and maintaining order among patients seeking basic supplies or health care. Although health workers may not directly establish security measures, they can play a pivotal role in facilitating the safety and protection of disaster-affected populations from crime, looting, and exploitation by relaying information about criminal activities to security forces. Furthermore, health workers can ensure the safety of unaccompanied minors, protecting them from potential exploitation until family reunification or other permanent solutions are arranged.

(C) *Epidemic Preparedness and Outbreak Response*

Recent epidemics, particularly the COVID-19 pandemic, have underscored the necessity of robust epidemic preparedness plans [7]. It is crucial to evaluate whether your facility has an updated plan and how it aligns with regional strategies. Additionally, contingency plans should address personal considerations for health-care workers, such as childcare or family care in the event of illness. As the demand for staffing may increase significantly during an outbreak, it's important to ascertain whether vaccination is mandatory for all health-care workers and to establish procedures for those who decline vaccination, such as assigning non-clinical roles or implementing specific mask-wearing protocols.

Epidemics can affect certain populations disproportionately, leading to varying numbers of mild versus critical cases. Therefore, establishing effective triage systems is imperative for sorting patients according to their needs. Daily surveillance of patient demographics and illness severity, along with monitoring hospital bed availability, will inform ongoing response plans.

The resources necessary to address these challenges will differ depending on the situation. Proactive planning for essential equipment and medical supplies—including ventilators, antibiotics, antimalarials, intravenous fluids, safe blood masks, vaccines, antivirals, and personal protective equipment—is crucial. Additionally, creating "alternate care guidelines" will provide a structured approach for managing a potentially high volume of patients within an overwhelmed health-care system. To ensure their effectiveness, these guidelines should clearly outline resource allocation, ethical considerations, and the legal frameworks required to implement them in advance.

Establishing Critical Priorities in Disaster Response: A Roadmap to Effective Action

Objectives

- Determine emergency intervention priorities following a disaster.
- Explain how modes of disease transmission influence intervention priorities after a disaster.

Pathways of Disease Transmission in Disaster Settings: Protecting Vulnerable Populations

Post-disaster living conditions often exacerbate the spread of infectious diseases. Understanding how these conditions pose health threats is crucial for prioritizing public health interventions. The primary modes of disease transmission following a disaster include fecal-oral, respiratory, and vector-borne pathways [11].

Infectious diseases are typically categorized by their mode of transmission, as this approach simplifies the study and management of these diseases. Conversely, establishing the epidemiological evidence for non-infectious diseases is more complex. For instance, while the link between lung cancer and cigarette smoking is well known, demonstrating causality in non-infectious diseases presents greater challenges.

Transmission modes can be divided into two main categories: direct and indirect. To illustrate the difference, consider the analogy of handing a note to a friend in person versus leaving it on a dry erase board for them to read later. In both scenarios, your friend receives the message, but the first instance represents direct transmission, while the second involves an extra step, thus characterizing it as indirect.

Direct Transmission

In the direct mode of infection transmission, there is direct contact or proximity between an infection source and host [11]. Examples of this are as follows:

(A) *Direct Contact*: This involves physical contact between the source and reservoir, such as an infected person or animal, and a susceptible host. Another example of spread by direct contact is that caused by contact with an infected wound such as *Staphylococcus aureus*. For agents in the soil such as tetanus, this could be contact with contaminated soil, which can enter through a break in the skin.

(B) *Direct droplet*: Droplet transmission occurs via respiratory droplets produced by coughing, sneezing, singing, shouting, or even breathing. These droplets are larger than 5 microns, thereby traveling only a short distance (less than 3 yards) and directly entering the mouth, nose, or eyes of a new potential host. This route for infection spread is enhanced by crowded conditions that frequently follow a disaster. Examples are illnesses such as chickenpox and streptococcal disease.

Indirect Transmission

For indirect transmission to occur, the source or reservoir and susceptible host don't need to be near each other, and it may not happen immediately. There are three types of indirect transmission, and they are categorized by the extra step involved.

(A) *Indirect airborne*: This transmission can happen through airborne particles. These particles are much smaller than the droplets involved in direct droplet transmission (less than 5 micron) and can stay afloat in the air for a longer time before falling to the ground. With direct droplet transmission, the potential new host is in the direct path of a sneeze or cough, but with indirect airborne transmission, the host needs to be in the vicinity of the floating airborne particles and breathe them in, even after the source is no longer present. Measles is an example of a disease spread by indirect airborne transmission. Respiratory particles containing the measles virus exhaled by an infected person can remain suspended in the air and be inhaled by a susceptible person several minutes later, leading to infection. Other examples of infection that occur through airborne transmission are tuberculosis, influenza, and COVID-19.

(B) *Indirect vector-borne*: Vector-borne transmission happens through arthropods such as mosquitoes, ticks, or flies to transfer the infectious agent from one host to another. For example, mosquitoes become infected with the malaria parasite by taking a blood meal from an infected person. After a period of parasite development, mosquitoes spread the agent to the next host through a bite. Vector-borne illnesses such as malaria and dengue frequently increase following disasters, particularly floods or hurricanes, because standing water increases mosquito breeding. Fecal-oral transmission is also a type of indirect vector-borne transmission that occurs when flies carry feces on their feet and transmit them to food sources.

(C) *Indirect vehicle-borne*: Unlike vectors that are living, a vehicle is a non-living object that can carry an agent from its reservoir to a susceptible host. This vehicle may be food, water, or fomites such as clothes, utensils, or a surface of furniture. Vehicle-borne transmission can happen when someone who is infected shares food, drink, towel, or other inanimate objects with another person. Depending on the agent and the vehicle, the agent may continue to grow and multiply between hosts. For example, if a person coughs or sneezes into their hand and then grabs a doorknob, the latter can become a vehicle to pass the agent. The next person who uses the doorknob and subsequently touches their mouth, nose, or eyes may get infected. Another example of indirect vehicle-borne transmission is when a food item becomes contaminated with bacteria such as *Salmonella* causing gastroenteritis.

An important example is the fecal-oral route, which can both cause vector and vehicle-borne transmission. Fecal-oral transmission is vehicle-borne when human waste enters the water supply by defecation into the water source, by flooding, or by unwashed hands. When flies carry feces on their feet to food sources, it represents a vector-borne indirect transmissions. Fecal-oral transmission has the greatest potential for the rapid spread of infection among a displaced population, particularly if the water supply becomes contaminated [11] (Box 2.8).

Box 2.8 Fecal-Oral Transmission
- Fecal-oral transmission as indirect transmission:

1. Vector-borne transmission: Occurs when flies carry feces, transferring pathogens to food sources.
2. Vehicle-borne transmission: Happens through contaminated water, where human waste enters the water supply.

Fecal-oral transmission is particularly concerning in post-disaster scenarios, as it often leads to the rapid spread of infections, exacerbated by poor hygiene conditions and a contaminated water supply.

Urgent Public Health Priorities in Disaster Settings: Safeguarding Communities Amidst Crisis

The primary aim of health interventions following a disaster is to reduce mortality, prevent the onset of disease, and prepare communities for future emergencies [6, 7 9, 10, 17]. These interventions should ideally be guided by a comprehensive emergency needs assessment and ongoing evaluations to assess their effectiveness throughout the crisis.

Among the survivors of a disaster, the leading causes of illness typically include diarrhea and acute respiratory infections. Immediate public health interventions should focus on the following priorities.

1. *Ensure Access to Safe Drinking Water*

Ensuring access to clean drinking water is the top priority in disaster relief efforts. Each individual requires approximately 3–4 liters of water daily [19]. Effective water purification initiatives significantly reduce community morbidity and mortality rates. For these programs to be successful, they must be accepted by the community, considering factors such as taste and convenient access to purified sources. Furthermore, sustainability is crucial; water purification programs should be designed to be maintained by the community long after the immediate disaster response is over.

Basic field treatments can enhance water quality and reduce the risk of waterborne infections. Techniques such as covering water containers and allowing sediments to settle can improve water quality while minimizing the chlorine required for purification. Sand filtration, which involves passing water through layers of stones and sand contained in a barrel, can also be beneficial. In larger-scale efforts, bulk chlorination is effective for supplying clean water to many people. Reverse osmosis units can produce thousands of gallons of pure water but are costly, require specialized knowledge to operate, and may take days to deploy, delaying urgent access to clean water.

Relying on individuals to purify their own water, whether by boiling or adding chlorine, is generally the least effective approach. Boiling is time-consuming, and household-level chlorination depends on individual understanding of water safety, motivation, and adequate distribution of purification supplies, along with proper educational guidance on their use.

In addition to ensuring water quality, establishing an effective distribution system is critical. If a community has access to high-quality water but uses contaminated pipes or containers for transport, the effort becomes ineffective. Therefore, clean, covered storage tanks and reliable methods for distributing water to community members are essential.

2. *Manage Human Waste*

A family-centered approach is vital in the establishment of portable lavatories. It is crucial to consider the needs of children when designing community sanitation programs, as they are more likely to defecate indiscriminately. Portable lavatories should be conveniently located and safe for children to use, as a frightening or inaccessible facility may discourage usage.

While access to soap and water for personal hygiene is important, it is a lower priority than ensuring clean drinking water and proper sanitation to eliminate feces. Once the water supply is secure, providing soap and water for hygiene is essential to prevent the spread of infectious diseases. A minimum of 7 liters of water per person per day is required for hygiene purposes, in contrast to the 3–4 L needed for drinking.

3. *Safeguard the Food Supply*

Planning for food supply protection should be an integral part of disaster preparedness. This involves securing community resources and safely storing emergency rations, with input from all relevant disaster planning agencies. Preventing contamination of food preparation areas is paramount, and basic measures to avoid foodborne illness include:

- Using clean drinking water for food preparation
- Ensuring strict hand hygiene among food handlers
- Keeping food preparation areas and utensils as clean as possible
- Controlling vectors such as flies
- Employing proper cooking, storage, and serving techniques

Additionally, providing health education to community members can help them safely prepare and utilize food resources.

4. *Implement Vector Control Measures*

Vector control is critical in managing diseases like malaria, dengue, leishmaniasis, and gastroenteritis, which contribute significantly to global morbidity and mortality. An integrated approach to vector control encompasses several strategies, including indoor residual spraying, eliminating breeding sites, and reducing human-vector contact through methods such as insecticide-treated nets (ITNs). As the threat from insecticide-resistant vectors and global environmental changes increases, incorporating a range of locally appropriate insecticide and non-insecticide-based interventions is essential for effective and sustainable vector control.

5. *Provide Adequate Shelter*

The World Health Organization (WHO) recommends a minimum of 3.5 square meters of floor space per person in emergency shelters. Shelters are most effective when they allow families and traditional community groups to stay together. They should be located close to essential resources such as food, water, sanitation facilities, medical care, and transportation. When homes are destroyed, establishing shelters within or near the preexisting community is ideal.

Guiding Use of Resources in Disaster Via Surveillance Cycles

Objectives

1. Utilize the surveillance cycle to inform rational health-care decisions
2. Recognize the essential role that primary care doctors and pediatricians have in gathering quality information while caring for individual patients
3. Apply this information appropriately in the decision-making process

Surveillance Cycle: A Critical Tool for Strengthening Public Health Systems

Once the emergency assessment is complete and disaster recovery operations are underway, ongoing surveillance becomes essential for evaluating the evolving needs of the affected population. The US Centers for Disease Control and Prevention (CDC) defines surveillance as "the ongoing, systematic collection, analysis, and interpretation of health-related data essential to the planning, implementation, and evaluation of public health practice, closely integrated with the timely dissemination of these data to those responsible for prevention and control." [10] The critical final step is applying this data for effective prevention and control measures. A robust surveillance system comprises the capacity for data collection, analysis, and dissemination that is directly linked to public health initiatives.

According to the CDC's definition, the surveillance cycle encompasses several key stages: gathering data crucial for monitoring health needs, analyzing and interpreting this data promptly, providing feedback to stakeholders, and implementing actions based on the findings (see Box 2.9). In essence, the surveillance cycle consists of a data collection phase followed by analysis, culminating in targeted interventions. This cycle is then repeated to assess the effectiveness of the implemented strategies.

To ensure the success of this process, efficient and reciprocal communication between field staff and public health leadership is vital. For instance, if clinicians perceive that maintaining a patient logbook merely increases their workload without offering tangible benefits for patient care, they may quickly abandon data collection efforts. Such a breakdown in communication between clinicians and public health services can hinder the optimal use of the surveillance cycle.

> **Box 2.9 Important Data for Surveillance Cycles**
> - Deaths: Tracking mortality rates to assess the overall impact of the disaster.
> - Severe morbidity: Identifying diseases that are prevalent within the community, focusing on those causing significant health issues.
> - Rapid detection: Monitoring for specific conditions or infections, such as cholera, malnutrition, malaria, and severe trauma, to enable timely responses.
> - Infection spread documentation: Collecting lists of affected individuals to understand and track the transmission of infections within the community.

Guiding Hope and Health: The Vital Role of Pediatricians in Community Disaster Prevention and Recovery

Pediatricians, whether working in public or private sectors, play a crucial role in disaster recovery within their communities. Their contributions extend beyond routine consultations; with proper preparation, pediatricians, alongside other healthcare professionals, can engage in a variety of important activities, from supporting search and rescue operations to conducting population surveys. Their effectiveness in these roles largely hinges on personal readiness and their integration into community disaster planning strategies.

Given that children represent a significant portion of the population and are among the most vulnerable groups during disasters, pediatricians can take on leadership roles in disaster response and preparedness initiatives. It is essential for drills to include children as mock victims, accurately reflecting the age range and numbers representative of the overall population. Effective disaster plans must address children's unique nutritional, psychological, and developmental needs, which will be more likely to occur if pediatricians are involved in every stage of the planning process [1]. By educating other health-care workers, such as nurses, general practitioners, and new community health workers, pediatricians can share their expertise regarding the specific needs of children across the disaster response network.

Despite their busy clinical schedules, pediatricians should prioritize establishing connections with public health officials to engage in pre-disaster planning efforts. Even within their conventional role of providing clinical care, pediatricians have a significant part to play in preventive medicine by ensuring that an effective surveillance cycle is operational. Key components of this cycle include the establishment of a comprehensive patient logbook that captures essential disease data and organizes it by specific age and sex groups. This marks the beginning of the surveillance cycle, initiated through clinicians' interactions with individual patients. If relevant data is not collected, public health decisions will rely on conjecture rather than factual information.

Once data is gathered, it is imperative for clinicians to promptly share this information with public health services. Doing so enables timely analysis and a swift response to emerging public health needs. By fostering strong communication between clinicians and public health officers, optimal interventions can be devised and effectively executed for the benefit of children within their communities.

Summary

Pediatricians play a vital role in disaster preparedness and response within their communities. Their expertise in children's medical needs, combined with their advocacy for pediatric health, makes them essential during crises. Following a disaster, prioritizing basic preventive medicine and public health measures becomes crucial, often taking precedence over direct clinical care. This underscores the importance of training pediatricians, family physicians, and nurses in disaster management and effective community response strategies.

Preventive medicine in disaster situations necessitates a comprehensive population evaluation and needs assessment [15]. The data gathered during this process is instrumental in guiding the initial disaster response efforts. Additionally, establishing a functional surveillance system is essential for evaluating the effectiveness of disaster interventions. Clinicians and public health professionals can utilize this data to identify emerging threats to the community, ensuring the best possible outcomes in the aftermath of a disaster.

Acknowledging Former Author Contributions
Douglas Lougee
Sathyanarayanan Doraiswamy
Angela Gentile

Resources

1. Umphrey L, Brown A, Hiffler L, et al. Delivering paediatric critical care in humanitarian settings. Lancet Child Adolesc Health. 2018;2(12):846–8. https://doi.org/10.1016/s2352-4642(18)30284-0.
2. Abu-Ghaida D, Silva K. Educating the Forcibly Displaced: Key Challenges and Opportunities. 2021:1–34. March 2021. https://www.unhcr.org/people-forced-to-flee-book/wp-content/uploads/sites/137/2021/10/Dina-Abu-Ghaida-and-Karishma-Silva_Educating-the-Forcibly-Displaced-Key-Challenges-and-Opportunities-1.pdf

3. Jayasinghe S. The 12 dimensions of health impacts of war (the 12-D framework): a novel framework to conceptualise impacts of war on social and environmental determinants of health and public health. BMJ Glob Health. 2024;9(5) https://doi.org/10.1136/bmjgh-2023-014749.

4. Kampalath V, MacLean S, AlAbdulhadi A, Congdon M. The delivery of essential newborn care in conflict settings: a systematic review. Front Pediatr. 2022;10:937751. https://doi.org/10.3389/fped.2022.937751.

5. Poverty and Child Health in the United States. Pediatrics. Apr 2016;137(4), https://doi.org/10.1542/peds.2016-0339.

6. US Department of Health and Human Services. Accessed 5 Oct 2024. https://www.hhs.gov/programs/emergency-preparedness/index.html

7. Administration for Strategic Preparedness and Response. US Department of Health and Human Services. Accessed 5 Oct 2024. https://aspr.hhs.gov/Pages/Home.aspx.

8. WHO (2017) A strategic framework for emergency preparedness. Accessed 10 Oct 2024. https://iris.who.int/bitstream/handle/10665/254883/9789241511827-eng.pdf?sequence=1

9. Health emergency and disaster preparedness. PAHO. Accessed 10 Oct 2024. https://www.paho.org/en/topics/health-emergency-and-disaster-preparedness

10. Jamison DT. et al. Public Health Surveillance: A Tool for Targeting and Monitoring Interventions: Disease Control Priorities in Developing Countries. 2nd edition. Washington (DC): The International Bank for Reconstruction and Development / The World Bank, https://www.ncbi.nlm.nih.gov/books/NBK11770/ (2006).

11. Lesson 1: Introduction to Epidemiology, Section 10: Chain of Infection, CDC, https://www.cdc.gov/csels/dsepd/ss1978/lesson1/section10.html (2023).

12. Principles of Epidemiology | Lesson 3- Section 2: Measures of Risk, CDC, https://www.cdc.gov/csels/dsepd/ss1978/lesson3/section1.html (2023).

13. Post-Disaster Needs Assessment, UNDP, https://www.undp.org/publications/post-disaster-needs-assessment (2015).

14. WASH Needs Assessment in Refugee Emergencies, UNHCR, https://emergency.unhcr.org/emergency-assistance/water-sanitationand-hygiene/wash-needs-assessment-refugee-emergencies (2023).

15. (2024) Clinical Preventive Medicine Integrative Medicine and Lifestyle Medicine: Current State and Future Opportunities in the Development of Emerging Clinical Areas AJPM Focus 3(1) 100166-10.1016/j.focus.2023.100166

16. Under-five mortality, UNICEF, https://data.unicef.org/topic/child-survival/under-five-mortality/ (2024).

17. (2019) Emergency health evaluation of affected population during disasters: Are there new approaches? Journal of Education and Health Promotion 8(1) 2-10.4103/jehp.jehp_115_18

18. Emergency Shelter Solutions and Standards, UNHCR, https://doi.org/https://emergency.unhcr.org/emergency-assistance/sheltercamp-and-settlement/shelter-and-housing/emergency-shelter-solutions-and-standards (2024).

19. Food and Water in an Emergency, FEMA, https://doi.org/https://www.fema.gov/pdf/library/f&web.pdf (2004).

Chapter 3
Disaster Planning and Considerations for Children

Tien Vu, Nithin Ravi, Andrew Oh, and Cory McEvoy

Introduction

Emergency preparedness planning is essential for minimizing the impact of disasters. Disasters are events where natural or human-made incidents escalate into catastrophic situations, overwhelming local capacities to respond. Without thorough planning, responses to such incidents typically focus on the immediate rescue and hospital transfer of victims. This strategy, however, often shifts the burden from the disaster site to nearby hospitals, potentially overwhelming their resources and disrupting healthcare services.

Some disasters occur with little or no warning, while others, like floods or hurricanes, provide some forewarning, allowing for preventative measures to reduce their impact. In any situation, it is crucial to plan and prepare effectively to alleviate the suffering caused by disasters, especially for vulnerable groups like children. Children are particularly at risk due to their unique physiological, psychological, and developmental needs. It is vital for pediatricians and communities to evaluate

---

Contributors to former editions: Ciro Ugarte, Jacobo A. Tieffenberg, Lou Romig.

T. Vu (✉)
University of Colorado School of Medicine/Children's Hospital Colorado, Aurora, CO, USA
e-mail: Tien.Vu@childrenscolorado.org

N. Ravi
University of Colorado School of Medicine, Department of Pediatrics, Aurora, CO, USA

A. Oh
75th Ranger Regiment, United States Military, Fort Moore, GA, USA

C. McEvoy
CU Anschutz Center for COMBAT Research, University of Colorado School of Medicine, Aurora, CO, USA

how preparedness plans at local, regional, and national levels can protect children. Ignoring children's needs in disaster preparedness jeopardizes their safety and well-being. Lessons learned from the impact of previous disasters on children can enhance and improve our future responses.

The chapter's information serves as a guide for creating an emergency preparedness plan that fosters coordination among various agencies involved in disaster response. Active involvement from all relevant parties in plan development is key to breaking down silos, promoting understanding, and encouraging cooperation. The process of inclusive, multidisciplinary planning is more critical than the plan itself. It ensures that all agencies and personnel involved have a shared understanding, which is crucial for effective implementation when necessary. Planning should encompass both short-term and long-term strategies for reducing disaster risks, educating community organizations on preparedness, and establishing coordination methods across local, regional, national, and international levels. Understanding regional and national response systems enables local planners to align their efforts with these broader systems.

Local Emergency Plan

Objectives
- Outline the key elements of a disaster preparedness plan and detail the role pediatricians play within it
- Identify and evaluate the risk factors that must be considered during disaster planning
- Describe the essential requirements for developing and coordinating a local disaster plan

General Terminology

Disaster management is a critical component of the social system, tasked with planning, organizing, directing, and controlling across all phases of emergency management. The general phases of disaster management are shown in Fig. 3.1 and include preparedness, prevention, response, and recovery.

The objectives of an emergency plan vary depending on the response phase. Disaster preparedness involves creating the plan, training and coordinating those who will carry it out, and ensuring the availability of necessary resources. A plan designed for multiple adverse events is known as an emergency or disaster plan (also referred to as an emergency operations plan). In contrast, a contingency or hazard-specific plan is tailored to address a specific event, such as a tornado, flood, or pandemic. See Box 3.1 for details. Any disaster plan should clearly outline the objectives, strategies, and activities, including a detailed timeline, assigned personnel, and an estimated budget.

Fig. 3.1 Phases of disaster management

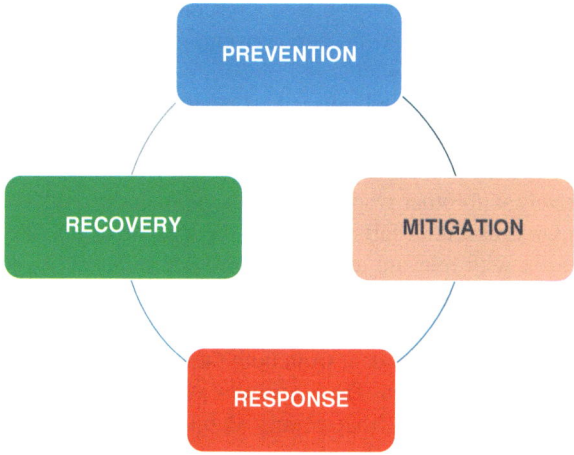

Box 3.1: Planning Definitions
- *Emergency or Disaster Plan (e.g., Emergency Operations Plan)*: A comprehensive plan designed to address a wide range of potential emergencies
- *Contingency or Hazard-Specific Plan*: A targeted plan developed to address specific threats or hazards

---

During the first two phases of disaster planning, prevention and mitigation, the primary goal is to avoid or mitigate the effects of a disaster by focusing efforts on reducing both risk and vulnerability. Despite these efforts, some damage from a disaster may still occur, which is referred to as *residual risk*.

The response phase involves implementing medical and humanitarian assistance according to the preparedness plans, as well as any spontaneous actions deemed necessary, even if they are not part of a formal plan.

Following the response phase is the recovery phase, where the focus shifts to repairing damaged services. Reconstruction and recovery aim to restore goods and services to their pre-disaster levels, if possible, and include measures to reduce future risks. Preparedness and lessons learned are essential for enhancing the capacity for future disaster response.

Pediatric Considerations

Each stage of a disaster involves critical planning elements that are essential for pediatricians. These planning activities engage various social agents and operate at different levels, including the family, local community organizations, emergency services, community physicians, hospitals, government bodies, and agencies like the local Red Cross and Red Crescent societies. Typically, town or district public health offices serve as the convening bodies for local disaster preparedness and response planning.

Pediatricians and other child healthcare providers should actively participate in all local committees focused on risk management, preparedness, and response. They must familiarize themselves with existing regional plans to collaborate effectively with other response system members and advocate for children's needs. If a plan is absent or fails to address the specific needs of children, pediatricians should work with relevant agencies to provide input or suggest enhancements. This may require gathering and analyzing data, conducting field visits, and meeting with representatives from various institutions and agencies.

Active involvement from both the healthcare sector and the community is essential for preparation. These efforts should culminate in the creation of concise operational documents that clearly define each participant's responsibilities and the agreements made. Regular drills are important to test the system's functionality and ensure coordination among all participants.

Risk Evaluation

A risk evaluation involves conducting an honest and critical analysis of both threats and vulnerabilities. It examines the characteristics of potential threats to a community and assesses their likely impact. This process includes identifying possible natural events that could pose a risk to a specific community, such as earthquakes, hurricanes, floods, volcanic eruptions, landslides, or pandemics. In some regions, climatic events that threaten the population have a seasonal pattern, and understanding these cycles can enhance preparedness efforts.

Disasters may also result from human activities, including technological failures that disrupt infrastructure, incidents at factories or chemical plants, fires (whether intentional or accidental), radioactive or nuclear accidents, armed conflicts, wars, or terrorism. In summary, risk evaluation involves pinpointing the regions and communities most vulnerable to these identified threats and detailing the specific characteristics that increase their susceptibility.

Community-Level Emergency Planning

Every community should develop its own emergency plans, in partnership with local institutions and agencies. The plans should clearly outline the responsibilities of each institution and establish methods for effective coordination and collaboration. It is crucial to analyze the risks that threaten different sectors of the community and to develop immediate interventions, considering the geographic and climatic conditions unique to various regions. Additionally, input from national and regional health officers should be incorporated into the planning process to ensure comprehensive preparedness.

Clinic- and Hospital-Level Emergency Planning

The emergency plan for hospitals should fulfill four essential characteristics: clarity, conciseness, completeness, and wide dissemination.

- *Clarity*: The language of the plan should be straightforward and free of ambiguity. Every instruction should be easily understood by all stakeholders, leaving no room for misinterpretation. Simplicity in wording ensures that everyone, regardless of their role, can quickly grasp the plan's directives.
- *Conciseness*: The plan should be succinct, making it quick to read and easy to implement. A plan that is too lengthy is less likely to be read in full and can be challenging to keep updated. The more concise the document, the easier it will be to regularly review, revise, and distribute.
- *Completeness*: The plan must encompass all the necessary components for effective action and coordination. This includes detailed protocols, resource allocation, communication channels, and contingency measures. A comprehensive plan ensures that no aspect of the response is overlooked, enabling a coordinated and efficient response to emergencies.
- *Dissemination*: The plan should be widely distributed to all key stakeholders and be easily accessible. It's essential that the plan is not only available in full but also summarized in a visually appealing and easy-to-understand format. This summary should be displayed in strategic locations such as office spaces, hospitals, and community centers to ensure that it is seen and remembered by those involved.

An effective emergency plan for hospitals clearly outlines each participant's responsibilities, identifies potential risks, and specifies the range of interventions required. It is vital that the organizations responsible for implementing the plan are actively involved in its development. For healthcare agencies, the emergency plan should detail the objectives, actions, and organizational structure of the hospital and its departments, including specific staff responsibilities. To ensure its effectiveness during an emergency, the plan must be well-known to all involved parties and regularly rehearsed.

Essential Elements of an Emergency Plan

A. *Situation Analysis*

To effectively prepare for disasters, it is crucial to identify and describe potential threats, whether natural or human-made. This involves assessing both structural and non-structural vulnerabilities within the community, which could be impacted by these threats. Evaluating how agencies would function and provide essential services with their existing resources, or operational capacity, is equally important. The disaster plan should clearly specify the types of events it addresses, estimate their likely impact on the community, and determine the expected timeframe for their occurrence. Additionally, it is necessary to analyze potential damages and the maximum demand for health services by correlating identified threats with community vulnerabilities. Finally, cultural and political factors, such as tribal or political dynamics, that may hinder the plan's implementation must be considered to ensure the plan is both comprehensive and feasible.

B. *Objectives and Goals*

The objectives and goals define the expected outcomes of the emergency plan based on the realistically available human, economic, and material resources. A common mistake is including resources that are not available, with the hope of acquiring them later. Since obtaining all desired resources may be impossible, prioritize actions based on the population and geographical area to be served. Include an outcome prediction that describes the measurable impact of implementing the plan.

C. *Organization*

Structure the institution's various sectors and departments so that authority, responsibility, and coordination methods for plan activation are clear and well-defined. Establish an Emergency Operations Committee (EOC) to oversee and coordinate response actions. Determine how and when to seek government support, as a national response framework can augment local efforts in emergencies.

D. *Roles and Responsibilities*

Clearly defining roles and responsibilities is essential to ensure an effective response to a disaster. This involves specifying who is responsible for performing each task, when these tasks should be carried out, how they should be executed, and the resources required. Additionally, it is crucial to establish a clear command chain for communication, supported by backup systems such as radios, megaphones, and mobile sound systems, to maintain effective communication during emergencies.

E. *Communication and Coordination*

Detail a notification chain from a central point to all necessary individuals. Establish communication means, including radio bands and frequencies, telephone numbers, and rendezvous locations. Each location should have an identified team leader who can conduct household counts and identify missing individuals needing rescue. Appendices should include an updated directory of participants, threat maps, vulnerable areas, a population database, a health profile, a directory of basic services (e.g., water, electricity, telecommunications, security), assistance agencies, and an inventory of available resources.

F. *Training*

After developing the emergency plan, conduct training sessions. These should cover the situation, expected damages, roles and responsibilities, and coordination methods, including various simulation exercises. Participants should engage in theoretical (tabletop) exercises to assess their knowledge and identify gaps. Later, organize disaster drills with prior notice to staff and key community members, and assess these drills with feedback from external observers. Use insights from drills to update the emergency response plan. Unannounced simulations without prior training are usually less effective and can lead to frustration.

G. *Resources*

Perform a requisite analysis to determine the resources needed for the emergency plan. Compare these needs with available resources and identify what still needs to be obtained. Ensure the plan is based on actual resources rather than wishful thinking.

H. *Coordination of the Local Emergency Plan*

The response mechanisms will vary based on community size and specific risks. Coordinators from hospitals, rescue services, and emergency medical services should report to an incident commander who directs the local emergency plan. For incidents involving multiple jurisdictions and agencies, a unified command system like an Emergency Operations Committee (EOC) may be established. This system allows representatives from different jurisdictions to collaborate on priorities, resource allocation, and strategies. A coordinated response may also involve local, state, and federal government levels, as well as non-governmental agencies providing humanitarian aid.

Box 3.2: Disaster Planning Resources

Federal Emergency Management Agency (FEMA) – National Incident Management System (NIMS) publications at http://www.fema.gov/emergency/nims/

Centers for Disease Control and Prevention—software planning model tools for governments at http://emergency.cdc.gov/cdcpreparedness/science/planningtools.asp

Your state's homeland security office, local government affairs office, or county government office, listings at http://www.fema.gov/about/contact/statedr.shtm.

Disaster Planning Levels

Objectives

- Identify the various levels of disaster planning, including local, regional, and national and their specific roles.
- Assist families in creating a family emergency plan, incorporating safety procedures, communication strategies, and emergency contacts.
- Recognize the importance of both personal preparedness and the planning efforts of healthcare professionals and health centers.

- Support elementary and high schools in developing their emergency plans and ensure these plans are integrated with the local community's emergency response framework.
- Identify and address special needs in disaster shelters, such as those related to disabilities or medical conditions.
- Describe the role of Emergency Medical Services (EMS) in disaster response, including their key responsibilities and functions.
- Discuss state and federal emergency response plans and understand their procedures and frameworks.

Preparedness Is Key to Disaster Survival

Disasters can vary in scale, affecting areas from a few blocks to entire cities, multiple counties, or even states and nations. Each type of disaster requires a unique approach and planning strategy. Consequently, preparation is essential at all levels, but individual and local preparedness is particularly crucial. Governmental and nongovernmental assistance takes time to mobilize, and even more time is needed to transport people and resources to the disaster site. Typically, the first 72 h of a disaster are managed by local officials, organizations, and individuals. Adopting a mindset that emphasizes local response is vital for effective early survival. Disaster response usually follows a bottom-up approach, where higher levels of response are activated if local resources are insufficient or overwhelmed. This section will cover planning levels in the following order: individual, local, hospital, and federal.

General Approach to Planning

As outlined in Section "Local Emergency Plan" (see Box 3.2), there are two primary approaches to disaster preparedness at all levels: disaster-specific (contingency) planning and all-hazards planning. It is crucial to understand the specific hazards that a community faces and the types of disasters that are most common in that area. For frequently occurring disasters—such as flooding in low-lying areas, hurricanes in coastal regions, or earthquakes near fault lines—contingency planning can effectively target anticipated needs and optimize the emergency response. However, it is impossible to prepare for every potential scenario, making it essential to incorporate flexible strategies. Therefore, adopting a general needs-based or all-hazards planning approach is vital. This approach prepares individuals, families, and local organizations to develop a single set of skills and concepts that can be applied to any disaster. In this section, we will explore disaster planning at different levels using the all-hazards planning approach.

Planning in the Family

Pediatricians can play a vital role in helping their patients and families prepare a comprehensive family emergency plan. These plans should be tailored to the specific needs of each household, considering the medical needs of family members, available resources, and the unique factors within the local community. For instance, families with children who have special needs may require early evacuation, as they often need more time and careful planning for equipment and medication. It is crucial to plan for evacuation before an area becomes inaccessible, especially for families with young children or those with additional medical needs.

When creating a family emergency plan, several important questions should be considered:

- What types of disasters are most likely to occur in your community?
- Is your home, your children's school, or your workplace located in a risk area?
- How well-prepared is your home to face the most likely disaster?
- Should your family be prepared to respond at any time, or can you be notified in advance?
- In the event of a disaster, how will you locate and reunite with your family members at a safe location?

It is important that all family members are familiar with evacuation routes and have printed maps that detail both primary and alternate routes, as well as a pre-established meeting point outside the risk area whenever possible. Families should also be aware of the location of command centers or community shelters in their area. Preparing a list of important contact telephone numbers in advance is also essential.

In situations where a family member must leave due to healthcare or other responsibilities during a disaster, having a clear, written plan that has been discussed and can be easily followed is critical. This is particularly important for those whose professional duties, such as healthcare providers, law enforcement officers, firefighters, and public officials, might limit their ability to assist their own families during a disaster.

For families with members who have special health needs, it is important to store and periodically renew necessary medications and supplies to ensure they are available during a disaster. In general, it is advisable to have 2 weeks' worth of medications and a week's supply of food and water. Additionally, consider having a small backup generator to keep a refrigerator operational for storing food and medications in the event of a power outage. If a disaster is anticipated, it is wise to stock up on shelf-stable foods and canned goods that can be consumed without cooking. Given the likelihood of limited access to potable water during a disaster, it is also important to have methods for purifying or filtering water.

Families should be provided with information on creating a contingency plan that allows for at least 3 days of self-sufficiency following a disaster. A list of supplies necessary for 3 days of self-sufficiency in a high-income country is provided in Box 3.3. This list should be adjusted based on what is appropriate and feasible for low- and middle-income countries. These items can typically be found in pre-made emergency kits available for purchase online, or families can assemble their own kits by purchasing the items individually. The emergency kit should be packed and ready to go in backpacks, so it can be taken immediately at the first sign of a disaster or the need for evacuation. Box 3.4 provides online resources for families to assist in their planning.

Box 3.3: Basic Disaster Supplies
Core supplies

Bottled drinking water: 4 L (1 gallon)/day/person
Identity cards and medical records of all family members
Well-equipped first aid kit and manual
Non-perishable food
Flashlight with batteries or hand-crank
Matches
Extra clothing for weather or outdoor stays
Blankets or sleeping bags
Money
Insect repellant
Personal hygiene products and sanitizer
Infant or child supplies (diapers, formula, baby food, bottles)
Portable radio, walkie-talkies, or cell phones with charging device
Map of the region
Essential medications
Emergency and family contact phone numbers

Complementary supplies

Manual can opener
Garbage bags
Two extra sets of home and car keys
Pet supplies
Extra glasses
Extra batteries and chargers

Box 3.4: Online Resources for Families
Federal Emergency Management Agency (FEMA) at https://www.ready.gov/collection/are-you-ready
American Academy of Pediatrics (AAP) Family Readiness Kit: Preparing to Handle Disasters at https://www.aap.org/en/patient-care/disasters-and-children/resources-for-families/

American College of Emergency Physicians (ACEP) Family
Disaster Preparedness at https://www.emergencyphysicians.org/globalassets/
   files/pdfs/acep-family-disaster-prep.pdf
American Red Cross Family Disaster Education Materials at
https://www.redcross.org/get-help/how-to-prepare-for-emergencies/make-a-
   plan.html
US Department of Education's resource, "Practical Information on Crisis
   Planning: A Guide for Schools and Communities" (https://www2.ed.gov/
   admins/lead/safety/emergencyplan/crisisplanning.pdf).
AAP and the American College of Emergency Physicians, emergency information form (EIF) for children with special needs, available at https://
   www.acep.org/globalassets/uploads/uploaded-files/acep/clinical-and-
   practice-management/resources/pediatrics/medical-forms/eifspecial-
   needs.pdf

Planning by Pediatricians and Medical Staff

Beyond creating a family emergency plan and educating the families of their
patients, pediatricians should also prioritize preparedness within their offices and
among their staff. This preparation involves several key areas: ensuring the safety of
both staff and patients, safeguarding essential equipment and materials, and securing patient records. Given the importance of maintaining the integrity of vaccines
and other temperature-sensitive medications, it is crucial to consider the need for a
backup generator to keep refrigeration systems operational during power outages.
Additionally, it's wise to plan for an alternative location where patients can be
treated if the primary office becomes unusable. Equally important is establishing a
reliable method for informing patients and callers about where they can receive care
during such emergencies. This could include setting up an automated phone message system, updating the office website, or using social media to disseminate information quickly. Furthermore, staff should be trained in emergency protocols and
know how to access patient records securely if electronic systems fail. Regular drills
and reviews of the emergency plan can help ensure that everyone is prepared to
respond effectively in a crisis.

Planning by Daycare Facilities and Schools

Any facilities where children spend their time must develop comprehensive emergency response plans. These plans should account for the most frequent incidents as
well as rare but potentially severe situations such as fires, school violence, terrorist
attacks, chemical exposures, and community violence. A crucial aspect of these
plans is detailing how urgent medical care will be provided onsite when needed. The

development of school emergency plans should involve key stakeholders, including parents, teachers, and staff, ensuring their concerns and insights are considered. Collaboration with external agencies, such as the police, fire departments, and health officials, is also essential to ensure a coordinated response during emergencies. Additionally, the plans should include specific provisions for training school staff in basic life support, first aid, and rescue techniques, with regular rehearsals and updates to refine the plan as needed.

School disaster plans must also address the identification and management of post-traumatic stress in both students and staff members, along with criteria for referring individuals for professional psychological intervention. After a disaster, children often benefit from the stability of a regular routine and the support of teachers and peers. Prolonged school closures can disrupt children's recovery and well-being, so efforts should be made to reopen schools as quickly as possible after a disaster. The use of school buildings as emergency shelters can delay or complicate their reopening, so coordination between schools and relief agencies, such as the Red Cross or local emergency management organizations, is vital to facilitate a smooth transition back to normal operations.

Childcare centers also need a well-prepared plan to ensure the safety of the children in their care, coordinate with community response agencies, and establish methods for reuniting children with their families during emergencies. Staff members at childcare centers should be thoroughly educated and trained to implement these emergency plans effectively.

In all cases, families, schools, and child care centers must carefully consider how to support children with special healthcare needs during emergencies, ensuring that their unique requirements are integrated into the overall planning process.

Medical Planning for Shelters

Shelters should designate staff members to coordinate with agencies and organizations for obtaining necessary supplies and assistance. Emergency planning must account for the possibility of extended shelter stays, which will necessitate additional resources and meticulous organizational management. Special attention should be given to the needs of pregnant women, infants, and young children, including their requirements for formula, diapers, basic first aid, hygiene products, and safety. Shelters must also accommodate children with special healthcare needs. For instance, children with asthma may require nebulizer treatments. While families are likely to bring their own nebulizers, a reliable source of electricity is crucial for their operation. Similarly, a refrigerator is essential for storing insulin for those with diabetes. Shelter staff should ideally have direct phone or radio access to emergency medical services to secure medical advice when needed. Furthermore, shelters should have protocols in place to isolate individuals with highly contagious diseases such as measles or chickenpox.

Shelter life must be structured to ensure that children are supervised and engaged in constructive play and entertainment. Such activities are important for coping with stress and fostering social development. They also provide necessary distractions and help mitigate the risk of adolescent violence and mischief. Safety within shelters is as critical as safety at home. Medications, medical supplies, and potentially hazardous items should be kept out of children's reach. Residents should be informed about the location and use of emergency exits. If shelters permit weapons, these must be securely stored away from children.

Emergency Medical Services Planning

Emergency Medical Services (EMS) are specialized emergency services focused on delivering out-of-hospital acute medical care and/or transporting patients with acute illnesses or injuries to definitive care facilities. EMS systems and their structures vary significantly from country to country, making it essential for national regulatory bodies to define the scope of practice for their EMS providers, especially in the context of disaster scenarios. See Fig. 3.2 for EMS's role in disaster planning.

The safety of EMS providers during disaster responses is paramount. As first responders, they are at high risk for serious injuries due to the hazards presented by the disaster itself. Consequently, it is crucial to provide appropriate training, materials, and resources to ensure a safe and effective prehospital response. While securing substantial public funding for safety supplies across various disaster scenarios can be challenging, it remains a critical consideration.

In pediatric care, EMS must ensure that providers are adequately trained to care for children, including knowledge of pediatric dosing, the use of pediatric equipment, and the specific needs of children during emergencies. EMS personnel should engage in mass-casualty incident drills and exercises that include pediatric patients. It is also important to be aware of regional pediatric resources, such as pediatric trauma and burn centers. Having established pediatric destination protocols, appropriate equipment, and memory aids to address the needs of children is a crucial component of an effective EMS response.

Fig. 3.2 EMS "DISASTER" Response		
	D	Detect
	I	Incident Command
	S	Scene security and Safety
	A	Assess hazards
	S	Support (determine needs and order resources early)
	T	Triage and Treatment
	E	Evacuation
	R	Recovery

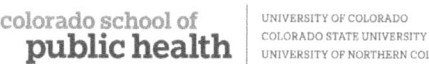

Emergency Planning By Hospitals

Hospital preparedness can be approached in two main ways, much like planning at other levels. The first approach is an all-hazards strategy, which involves creating an Emergency Operations Plan (EOP). This plan outlines the hospital's overall strategy for responding to any disaster, providing a general direction and response framework rather than focusing on specific types of disasters. To assist with this, the World Health Organization has developed a hospital emergency response checklist to guide administrators and emergency managers in addressing various types of emergencies effectively. The checklist includes several key components: command and control, communication, safety and security, triage, surge capacity, continuity of essential services, human resources, logistics and supply management, and post-disaster recovery.

Hospital and emergency department directors should have a fundamental understanding of local disaster plans and command levels. It is essential to appoint one or more staff members as liaisons to coordinate with other responding organizations and agencies outside the hospital environment. Some hospitals in the United States have adopted a modified system for managing mass casualty incidents or disasters that aligns with the external incident command system. Initially known as the Hospital Emergency Incident Command System (HEICS), it is now referred to as the Hospital Incident Command System (HICS) (see Fig. 3.3). This system enhances integration with external response plans and establishes a functional command structure within the hospital. It also acknowledges the importance of various ancillary services and functions that, while not directly involved in patient care, are crucial for emergency hospital operations. Furthermore, general hospitals should ensure that their emergency plans adequately address the specific needs of children.

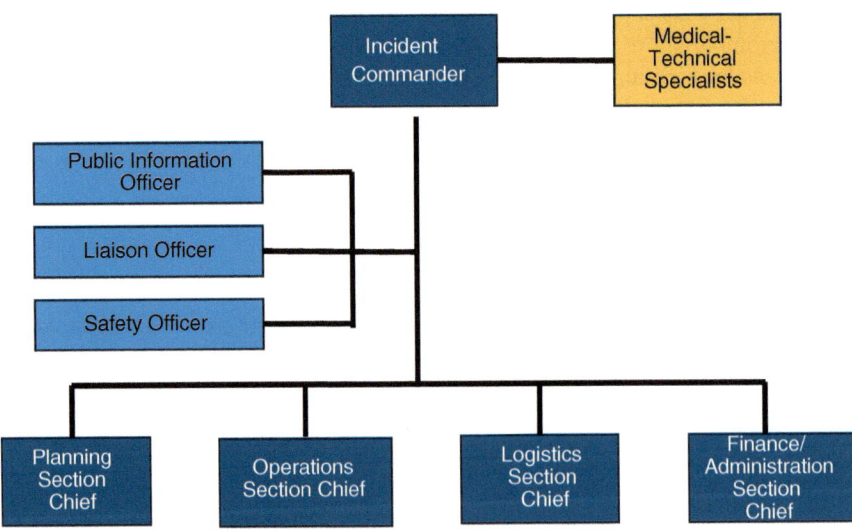

Fig. 3.3 Hospital incident command system (HICS)

The second approach to disaster preparedness involves developing specific contingency plans tailored to various scenarios. Hospitals should prepare for a range of potential situations based on a risk assessment that identifies the most likely hazards for the community. The Hospital Incident Command System (HICS) has created a set of Incident Planning Guidelines (IPGs) that can serve as a valuable template. These guidelines, detailed in Box 3.5, should address both hospital and pre-hospital events, including accidents and non-accidents such as structural collapses, fires, explosions, pandemics, and toxic exposures. Plans need to include detailed measures to safeguard staff, patients, and visitors. For cases involving infectious diseases or toxic exposures, it is critical to implement personal protective equipment and isolation procedures immediately. In incidents of structural damage, fires, or explosions, untrained hospital staff attempting rescue operations may face significant danger. Therefore, educating staff on basic safety protocols and when to wait for trained rescue teams is essential. Regular practice and evaluation of these plans are necessary to ensure that staff are well prepared for various emergency situations.

Hospitals and their personnel play a crucial role during disasters, but they are also at increased risk of harm, which can jeopardize the delivery of essential health services. To address this issue, the World Health Organization (WHO) developed the Safe Hospital Framework to guide hospitals in preparing for emergencies. A "safe hospital" is defined as a facility that maintains full functionality and infrastructure before, during, and immediately after emergencies or disasters. The continued functionality of a hospital relies on factors such as the safety of its buildings, critical systems and equipment, the availability of supplies, and the hospital's capabilities in emergency and disaster management, including response and recovery efforts. The WHO has also developed a hospital safety index, a global tool for evaluating a hospital's ability to remain operational during emergencies and disasters. This assessment provides valuable insights into a hospital's strengths and weaknesses and identifies necessary actions to improve its safety and emergency management capabilities.

Hospitals must also evaluate whether they need to enhance their surge capacity to manage a sudden influx of patients. Factors influencing this decision include the number of available inpatient, ICU, and emergency beds, surgical capacity, staffing needs across all departments, available supplies, and physical space for expanding treatment areas. It is important to ensure that current inpatients continue to receive appropriate care and that they are discharged or transferred to other facilities as needed. The plan should also include a method for mobilizing additional healthcare professionals and ancillary staff. Hospitals should develop a surge provider plan with an expanded network of community physicians who can be called upon for extra support. These additional physicians can assist regular hospital staff with patients who have less severe conditions, allowing core staff to focus on more critical cases.

Additionally, hospital plans should address stress management. Rotating providers and staff frequently during surge periods helps maintain performance and reduces psychological and physical fatigue. Plans should also consider the care of individuals experiencing acute stress reactions, survivor's guilt, material losses, or other psychological impacts related to the disaster. Post-traumatic stress disorder and other stress-related conditions are common following disasters, highlighting the need for comprehensive mental health support for both staff and patients.

Box 3.5: Resources for Hospital Planning
- World Health Organization—Hospital Emergency Response Checklist
  https://www.who.int/docs/default-source/documents/publications/hospital-emergency-response-checklist.pdf
- World Health Organization – Hospital Safety Index
  https://apps.who.int/iris/bitstream/handle/10665/258966/9789241548984-eng.pdf?sequence=1&isAllowed=y
- Centers for Disease Control and Prevention—Healthcare preparedness Toolbox
  https://www.cdc.gov/cpr/readiness/healthcare/toolbox.htm
- Occupational Safety and Health Administration at
  http://www.osha.gov/dts/osta/bestpractices/firstreceivers_hospital.html
- Agency for Healthcare Research and Quality (AHRQ)—Pediatric
- Hospital Planning
  http://www.ahrq.gov/prep/pedhospital/
- American Academy of Pediatrics – Pediatric Readiness in the ED
  https://publications.aap.org/pediatrics/article/142/5/e20182459/38608/Pediatric-Readiness-in-the-Emergency-Department?autologincheck=redirected&_ga=2.182689254.1550156137.1657835328-1483023652.1657835327
- Hospital Incident Command System (HICS)—Incident Planning Guidelines
  https://emsa.ca.gov/hospital-incident-command-system-incident-planning-guides-2014/

Government-Level Emergency Planning

Major public health organizations, such as the Centers for Disease Control and Prevention (CDC) in the USA, operate at both state and federal levels and play a crucial role in disaster preparedness. These organizations, alongside hospitals, work toward a unified goal during disaster situations, though their approaches to planning differ significantly. While hospitals focus on direct patient care after a disaster occurs, public health systems prioritize prevention on a population level before or during a disaster. Public Health Emergency Management (PHEM) is responsible for tasks such as epidemiologic surveillance, disaster prevention, creating and sharing guidance for preparedness and response, coordinating efforts across all levels, and distributing resources during a crisis.

Although disaster response typically begins at the individual and local levels, state and federal governments often provide additional support when local resources are exhausted. In some countries, the federal government maintains a strategic national stockpile, a reserve of critical medical supplies and equipment intended to support healthcare agencies during national emergencies. This stockpile is designed to be rapidly distributed to state and local communities as needed. While not all countries have a national stockpile, it is advisable for local healthcare workers and agencies to be aware of the resources that state and federal governments can mobilize in times of crisis. Additionally, federal and state governments frequently have medical teams composed of public health officials, medical professionals, and volunteers ready to assist local communities during disasters. A detailed national response plan should outline how these resources will be delivered to local communities to ensure swift and effective mobilization when needed.

Summary

Disaster preparedness is a continuous cycle that involves all individuals and groups involved in disasters, from people and families to governmental entities. For effective disaster response, planning needs to be cross-jurisdictional, include all response partners, and be coordinated across key stakeholders. Finally, children have unique needs during disasters, which requires further consideration, planning, and coordination.

References & Websites

Federal Emergency Management Agency (FEMA)

National Incident Management System (NIMS): https://www.fema.gov/emergency-managers/nims
National Response Framework (NRF): http://www.fema.gov/nrf
National Incident Management System (NIMS) publications: http://www.fema.gov/emergency/nims/
Family Disaster Readiness: https://www.aap.org/en/patient-care/disasters-and-children/resources-for-families/

Centers for Disease Control and Prevention (CDC)

Center for Preparedness and Response: https://www.cdc.gov/cpr/index.htm
Healthcare Preparedness Toolbox: https://www.cdc.gov/cpr/readiness/healthcare/toolbox.htm
Software Planning Model Tools for Governments: http://emergency.cdc.gov/cdcpreparedness/science/planningtools.asp

World Health Organization (WHO)

Strengthening National Emergency Preparedness: https://www.who.int/activities/strengthening-national-emergency-preparedness
Hospital Emergency Response Checklist: https://www.who.int/docs/default-source/documents/publications/hospital-emergency-response-checklist.pdf
Hospital Safety Index: https://apps.who.int/iris/bitstream/handle/10665/258966/9789241548984-eng.pdf?sequence=1&isAllowed=y

American Academy of Pediatrics (AAP)

Pediatric Readiness in the Emergency Department: https://publications.aap.org/pediatrics/article/142/5/e20182459/38608/Pediatric-Readiness-in-the-Emergency-Department?autologincheck=redirected&_ga=2.182689254.1550156137.1657835328-1483023652.1657835327

Family Readiness Kit: https://www.aap.org/en/patient-care/disasters-and-children/resources-for-families/

Emergency Information Form for Children with Special Needs: https://www.acep.org/globalassets/uploads/uploaded-files/acep/clinical-and-practice-management/resources/pediatrics/medical-forms/eifspecialneeds.pdf

American College of Emergency Physicians (ACEP)

Family Disaster Preparedness: https://www.emergencyphysicians.org/globalassets/files/pdfs/acep-family-disaster-prep.pdf

American Red Cross

Family Disaster Education Materials: https://www.redcross.org/get-help/how-to-prepare-for-emergencies/make-a-plan.html

Occupational Safety and Health Administration (OSHA)

First Receivers Hospital Best Practices: http://www.osha.gov/dts/osta/bestpractices/firstreceivers_hospital.html

Agency for Healthcare Research and Quality (AHRQ)

Pediatric Hospital Planning: http://www.ahrq.gov/prep/pedhospital/

Hospital Incident Command System (HICS)

Incident Planning Guidelines: https://emsa.ca.gov/hospital-incident-command-system-incident-planning-guides-2014/

U.S. Department of Education

Practical Information on Crisis Planning: https://www2.ed.gov/admins/lead/safety/emergency-plan/crisisplanning.pdf

Your State's Homeland Security Office, Local Government Affairs Office, or County Government Office

Contact Listings: http://www.fema.gov/about/contact/statedr.shtm

Chapter 4
Pediatric Triage in the Disaster Setting

Tien T. Vu, Nithin Ravi, Andrew S. Oh, and Cory McEvoy

Introduction

This chapter outlines fundamental concepts for emergency planning and response preparedness, covering various levels of planning, including families, health professionals, community organizations, healthcare facilities, and government bodies. The final section provides guidance on organizing community emergency services to effectively respond to mass casualty incidents.

Mass Casualty Management and Medical Care

Objectives

- Describe the fundamental components of a mass casualty management approach

---

Contributors to former editions: Ciro Ugarte, Jacobo A. Tieffenberg, Lou Romig.

T. T. Vu (✉)
Pediatric Emergency Medicine, University of Colorado School of Medicine/Children's Hospital Colorado, Aurora, CO, USA
e-mail: Tien.Vu@childrenscolorado.org

N. Ravi
Pediatric Emergency Medicine, University of Colorado School of Medicine, Aurora, CO, USA

A. S. Oh
75th Ranger Regiment, United States Military, Fort Moore, GA, USA

C. McEvoy
CU Anschutz Center for COMBAT Research, University of Colorado School of Medicine, Aurora, CO, USA

- Differentiate the various roles of individuals aiding during a disaster
- Describe the multisector rescue chain process from the incident site to the hospital

Mass Casualty Management

Mass casualty management (MCM), which is essential during a disaster, necessitates a departure from the conventional emergency care approach. Typically, first responders offer victims preliminary triage and medical care before transporting them to the nearest healthcare facility. This method often involves two distinct entities—field responders and receiving healthcare organizations—working somewhat independently with minimal coordination. In the context of a mass casualty event, this fragmented approach can quickly lead to disorder. To address this, a unified system was established to facilitate a more organized and effective response.

The MCM system is designed to address these challenges by integrating pre-established procedures for mobilizing resources, managing the field, and receiving patients at hospitals. It involves specific training for responders at various levels and ensures strong connections between field operations and healthcare facilities through a centralized command post. The system emphasizes the need for a coordinated multi-sector response, including triage, field stabilization, and patient evacuation to specialized healthcare facilities. MCM assumes the availability of substantial human and material resources and must be adapted to the resources available in the specific context of the emergency.

The MCM system relies on several core principles:

- Utilizing pre-established procedures that are adaptable for both routine emergency activities and major incidents
- Maximizing the use of existing resources
- Ensuring a multi-sector approach to preparation and response
- Establishing and maintaining strong, tested coordination among all involved parties

The system aims to:

- Enhance and expedite routine procedures to better utilize available resources
- Create a coordinated multi-sector rescue network
- Quickly restore disrupted emergency and healthcare services to normal operations

In practice, the MCM system involves a collaborative rescue chain that includes the health department, private hospitals, police, fire departments, non-governmental organizations (NGOs), transportation services, and communication networks (see Fig. 4.1). This chain begins at the disaster site, where initial activities include assessment, command and control, search and rescue, and field care. It progresses with the transfer of victims to appropriate facilities, guided by procedures for managing evacuation and ambulance traffic. The process continues with hospital reception,

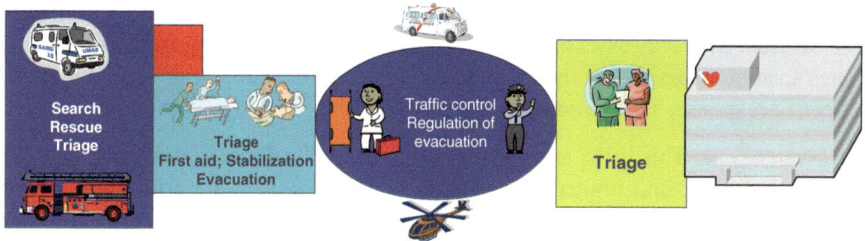

Fig. 4.1 A multi-sector rescue chain

where the hospital's disaster response plan is activated and concludes only when all victims have received the necessary emergency care to stabilize their condition.

To implement this rescue chain effectively, the following components are essential:

- A well-functioning emergency department
- A reliable basic radio communications network
- Coordination procedures among all sectors involved
- Skilled multi-sector rescue teams

The assignment and organization of resources in mass casualty management requires careful planning. As in any chain, the strength and reliability of the system depend on each link; if one fails, the entire system will be compromised.

Specific Activities at the Disaster or Mass Casualty Site

Objectives

- Appreciate the importance of patient documentation and accurate record-keeping during a disaster.
- Recognize key triage algorithms relevant to mass casualty management.
- Distinguish between the adult and pediatric triage algorithms (START and JumpSTART).
- Identify the key tasks involved in mass casualty management during humanitarian emergencies.
- Describe the planning tasks during the mitigation phase.

Specific activities at the site of a disaster or mass casualty event involve organizing the disaster zone through a series of critical steps and interventions. The process begins with an alert from any observer or bystander, who provides detailed information about the disaster. This includes the exact location where the event occurred, the time it happened, the nature of the disaster, the estimated number of injured individuals, associated risks, and the populations at risk from these dangers.

The initial assessment plays a crucial role in determining the resources needed at the disaster site. This assessment, carried out by the initial evaluation unit, designates specific zones within the incident area to streamline operations and ensure an effective response. These zones are (Fig. 4.2):

- *Impact Zone*: This is the area directly affected by the disaster, where the damage is most severe and immediate response is required. It is the primary focus for rescue and medical interventions.
- *Incident Command Post*: This central location serves as the hub for coordinating all disaster response activities. It is where leaders from various response teams meet to manage operations, make strategic decisions, and ensure effective communication between different sectors.

- *Advanced Medical Post*: Located near the impact zone, this post provides immediate medical treatment to casualties before they are transported to more comprehensive healthcare facilities. It is equipped with essential medical supplies and staffed by emergency medical professionals.

- *Evacuation Area*: This zone is designated for the safe and orderly evacuation of individuals from the disaster site. It ensures that there is a clear and organized process for moving people to safety away from the affected area.

- *Public Affairs and Press*: This area manages communications with the media and the public. It provides accurate information, updates on the situation, and instructions for the affected population to manage public perception and maintain order.

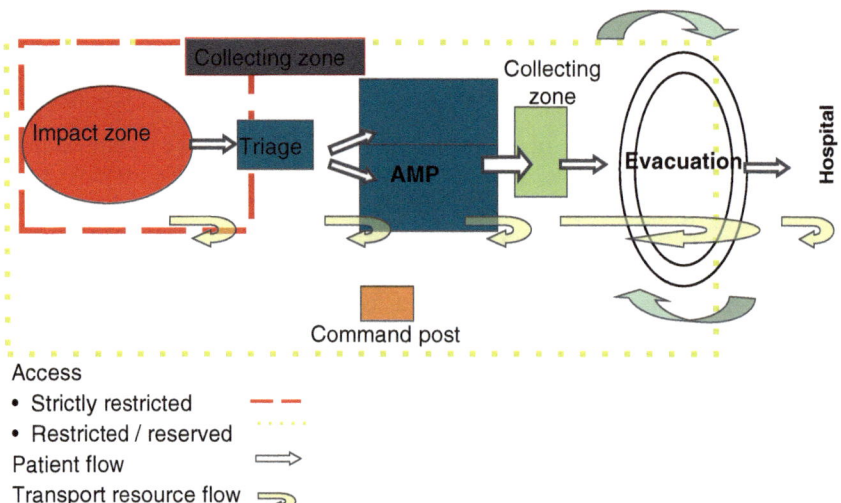

Fig. 4.2 Organization at the disaster site

- *Access Roads*: These are designated routes to and from the disaster site. They are kept clear for emergency vehicles and personnel to ensure rapid access and efficient movement of resources.

- *Restricted Areas*: Sections of the disaster zone that are off-limits to non-authorized personnel. These areas are controlled to prevent interference with emergency operations and to ensure the safety of both responders and the public.

Establishing and managing these zones effectively is vital for orchestrating a coordinated response and minimizing further risks to individuals and the community.

Safety

During rescue operations in a disaster, it is vital to ensure the safety of victims, rescue personnel, and the general public, with particular attention to the needs of children. Comprehensive safety measures should be in place to protect all individuals involved in the response efforts.

Communication and Documentation

Following a disaster, communication systems such as landline and cell phones may become overloaded. For effective emergency management, ultra-high frequency (UHF) and very high frequency (VHF) radios are recommended. UHF radios are used for local communication within the disaster area, while VHF radios are used for long-range communication and coordination with strategic centers.

Essential patient referral information should be communicated from the disaster site to the Incident Command Post and then to relevant agencies and nearby hospitals. Key details to document include:

- *Number of victims, categorized by triage level*: This helps prioritize care, especially for children who may need immediate attention.
- *Number of individuals requiring hospital transfer*: Ensuring that children and adults who need hospital care are properly accounted for.
- *Special medical equipment needed for transfer*: Identifying any specialized equipment, such as pediatric-specific supplies, ensures its availability.
- *Details of transportation logistics*: Information on the timing and methods of transportation helps in efficient resource management.
- *Relevant injuries of victims*: Documenting injuries helps determine the specific care needs of children and adults.

Care of Victims

Search and rescue operations should be carried out by trained professionals, including firefighters and specialized rescue teams, who are equipped to handle various types of disasters. It is crucial to ensure the safety of these frontline workers, including any personnel who may be specifically trained to address the needs of children. Before entering the disaster area, it is essential to assess whether rescue teams need protective clothing or breathing apparatus to safeguard against environmental hazards.

Once victims are located, including children, they should be transported to a designated casualty collection point for initial assessment (field triage). At this stage, first aid is administered based on the priority status of each victim. If the number of victims or the distance from the incident site makes direct hospital transport impractical, an advanced medical post should be set up nearby but outside the impact zone.

At the advanced medical post, all victims, including children, undergo a second round of medical triage to identify those who need immediate care. Victims are then stabilized at this post, where procedures may include:

- *Advanced airway management*: Ensuring proper breathing and ventilation, particularly critical for children who may have smaller airways.
- *Fluid therapy*: Maintaining circulation and treating shock, with dosages adjusted for pediatric patients.
- *Hemorrhage control*: Stopping bleeding and preventing further blood loss, including using pediatric-specific techniques if necessary.
- *Analgesics*: Managing pain effectively, considering the specific needs of children.

Documentation of the treatments administered at the advanced medical post is essential. This information should be included in the patient's evacuation documents, especially for children, to inform subsequent medical care decisions at the hospital.

In summary, the goals of the advanced medical post are to stabilize patients, reassess their condition (re-triage), and coordinate their transport to appropriate hospitals. This process is known as the 3 T's principle: typifying (classifying), treating, and transporting. Ideally, the advanced medical post should be staffed with emergency medicine physicians and nurses experienced in pediatric care. Additional medical specialists, such as pediatric surgeons and anesthesiologists, should be included if available and needed.

Patient Triage Rationale

Triage is a critical system used to prioritize care and transport during emergencies, aiming to maximize survival in situations with limited resources. This process is essential during the rescue phase of a disaster and involves assessing patients to determine who needs immediate stabilization and transport versus those who can be managed later. Triage helps identify individuals requiring emergency resuscitation and surgery, ensuring that resources are allocated effectively.

The initial step in managing a mass casualty incident (MCI) involves a rapid assessment to evaluate all victims quickly and make decisions about treatment priorities. Various triage algorithms exist, and their application may vary depending on regional or institutional protocols. During this evaluation, victims are tagged with color-coded identifiers—such as tags, tape, or markers—to signify the level of medical urgency. This color-coding system is generally consistent across different triage methods.

The primary principle of triage is to treat all victims with equal importance, regardless of age, gender, occupation, or other factors. Decisions are made based solely on the clinical condition of the patient. Victims are classified into categories based on the severity of their injuries:

- *Green*: These individuals are ambulatory, meaning they can walk and are either uninjured or have only minor injuries. This category includes victims who are not in immediate danger and can wait for treatment.
- *Yellow*: This designation is for those who are moderately injured or require urgent care but are not in immediate life-threatening conditions. This group may include children who need prompt but not immediate attention.
- *Red*: Individuals in this category are severely injured or in critical condition, requiring immediate intervention to survive. Children in this group may need specialized care and rapid transport to medical facilities.
- *Black*: This category is reserved for those who are deceased or have injuries that are incompatible with survival. Some triage systems may also use a *Grey* designation for victims who are in a state of expectant death, where recovery is unlikely but the patient is not yet deceased.

By implementing these triage categories, responders can ensure that medical resources are directed to those most in need, including providing urgent care for critically injured children and adults while managing less severe cases accordingly.

Patient Triage Methods

Triage is a crucial system for establishing care priorities and ensuring that resources are allocated to save as many lives as possible, especially in resource-limited situations. This process involves categorizing patients based on their medical needs, allowing for efficient treatment and transport. In a mass casualty incident, triage helps distinguish between those who require immediate intervention and those who can wait.

Adult Triage

For adults, the START (Simple Triage and Rapid Treatment) system is commonly used (see Fig. 4.3). This method employs a color-coding system to classify patients over 8 years old. START evaluates patients based on their respirations, pulse/perfusion, and mental status before initiating treatment. When victims arrive at the casualty collection point, a triage officer quickly assesses each individual, focusing mainly on controlling hemorrhage and repositioning airways without providing extensive treatment at this stage.

Field triage typically operates at three levels:

1. *Onsite Triage (Field Triage):* This initial assessment is conducted at the disaster scene by first aid providers or emergency medical technicians. Victims are classified to determine who needs immediate transport to the advanced medical post. For less experienced personnel, it may be helpful to group victims into "yellow" and "red" categories together to reduce errors and save time during the initial evaluation.

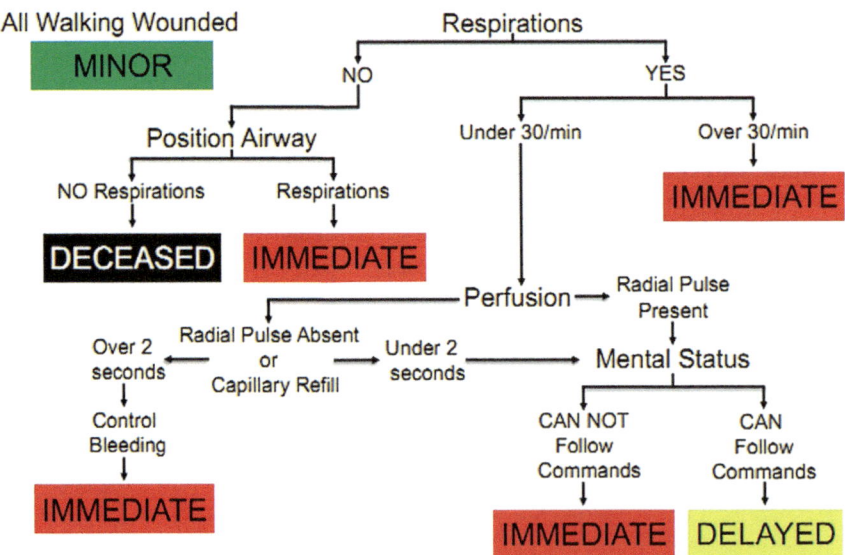

Fig. 4.3 Simple triage and rapid treatment (START) system

2. *Medical Triage:* Conducted by an emergency physician, anesthesiologist, or surgeon, this stage determines the level of medical care required. Victims are classified as follows:

- *Red:* Requires immediate stabilization and life-saving treatment within 4 hours. Includes patients with shock, severe breathing difficulties, extensive bleeding, or critical head trauma.
- *Yellow:* Requires delayed treatment, usually within 24 hours, with close monitoring. Includes those with risks of shock, open fractures, severe burns, or head trauma but who are responsive.
- *Green:* Can wait for treatment or have minimal injuries. Includes ambulatory patients with minor fractures or wounds.
- *Black:* Deceased or expectant, requiring transportation to the morgue or comfort care.

After initial field triage, victims should be transported to a medical facility based on their priority, and a secondary triage should be performed upon arrival to reassess their condition.

Pediatric Triage

The JumpSTART triage system is specifically designed for children aged 1 to 8 years old (see Fig. 4.4). It modifies the START system to accommodate pediatric physiological differences. Unlike the adult system, JumpSTART recognizes that children who are apneic may still have some degree of perfusion and can survive if their respiratory function is restored. Children unable to walk or those carried by adults should at least be categorized as "yellow" to ensure they receive appropriate attention.

Combined Adult and Pediatric Triage

The SALT (sort, assess, life-saving interventions, and treatment) system is another triage approach applicable to both adults and children (see Fig. 4.5). Developed by an interdisciplinary committee, SALT addresses the limitations of various existing triage systems by incorporating comprehensive features. This method includes:

- *Global Sorting:* Victims are prioritized based on their ability to follow commands and walk. Those who cannot follow commands or have obvious life-threatening conditions are prioritized first, followed by those who can follow commands but cannot walk.

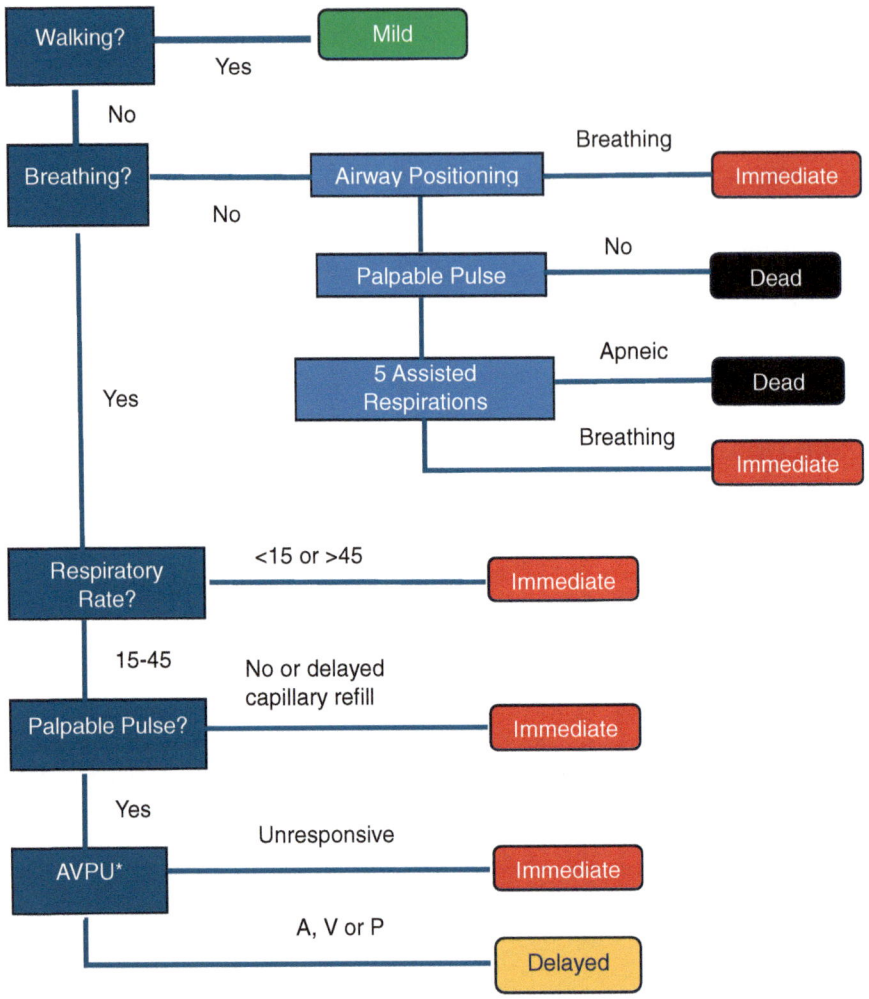

*A- Alert; V- Response to verbal stimulus; P - Response to painful stimulus; U - Unresponsive, or decerebrate/decorticate posturing

Fig. 4.4 JumpSTART pediatric triage system

Sort, Assess, Life-saving intervention, Treatment/Transport

Step 1: Global Sorting

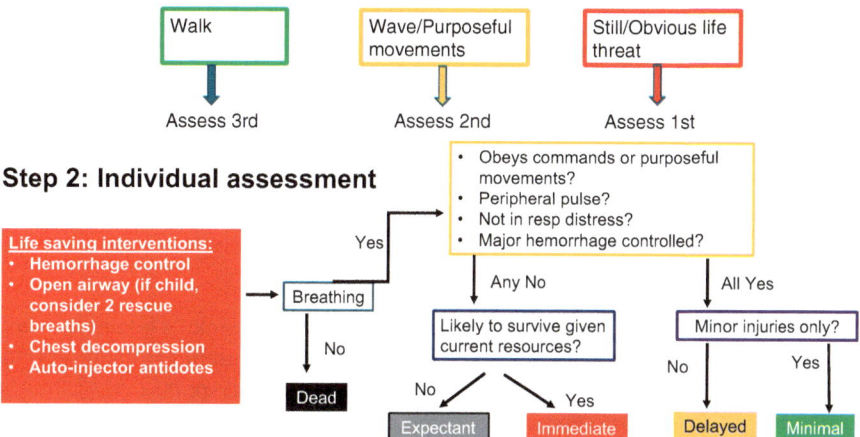

Fig. 4.5 Sort, asses, life-saving interventions, and treatment (SALT) triage system

- *Life-Saving Interventions:* Immediate interventions such as controlling major hemorrhage, opening airways, or administering antidotes are performed before assigning triage categories.
- *Triage Categories:* Patients are classified as delayed, immediate, or expectant based on their response to life-saving interventions. The "expectant" category is used for those with severe injuries but who may not receive adequate resources immediately.

Children are often over-triaged in this system due to their developmental stage, which affects their ability to follow commands. Despite this, SALT aims to integrate the best features of various triage systems and should be tested against the JumpSTART method to assess its effectiveness.

Regardless of the triage system employed, it is essential to perform thorough secondary evaluations of all victims both onsite and at the emergency department. Triage is a dynamic process that continues until each patient receives definitive care and treatment.

Organization of Patient Transfer

Transfer organization involves the procedures designed to ensure that victims of a mass casualty incident are transported safely, quickly, and efficiently to appropriate healthcare facilities.

Effective transfer is managed based on several key principles, including strict control over the rate and destination of evacuation to prevent overwhelming healthcare facilities. One important aspect of on-scene mass casualty management is to prevent untrained personnel from initiating spontaneous evacuations of unstable or minimally injured victims. Such unmanaged transport poses significant risks: it endangers the lives of victims, bypasses essential field decontamination procedures, and disrupts the overall mass casualty management system.

To ensure a safe and effective transfer, victims should only be moved from the advanced medical post to healthcare facilities when:

- *Stabilization*: They are in the most stable condition possible. This means that medical interventions have been applied to manage their injuries or conditions to a point where further stabilization is achievable during transport.
- *Preparation*: They are adequately equipped for the transfer. This includes ensuring that necessary medical equipment, such as monitoring devices or medications, is in place and ready for use during transport.
- *Communication*: The receiving healthcare facility has been properly informed and is prepared to receive the patient. This involves sharing relevant medical information and ensuring that the facility has the necessary resources and personnel to provide continued care.
- *Transportation*: The most appropriate vehicle and escort are available. This means using vehicles that are equipped for the specific medical needs of the victims and having trained personnel or escorts to accompany them during the transfer.

By adhering to these procedures, the safety of victims is enhanced, and the efficiency of the overall mass casualty response is maintained. This careful coordination is particularly critical for transporting children or individuals with severe injuries, as they may require specialized medical care and careful handling during transfer.

Control of Victim Flow: The Noria Principle

Effective patient movement during a mass casualty incident must follow a "one-way" direction to ensure efficiency and minimize confusion. This process involves a clear, linear progression from the impact zone to various stages of care, without any back-tracking.

Victims are moved through a series of stages in a sequential, unidirectional manner. Initially, patients are transported from the impact zone to the collection point. From there, they are moved to the entrance of the advanced medical post. After receiving initial treatment at the advanced medical post, patients are further transported to areas designated for treatment, evacuation, and ultimately, hospital care.

This organized movement creates a streamlined "conveyor belt" system that efficiently guides victims through increasingly sophisticated levels of care. By maintaining a one-way flow, the system prevents bottlenecks and ensures that each stage of care is reached in a systematic order, reducing the risk of delays or errors.

Key stages include:

- *Impact Zone to Collection Point*: Victims are initially assessed and stabilized in the impact zone before being moved to a designated collection point.
- *Collection Point to Advanced Medical Post*: At the collection point, victims are triaged and then transported to the advanced medical post, where stabilizing medical interventions can be provided.
- *Advanced Medical Post to Evacuation Areas*: After initial stabilization, patients are prepared for evacuation.
- *Evacuation Areas to Hospital Care*: Finally, patients are transported to hospitals equipped to handle their specific needs, where they receive ongoing care and treatment.

Maintaining this one-way flow is crucial for efficient mass casualty management, particularly for pediatric patients or individuals with severe injuries who may need specialized attention at each stage of their journey. Proper planning and coordination at each step ensure that victims receive the appropriate care in a timely manner, enhancing overall outcomes and minimizing additional risks.

Organization of Hospitals

For effective mass casualty management, hospitals must be well-organized to efficiently handle incoming victims. This organization enables the swift mobilization and management of available resources, ensures clear communication with prehospital providers, and facilitates the management of inpatients as well as the flow of new arrivals. Essential tasks include coordinating secondary evacuations and maintaining communication with victims' families and various public entities. Key departments such as emergency services, surgery, operating rooms, intensive care units, laboratory, radiology, blood bank, and pharmacy need to be reinforced. It's crucial to prepare for sequential reinforcements and staff augmentation in areas with the highest expected workload. This approach helps prevent overburdening the staff and supports a quick return to normal operations. Adding hallway beds or opening in-hospital clinics can increase surge capacity, while outdoor tents can provide additional treatment areas for minimally injured victims. Decontamination facilities should be ready if there is a risk of hazardous material exposure. Hospital security should be bolstered, with police officers stationed at entrances and reception areas. Each hospital should have a well-equipped command post ready for emergencies. Special attention should be given to the needs of children among the victims, ensuring that pediatric care is adequately integrated into the emergency response plan.

Reception of Victims

To manage the influx of new patients, those who can receive outpatient care should be discharged. If victims bypass on-scene medical triage and arrive at the hospital independently, they must undergo triage upon arrival, just like any other new patient. When prehospital management is efficient, an experienced emergency nurse can conduct the triage. If not, an experienced emergency physician, anesthesiologist, or surgeon should perform it. All arriving victims, regardless of previous triage, should be reassessed upon arrival. Continuous communication between the on-scene command post, advanced medical post, and hospital command post is essential for updating the number and severity of injured victims, transport times, and current hospital capacity. Special considerations should be given to children, ensuring they are prioritized and their specific needs are addressed during triage and treatment.

Treatment Areas

Designate and staff treatment areas within the hospital based on triage levels. For instance, a red treatment area should be reserved for victims classified in the red category. An emergency medicine physician or anesthesiologist should oversee the red treatment area and be prepared to handle severe, life-threatening injuries. Additional triage within the red area can prioritize patients for operative interventions. Victims in the yellow category should be reevaluated by a physician and provided with necessary care or observation. If their condition deteriorates, they should be moved to the red treatment area. Patients with no chance of survival should receive only supportive care and be placed in a separate ward. Prepare an area for deceased victims if the hospital morgue is overwhelmed, with special arrangements made for the handling of children's remains, ensuring sensitivity and proper care in these situations.

Summary

When responding to a mass casualty incident, a management system should be established that includes a command post, an advanced medical post, evacuation and transport logistics, and hospital care. This system must be activated in a coordinated manner, ensuring that each sector is prepared to manage patient care effectively. All lessons learned during the immediate response to the disaster should be integrated into future planning efforts.

Suggested Reading

1. Cicero M, et al. Comparing the accuracy of three pediatric disaster triage strategies: a simulation-based investigation. Disaster Med Public Health Prep. 2016;10(2):253–60. https://doi.org/10.1017/dmp.2015.171.
2. Purwadi H, Breaden K, McCloud C, Pranata S. The SALT and START triage system for classifying patient acuity level: a systematic review. Nurse Media J Nurs. 2021;11(3):413–27.
3. Romig LE. Pediatric triage: a system to JumpSTART your triage of young patients at MCIs. JEMS. 2002;27(7):52–63.
4. Romig LE. Disaster management. In: APLS course manual. Jones & Bartlett Publishers; 2006.
5. Safe Hospitals: a collective responsibility. A global measure of disaster reduction, Pan American Health Organization/World Health Organization, Available at: http://www.paho.org/spanish/dd/ped/SafeHospitals.htm.

Chapter 5
Pediatric Trauma

Kristin McAdams Kim, Ana Alejandra Ortiz Hernández, Conrad W. Wanyama, Celia Wanda Kariuki, Andrew S. Oh, and Joseph Wathen

Introduction

Several factors influence the response to disasters involving trauma, such as the type of disaster, the number of casualties, and the community's ability to organize a swift response. Proper preparation and planning are crucial for ensuring a coordinated and effective disaster response. Since pediatric patients are frequently involved in disasters, it is essential to include children in all plans and preparations for responding to such events.

Healthcare professionals who are trained in the assessment and treatment of pediatric patients play a vital role in caring for injured children. Medical facilities

K. M. Kim (✉)
Department of Pediatrics, Section of Emergency Medicine, University of Colorado School of Medicine Anschutz Medical Campus, Aurora, CO, USA
e-mail: kristin.kim@childrenscolorado.org

A. A. O. Hernández
Emergency Department, Instituto Nacional De Pediatría (INP), Mexico DF, Mexico

C. W. Wanyama
Kenya Medical Research Institute (KEMRI)/Wellcome Trust Research Programme, Kilifi, Kenya

Department of Nursing Sciences, University of Nairobi, Faculty of Health Sciences I, Nairobi, Kenya
e-mail: CWanyama@kemri-wellcome.org

C. W. Kariuki
Mama Lucy Kibaki Hospital, Nairobi, Kenya

A. S. Oh
Fort Moore U. S. Army, GA, USA

J. Wathen
Department of Pediatrics, Section of Emergency Medicine, University of Colorado School of Medicine, Anschutz Medical Campus, Aurora, CO, USA
e-mail: Joseph.wathen@childrenscolorado.org

© The Author(s), under exclusive license to Springer Nature Switzerland AG 2025
L. Umphrey et al. (eds.), *Pediatric Considerations in Disaster Settings*,
https://doi.org/10.1007/978-3-031-85501-6_5

and communities must be equipped to care for both adults and children during a disaster.

Key strategies for managing a disaster or mass casualty event begin with identifying the location of the incident, classifying and sorting affected individuals based on the severity of their injuries (triage), and providing treatment for injuries, some of which may be uncommon outside large-scale disasters. Treating pediatric patients poses unique challenges. Children may be unable to communicate effectively, may experience fear, or may have been separated from their families. While pediatric patients often suffer from the same types of injuries as adults, rescue personnel may lack familiarity with child-specific treatment methods. Providing medical care and transportation for injured children should follow established priorities and available resources. Those with severe trauma often require immediate first aid before being transferred to more advanced healthcare facilities.

Response to a Disaster

Objectives

- Describe the critical role of safety and secure transportation for the wounded to ensure timely and effective medical care, minimizing further injury during transit
- Describe the importance of having a well-prepared hospital disaster plan to guide medical facilities in managing large-scale emergencies efficiently and ensuring the best possible patient outcomes

Planning for a Disaster

Effective disaster response requires thorough planning, particularly for trauma-related incidents and mass casualty events. These emergencies often demand rapid, coordinated, and unanticipated action. Except in cases of ongoing conflict, most mass casualty incidents, such as bombings, shootings, earthquakes, and floods, occur suddenly and within a limited timeframe. Having a response plan in place beforehand allows local resources to respond efficiently and cohesively. It is essential to anticipate that local resources, including healthcare facilities, may need to operate independently for an extended period before external assistance arrives. Depending on various factors such as location and resource availability, this could range from hours to weeks. A disaster response plan should address the management of traumatic injuries and include the following basic components:

- *Staff*: Ensure the availability of personnel for immediate and on-call responses, identifying local experts and potential responders before the event.

- *Supplies*: Pediatric care requires specialized equipment due to the unique needs of children. Ensuring access to pediatric-specific airway devices, vascular access tools, and transport equipment is essential.
- *Safety:* Particularly in cases of violent incidents, measures must be in place to protect both responders and patients, both at the disaster site and after transportation.
- *Space:* Establish designated areas for treating a surge of patients, which may include repurposing non-clinical spaces for medical use. These areas should also provide a safe environment for pediatric patients to protect them from further psychological trauma.
- *Sorting:* Implement triage both at the scene and upon arrival at the healthcare facility to ensure that resources are allocated to those most in need.

Effective communication is vital during a disaster response and may require non-traditional methods. Communication is essential not only between medical personnel but also with the broader community. A coordinated response is necessary to handle the large influx of patients. Ideally, personal radios or cell phones should be available so healthcare personnel can communicate with each other and with the central command. However, in cases where resources are overwhelmed or unavailable, secondary communication systems, such as hospital-wide radio networks, can be crucial. Multiple communication options should be in place as backups, as cell phone networks may fail, and handheld radios can be unreliable in difficult terrain or through thick walls.

Disaster Planning for Traumatic Injuries

Disasters involving large numbers of traumatic injuries require advance planning and specific preparations. Simply developing a plan is not enough—regular drills and training exercises are essential to ensure an effective response, refine procedures, and address unforeseen challenges.

Staff

In a disaster setting, the first healthcare provider on the scene may not be specialized in pediatrics. In such cases, surgeons or personnel with surgical training may be necessary. Responding staff should be able to stabilize patients until specialized teams arrive. Additionally, the sheer number of casualties may necessitate additional staff. Identifying available resources, including retired or mid-level providers with pediatric experience, is a key part of preparation. Keeping a list of available personnel and a system to contact them quickly is crucial. Establishing a central communication system that can activate a call-up roster ensures timely assistance. If transportation is challenging due to distance or terrain, bringing expert staff to the disaster area may be more practical than transferring large numbers of patients to other facilities.

Once staff are onsite, it is important to organize them effectively and provide clear job descriptions. Having easy-to-follow guides for procedures like chest decompression, tourniquet application, and chest tube placement can help extend resources in critical moments.

Supplies—Pediatric-Specific Equipment

In emergency situations involving children, having the right equipment is crucial. Trauma-specific supplies include hemorrhage control devices, such as tourniquets, clotting agents, hemostatic and pressure dressings; see Box 5.1 for details. Blood products and fluids may be needed in larger quantities than usual and burn dressings and pain control measures will be required. Decontamination supplies for small children can be simple, such as a plastic laundry basket, but must include provisions for preventing hypothermia, such as blankets or heating devices. Pediatric-sized airway and IV supplies are also essential.

Box 5.1 Recommended equipment for pediatric emergencies in disaster situations

Airway management

- Oxygen source with flow meter*
- Simple face masks—infant, child, adult sizes*
- Face masks for assisted ventilation—infant, child, adult sizes*
- Self-inflating bag with 250 cc/1000 cc reservoir for ventilation*
- Suction catheters (Yankauer)—8, 10, 14 Fr*
- Oropharyngeal airway tubing—infant, child, and adult sizes
- Nasal oxygen delivery tubing—infant, child, adult sizes
- Optional for intubation:

  - Laryngoscope handle with batteries
  - Miller blades—0,1,2,3
  - Endotracheal tubes (cuffed preferred)—3.0, 3.5, 4.0, 4.5, 5.0, 6.0, 7.0, 8.0
  - Adhesive tape to secure endotracheal tube

Intravascular access/fluid management

- IV catheters—18,20, 22, 24 g
- Intraosseous (IO) needles—15 or 18 gauge (with insertion device)
- Supplies to secure the IV—arm boards, tape
- Pediatric sized drip chambers and tubing
- Fluids:

- 5% Dextrose in 0.9% NS or 5% dextrose in lactated Ringers (for maintenance fluids)
- Isotonic fluids—0.9% NS and/or lactated Ringer's solution
- Ideally in 250 cc, 500 cc, 1 L bags to allow safer administration for small children

Monitoring Equipment

- Blood pressure cuffs—infant, child, adult
- Portable monitor/defibrillator (with pediatric settings <10 J)
- Pediatric-sized defibrillator paddles/patches
- Pediatric-sized ECG skin contact electrodes
- Pulse oximeter with reusable (for older children) and non-reusable sensors (for small children)

Miscellaneous

- Tool to estimate weight (Broselow tape, Hand Tevy, other tools as available locally)
- Splints and gauze padding
- Portable/rolling carts with extra supplies such as linens, blankets
- Potable water source with warming
- Portable shower for decontamination—ideally with warming capability
- Thermal control—portable heaters, warming cradles, warming lights
- Geiger counter—to measure radioactive contamination
- Personal protective equipment

These are key pieces of equipment for pediatric resuscitation as airway management in children is crucial.

Safety

Most physicians and nurses are not trained for on-scene rescue operations, which are typically managed by local police, firefighters, and hazardous materials teams. However, in some cases, healthcare providers may need to operate close to the disaster site, especially in confined spaces. The risks vary depending on the nature of the disaster and may include structural instability, fires, toxic gases, and the potential for coordinated attacks targeting responders (Box 5.2). Hospitals may also become secondary attack sites and should have appropriate security measures in place. Crowds of family members searching for their loved ones can create chaos, so it is essential to plan for their needs to help maintain order.

> **Box 5.2 Risks at the scene of a disaster**
> - Structural instability and further collapse
> - Fires, carbon monoxide, cyanide
> - Dirty bombs: chemical and/or radioactive contamination
> - Biohazards: sewage, bodily fluids, blood exposure, intentional pathogen contamination
> - Infectious agents
> - Active shooter
> - Secondary attack/secondary bomb risks

Space

Establishing locations for both on-scene triage and patient care is crucial. Hospitals should prepare by clearing non-emergent patients and making operating rooms available. Spaces should be safe for children, who may not have adequate supervision. Childproofing areas and creating dedicated spaces for pediatric care can help minimize the trauma of seeing medical procedures.

Triage

Using an established triage system is essential to prioritize treatment and transportation of patients. Implementing a triage guideline at the scene helps ensure that those who can benefit most from higher levels of care receive it promptly. At the receiving hospital, more detailed triage by staff trained in pediatric injury management can be performed.

Patient Transport

Patients should be promptly transported to medical facilities once they have been rescued. At the disaster site, initial interventions include airway support, hemorrhage control, and spinal immobilization if needed. Airway management includes positioning, supplemental oxygen, and the use of airway adjuncts like oropharyngeal or nasopharyngeal airways. Supraglottic devices like laryngeal mask airways (LMAs) or endotracheal tubes may also be used, depending on the resources available during transport.

Maintaining a clear airway during transport is a top priority, and this can often be managed effectively with bag-valve-mask ventilation (BVM). Intubation before transport is generally unnecessary and can lead to complications. A large study comparing intubation to BVM in children over 13 years old found no significant advantage to intubation before transport. Intubation commits the patient to mechanical ventilation, which can introduce further complications during transport. Therefore, proper airway positioning and BVM technique remain essential skills for first responders.

Hemorrhage Control

Controlling bleeding before transport is critical to reducing mortality and preventing further complications. Initial measures include applying direct pressure, pressure dressings, packing wounds, and using tourniquets for severe limb injuries. Recent studies have shown that tourniquets can be lifesaving without increasing the risk of limb loss.

Spinal Immobilization

Spinal immobilization helps prevent further injury in cases of blunt or blast trauma. However, most simple penetrating injuries, such as gunshot or stab wounds, do not require full spinal immobilization unless the injury affects the spine. Immobilization should aim to keep the spinal column in a neutral position. Infants and toddlers may need extra padding to prevent flexion of the cervical spine. Specialized pediatric backboards are available for this purpose. Immobilization is mainly used during transport and should be discontinued as soon as possible to avoid pressure injuries.

Conclusion

Injured individuals at high risk for morbidity or mortality, including those affected by fires, explosions, or severe trauma, should be transported to medical facilities as quickly as possible for further care.

Pediatric Trauma Assessment

Objectives

- Identify the unique aspects of global trauma management in pediatric patients
- Evaluate pediatric trauma cases based on prioritized assessments
- Describe the most common types of traumatic injuries in children

Effective Global Practices for Pediatric Trauma Care

Globally, traumatic injuries account for 33% of all deaths among children aged 5–19 years. Of these deaths, 1.5% result from natural disasters or collective violence such as war. Timely and skilled treatment for injured pediatric patients can be lifesaving.

Trauma mortality can be categorized into three distinct peaks. The first peak occurs within seconds or minutes following a traumatic event and is primarily due to severe injuries affecting the brain, spinal cord, heart, or major vessels like the aorta. Injuries in this category are typically non-survivable, even with immediate intervention.

The second peak in mortality happens from minutes to hours after the trauma. Patients in this timeframe have a significantly improved chance of survival if treated during the critical "golden hour" immediately following the incident. Injuries associated with this peak include epidural or subdural hematomas, hemothorax or tension pneumothorax, and significant intra-abdominal bleeding, such as spleen lacerations or ruptures, as well as complex pelvic fractures.

The third peak of trauma mortality occurs days to weeks post-injury and is often the result of multisystem failure stemming from inflammation, infection, or sepsis.

Effective management of pediatric trauma necessitates a systematic approach. Employing the primary, secondary, and tertiary evaluation/survey framework allows for the rapid and thorough identification and treatment of injuries. The (X)-ABCDE method is widely accepted for initial assessment, stabilization, and immediate intervention when necessary, and it is typically followed by a secondary evaluation. This process usually occurs before comprehensive personal history or detailed physical examination data is available.

The Advanced Trauma Life Support (ATLS) course was developed in the United States to equip hospital-based health personnel with a systematic framework for managing injured patients. Similar courses exist globally and adhere to comparable guidelines. These guidelines are also applicable in disaster scenarios involving large numbers of victims. The primary aim for each patient is to identify and manage life-threatening conditions using the (X)-ABCDE approach, particularly during the second mortality peak and ideally within the first hour of critical care. This strategy can be effectively employed for both adults and children, provided that pediatric-specific considerations are considered.

Identifying Features Unique to Pediatric Trauma Patient

In emergency settings, it is essential to recognize the specific differences between children and adults. Children face a disproportionately higher risk of traumatic death for various reasons:

- **High Respiratory Rate:** Children are more vulnerable to aerosolized agents, chemicals, and carbon monoxide.
- **Reduced Fluid Reserve:** They are more susceptible to dehydration.
- **Lower Circulating Blood Volume:** Even small amounts of blood loss can lead to hypovolemic shock.
- **Underdeveloped Musculoskeletal Strength:** Their thoracic and abdominal organs are less protected by ribs and abdominal muscles.
- **Developmental Vulnerabilities:** Infants and toddlers struggle to escape disasters as they cannot follow directions or make quick decisions. Younger children may not recognize or respond appropriately to risky situations.
- **Anatomic and Physiologic Differences:**
  - **Prominent Occiput:** This can lead to neck flexion when placed on flat spine boards.
  - **Increased Oral Secretions:** More suctioning may be necessary.
  - **Obligate Nose Breathers:** Infants under 3 months are particularly susceptible to anatomical obstructions and infections.
  - **Relatively Larger Tongue:** This can complicate the use of bag-valve-mask ventilation or intubation.
  - **Large Adenoids:** Bleeding is common, especially with nasal intubations.
  - **Flexible, Omega-Shaped Epiglottis:** Its anterior location requires the use of a straight blade to lift the epiglottis for intubation and visualization of the larynx.

Methods for Assessing Injured Children

The assessment of pediatric trauma employs an (X-)ABCDE approach tailored to the unique characteristics of children. This method focuses on identifying and managing pediatric trauma, including traumatic brain injuries, respiratory and thoracic trauma, and blunt abdominal injuries.

Primary Survey

The primary survey serves as the initial evaluation of the patient, aimed at identifying and addressing life-threatening issues. It systematically assesses the following components in a specific order:

- X—Control of Exsanguinating Hemorrhage: This step is often added for on-scene evaluations.
- A—Airway Maintenance: This includes restricting cervical spine motion.
- B—Breathing and Ventilation
- C—Circulation with Hemorrhage Control

- D—Disability: Neurological status assessment
- E—Exposure/Environment

At each stage, a quick assessment is conducted, and if life-threatening issues are identified, the patient is stabilized before proceeding to the next step. For instance, if there is active massive hemorrhage, bleeding control must be initiated before evaluating the disability.

Exsanguinating Hemorrhage

The initial on-scene evaluation starts with the identification and immediate control of significant life-threatening hemorrhage. Massive arterial bleeding should be managed using tourniquets, compression bandages, or wound packing. It is advisable to mark the time of tourniquet application. If a non-commercial tourniquet is used, writing directly on the extremity with a marker or pen is appropriate.

Airway

The airway assessment determines if it is stable. If the patient can speak without difficulty, this indicates that the airway is patent. Signs of upper airway obstruction, such as gurgling, stridor, or respiratory distress, require interventions like jaw thrust maneuvers and nasal or oral suctioning to maintain airway patency. Consider using oral or nasal airway adjuncts (oropharyngeal or nasopharyngeal airways) to keep the airway open. While managing a trauma patient's airway, potential cervical spine injuries must be considered by maintaining mid-line positioning and using a jaw thrust maneuver without tilting or lifting the cervical spine.

In some cases, maintaining the airway may be impossible, necessitating the placement of a supraglottic airway (e.g., laryngeal mask airway, LMA) or an endotracheal tube (ETT). If securing the airway is unsuccessful, a surgical airway (e.g., cricothyrotomy) may be required (Box 5.3). In disaster situations, it is crucial to consider the need for ongoing ventilation if an LMA, ETT, or cricothyrotomy is performed. If resources for continued ventilation are unavailable, the patient may require expectant care. Judicious use of other airway adjuncts can delay respiratory compromise, allowing time for additional resources to facilitate mechanical ventilation for patients with tenuous airways.

Box 5.3 Airway assessment in children
Stable airway—it is possible to keep the airway open

- Use airway opening maneuvers (jaw thrust, positioning)
- Use airway adjunct devices—oral/nasal airway devices

Unstable airway—it is NOT possible to keep the airway open (note that this will commit patient to mechanical ventilation and may not be appropriate if resources are not available)

- Bag-Valve-Mask (BVM) ventilation
- Laryngeal mask airway (LMA)
- Endotracheal tube placement (ETT and rapid sequence intubation)
- Cricothyrotomy

Breathing

After ensuring that the airway is open, the next step in the primary survey is to assess breathing, which evaluates oxygenation and ventilation (chest wall rise, air entry, oxygen concentration in inspired air, and skin color). This includes auscultation of breath sounds and physical examination of the chest wall to check for conditions such as tension pneumothorax or flail chest. Treat any significant or suspected life-threatening injuries. If tension pneumothorax is suspected, consider needle decompression, apply a three-sided dressing for sucking chest wounds, and provide oxygen supplementation for poor oxygenation. Patients with pulmonary contusions may require positive pressure ventilation if resources allow, initially provided through bag-valve-mask (BVM) ventilation until a definitive airway is established. End-tidal CO_2 monitors and pulse oximetry can serve as effective adjuncts to assess the efficacy of breathing.

Circulation

Following the stabilization of the airway and breathing, the next step involves assessing circulation. Adequate circulation can be evaluated by checking pulse strength and rate both centrally and peripherally. Although environmental factors like temperature can influence them, capillary refill and the color of the skin/mucous membranes can also provide insights into peripheral perfusion. Blood pressure should be measured, but it's important to note that compromised circulation in children may not be evident until 25–30% of blood volume is lost, which is a concerning sign.

Tachycardia is an early indicator of hypovolemia in children and should not be disregarded, as it reflects a compensatory mechanism for blood loss and is typically more pronounced in children than in adults. Once hypotension occurs, the child's condition becomes critical.

If external hemorrhage is present, control the bleeding by applying direct pressure to the wound, placing a tourniquet proximal to an extremity wound when possible, or packing a trunk or abdominal wound when direct pressure cannot be applied. It is vital to assess for hemorrhage on the patient's back, which may be obscured by clothing, as head injuries can often result in significant bleeding. Generally, use thin compression dressings instead of bulky ones to apply adequate pressure to the bleeding site. If available, consider using hemostatic agents (e.g., QuikClot, Surgicel). Quickly establish vascular access (IV or IO), as volume resuscitation may be necessary. Be cautious with significant crystalloid volume administration, as it may worsen hemorrhage by dislodging clots and lead to further injury due to fluid overload. If available, administering blood products is recommended for ongoing hemorrhage with signs of hypovolemia, as it has been shown to reduce mortality in cases of hypotension due to blood loss.

Disability—State of Consciousness

The state of consciousness is assessed through a rapid neurological evaluation. Determine if the child is alert, responsive to verbal or painful stimuli, or unresponsive (using the AVPU scale). Recent literature suggests that AVPU may be more sensitive to acute neurological dysfunction compared to the Glasgow Coma Scale (GCS). Additionally, evaluate the pupils for size, equality, and light response. A quick motor examination can assess motor activity in all four extremities. A detailed neurological examination can be conducted during the secondary survey. Some medical facilities will assign a score to the child at this point using the adult/child and infant versions of the GCS (see Table 5.1). A GCS score of 8 or lower indicates significant neurological impairment and may suggest the need to secure the airway with an ETT, LMA, or another device. In disaster settings, it is essential to consider the availability of ongoing ventilation before compromising the patient's ability to breathe independently.

Exposure/Environment

The assessment of exposure and environmental factors requires a thorough examination of the entire body, necessitating the removal of clothing for a complete evaluation. One critical concern related to the environment is maintaining proper body temperature. Hypothermia significantly increases the mortality rate associated with traumatic injuries and is one of the three components of the lethal triad in trauma. Preventing hypothermia is often overlooked but requires minimal resources. To mitigate heat loss, remove any wet or contaminated clothing. After a visual

Table 5.1 Glasgow coma scale

Best response	Child/adult	Infant	Score
Eye opening	Spontaneous		4
	To speech		3
	To pain only		2
	No response		1
Verbal response	Oriented, appropriate	Coos, babbles	5
	Confused	Cries but consolable	4
	Inappropriate words	Cries to pain	3
	Incomprehensible sounds/moans/grunts	Moans/grunts to pain	2
	No response		1
Motor response	Obeys commands	Moves spontaneously/purposefully	6
	Localizes painful stimulus	Withdraws to touch	5
	Withdraws to pain		4
	Abnormal flexion		3
	Abnormal extension		2
	No response		1

[a]Use best response in each category. If intubated, motor score is most useful. A score <8 or worsening rapidly may indicate need for further airway management

inspection of the entire body, cover the patient with warming measures as needed (blankets, sheets, or external warming devices). It is particularly important to note that infants can rapidly become hypothermic due to their large surface area-to-volume ratio, especially if they are wet.

Secondary Survey

The secondary survey begins once the ABCDE assessment has been completed and initial management of any life-threatening conditions has occurred. This examination involves a systematic physical assessment aimed at identifying all significant injuries without being sidetracked by visibly dramatic injuries.

Vital signs are monitored, and appropriate equipment is attached as available. The secondary survey entails a comprehensive head-to-toe examination, including a history of the traumatic event and a brief medical history. The AMPLE mnemonic is utilized to gather this information: Allergies, Medications, Past Medical History, Last Meal or Oral Intake, and Events Leading Up to the Trauma. Throughout this survey, the patient should be continuously monitored, and relevant laboratory and radiologic studies should be conducted. Definitive care can commence with the splinting of fractures and the application of wound dressings. Additionally, it is important for a staff member to provide emotional support to the child until family members arrive.

Common Traumatic Injuries in Children

Traumatic injuries in children can be severe and often differ in nature and presentation from those seen in adults. The unique anatomical and physiological characteristics of children make them particularly vulnerable to specific types of injuries. Below, we outline the most common traumatic injuries in children, including head, thoracic, abdominal, and extremity injuries, and discuss their management.

Head Injuries

Pediatric head injuries are among the most prevalent traumatic lesions in children. Due to their thinner and more flexible skulls, children can transmit trauma forces to the brain more intensely than adults. Additionally, younger children have disproportionately larger heads and weaker neck muscles, which often results in them "leading with their heads" during trauma events.

When assessing a child with a significant brain injury, or traumatic brain injury (TBI), it is crucial to ensure adequate cerebral perfusion pressure (CPP) and consider supplemental oxygen delivery. CPP is determined by the difference between the mean arterial pressure and intracranial pressure (ICP). Maintaining an adequate mean arterial pressure while implementing measures to decrease ICP is vital. Some interventions, such as elevating the head to 30 degrees, ensuring proper ventilation, and avoiding hypercarbia, can be performed with limited resources.

Elevated ICP can lead to altered vital signs, with Cushing's triad—characterized by hypertension, bradycardia, and irregular breathing patterns—indicating significant pressure increases. In children, bradycardia is often the first sign and may suggest impending brain herniation; thus, it should be regarded as a concerning finding.

TBIs can be classified into primary and secondary categories. Primary injuries occur at the time of trauma and may involve brain contusions, diffuse axonal injuries, or intracranial hemorrhages (Fig. 5.1). Secondary injuries emerge later due to metabolic effects like cerebral ischemia and edema, typically appearing hours to days after the event. Proper medical care can mitigate these secondary injuries.

Management of a child with TBI begins with the X-ABCDE approach, which emphasizes airway, breathing, circulation, disability, and exposure/environment. Ensuring airway patency requires cervical spine immobilization, and hypoxemia should be avoided. All children should receive 100% oxygen when available, and intubation should be considered if the Glasgow Coma Scale (GCS) score is below 8 or if maintaining a stable airway is impossible. Ideally, ventilation should be assisted to maintain a PCO_2 of 35–40 mm Hg; in cases of brain herniation or neurologic decline, a lower PCO_2 may be necessary. Elevating the patient's head (30–40 degrees) is advised while maintaining spinal immobilization.

Osmotic agents such as mannitol (0.5–1 g/kg) or 3% hypertonic saline (3–5 cc/kg) can be administered to reduce ICP. Managing hypotension is essential to prevent anoxic brain injury; in cases of hypovolemia, consider administering available

HEAD INJURY

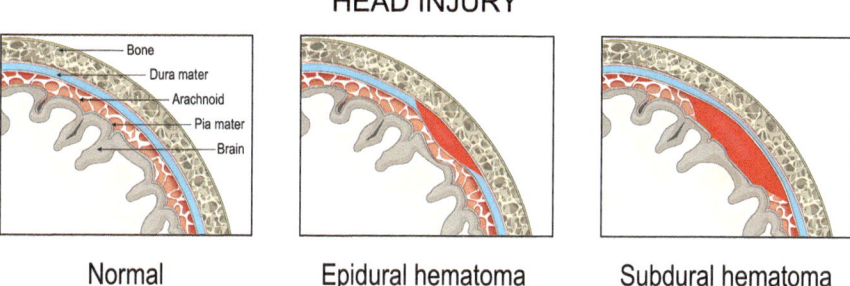

Fig. 5.1 Types of intracranial hemorrhage

blood products or crystalloid fluids (preferably 0.9% normal saline). If hypotension persists despite fluid resuscitation, medication with cardiovascular pressors may be indicated. Once the child is euvolemic, intravenous fluids can be given at maintenance rates: 4 mL/kg/h. for the first 10 kg, 2 mL/kg/h. for the next 10 kg, and 1 mL/kg/hr. for children over 20 kg.

If resources permit, trauma laboratory studies, radiographs, and cross-sectional imaging can be obtained as needed. Useful laboratory tests may include serum electrolytes, glucose levels, complete blood counts (CBC), partial thromboplastin time (PTT), prothrombin time (PT), international normalized ratio (INR), and blood type cross-matching. Maintain the head in a neutral position using a rigid cervical collar or other immobilization devices to prevent further spinal injury if cervical spine damage is suspected.

Short-term sedation and analgesia can be provided with medications like midazolam (0.1 mg/kg) and fentanyl (1–2 mcg/kg). If signs of increased ICP appear, such as unequal pupil dilation, abnormal posturing, or Cushing's triad, additional interventions may include hypertonic saline (3% normal saline, 3–5 cc/kg), sedation, mannitol (0.5–1 g/kg), and mild hyperventilation (targeting a PCO_2 of 25–30 mm Hg) until clinical conditions improve. Hyperventilation should be reserved for severe injuries that do not respond adequately to other interventions or in scenarios where resources are limited.

Thoracic Injuries

Thoracic injuries in children carry a high mortality risk. The greater elasticity of the ribs and sternum results in fewer fractures than in adults, yet these injuries can lead to significant energy transfer to underlying structures.

Pulmonary contusions are the most frequent injury associated with thoracic trauma and may initially present with subtle clinical signs. Essentially a bruise of the lung, a pulmonary contusion can lead to alveolar and interstitial hemorrhage and edema, with severity linked to the extent of lung tissue involved. Clinical signs may include bruising and abrasions on the chest wall, tachypnea, use of accessory

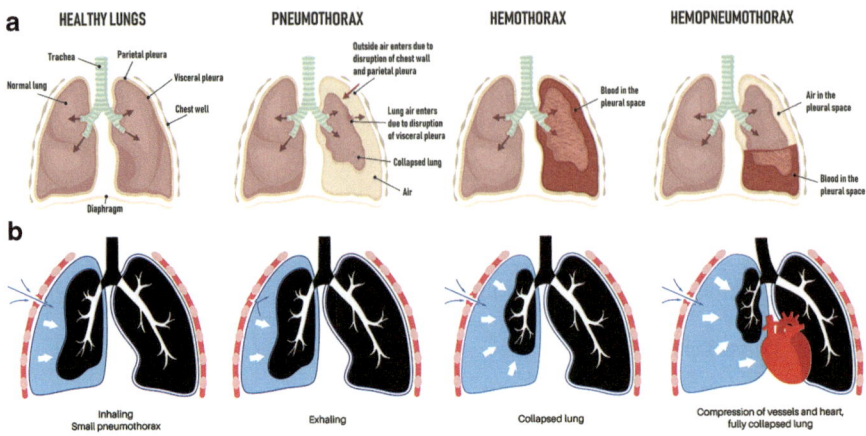

Fig. 5.2 (**a**) Pneumothorax, hemothorax, and hemopneumothorax. (**b**) Tension pneumothorax

respiratory muscles, and hypoxia. Continuous pulse oximetry and end-tidal CO2 monitoring can help assess ventilation. Treatment for lung contusions typically involves supplemental oxygen, close monitoring, and intubation if needed, along with positive end-expiratory pressure (PEEP) if resources allow.

In pneumothorax cases, air enters the pleural space, leading to the collapse of the lung due to loss of negative pressure (Fig. 5.2a) An open pneumothorax, often referred to as a "sucking chest wound," occurs when there is a breach in the chest wall. Immediate treatment includes applying an occlusive dressing with one side left open to prevent tension pneumothorax development.

Hemothoraces and pneumohemothoraces occur when blood accumulates in the pleural space, potentially compressing the lung (Fig. 5.2a). A massive hemothorax suggests a significant lung injury and involvement of large vessels. Therapy focuses on draining the blood with a chest tube (inserted posteriorly) and addressing hypovolemia.

Differentiating between simple and tension pneumothorax involves assessing tracheal position; tension pneumothorax (Fig. 5.2b) is diagnosed clinically through signs like tracheal deviation away from the affected side, absent breath sounds, hypotension, and potentially distended neck veins. In children, identifying jugular venous distension and tracheal deviation may be challenging. Tension pneumothorax requires immediate needle decompression at the second intercostal space, mid-clavicular line, or chest tube placement in the fourth or fifth intercostal space, anterior axillary line.

Pericardial effusion arises when fluid, typically blood in trauma cases, accumulates in the pericardial sac; pericardial tamponade is caused when the effusion causes myocardial restriction and decreased cardiac output (Fig. 5.3). Clinically, Beck's triad—reduced pulse pressure, neck vein distension, and muffled heart sounds—suggests pericardial tamponade. However, these classic findings may be difficult to identify in pediatric patients. Arrhythmias, including bradycardia,

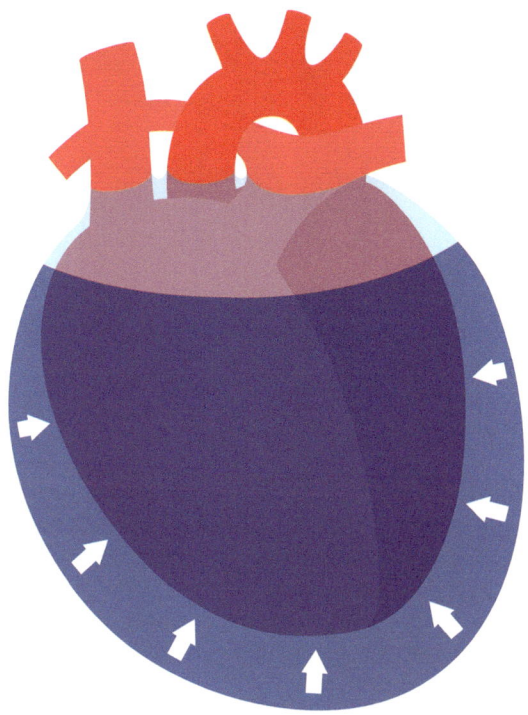

The buildup of fluid in the pericardial cavity.
It can compress heart and cause cardiac tamponade

Fig. 5.3 Pericardial effusion and tamponade

pulseless electrical activity (PEA), and asystole, may also occur. Treatment involves pericardiocentesis and increasing cardiac preload with intravenous fluids or blood products, especially in cases of penetrating trauma to the trunk.

Ultrasound can be a valuable adjunct for diagnosing pericardial tamponade, as portable ultrasound devices become more accessible. Note that penetrating injuries to the heart may allow pericardial blood to drain, complicating ultrasound evaluation.

Abdominal Trauma

Abdominal injuries rank as the third leading cause of traumatic death in children, following head and thoracic injuries. Such injuries can affect both solid and hollow organs, with splenic injuries being the most common in pediatric trauma patients. Unique anatomical features in children, including a thin abdominal wall and reduced adipose tissue, contribute to their increased risk for abdominal injuries. The

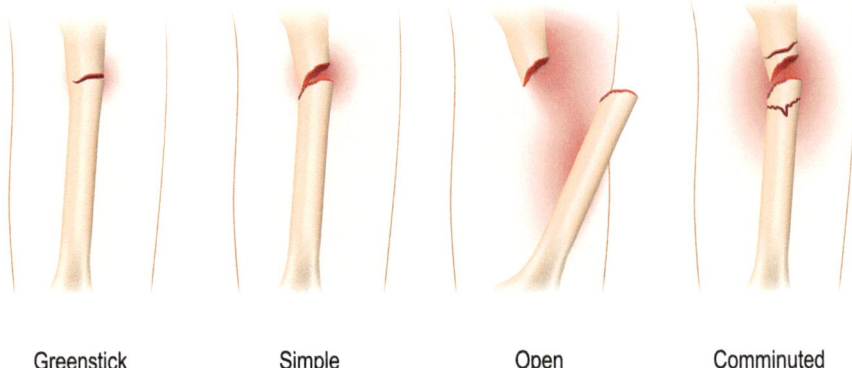

| Greenstick | Simple | Open | Comminuted |

Fig. 5.4a Types of fractures

abdomen in children is often a site of "silent" hypovolemia, with other sites of silent hemorrhage potentially including the pelvis and retroperitoneum.

Prompt treatment involves blood products and/or careful IV fluid replacement, especially if blood products are unavailable, with ongoing assessments of the patient's hemodynamic status. Many significant liver and spleen injuries can be managed conservatively, often negating the need for surgical intervention.

Extremity Trauma

Extremity trauma is prevalent in children, with fractures of the radius, ulna, and femur being the most common, classified as either open or closed. Assessing neurovascular status distal to the injury is crucial. Initial management involves recognizing the injury, splinting to prevent further damage, conducting a neurovascular assessment, and providing pain control. In cases of open fractures, it is essential to clean and cover the area (Fig. 5.4a). Current literature suggests that potable tap water is as effective for infection prevention as sterile saline or distilled water.

Various splinting devices can be utilized, and at the disaster scene, improvised materials (such as wood, magazines, or the other leg) may suffice. Upon reaching a medical facility, fiberglass splints are preferred due to their strength and water resistance (Box 5.4b).

Box 5.4b Keys to proper splinting
- Clean and cover any skin wounds before applying splint.
- Apply padding in layers, ensure padding is smooth, and apply extra layers at any pressure points.
- Splint the joint above and below the fracture (for most fracture types).
- Fiberglass is preferred material; however, use locally appropriate material as fiberglass saws, etc., may not be available.

Open fractures add the concern of infection to the medical management. Open fractures also imply that a significant force has been involved. It is therefore important to look for other injuries. In addition to infection, other complications of open fractures include nerve entrapment and compression. Treatment of an open fracture includes cleaning with copious amount of available irrigation, covering without suturing the opening, early administration of intravenous antibiotics, and immobilization. Ideally, these injuries will need surgical debridement (Fig. 5.4a).

Pelvic and hip fractures are a concern because they are generally the result of high-impact blunt trauma, and blood loss can be significant. The pelvic ring may be fractured in a single place, which would be a stable fracture, or more commonly in multiple places, which could be an unstable fracture. Additional injuries associated with pelvic fractures include genitourinary and abdominal lesions, and vascular abnormalities (i.e., pelvic vein disruption). A sheet tightly wrapped around the pelvis, at the level of the femoral greater trochanters may be the only temporizing measure for the unstable, bleeding pelvic fracture until operative treatment is arranged. In children, "open book" pelvic fractures are rare and shear injury fracture morphology is more commonly seen. Hence, use of a pelvic binder should only occur if hemodynamic instability or significant hemorrhage from the pelvis is suspected.

If orthopedic specialists are available, consultation is recommended before reducing displaced or angulated fractures. In resource-limited scenarios, closed reduction of fractures may alleviate pain and reduce ongoing hemorrhage. Simple reduction can limit blood loss from long bone fractures. After splinting, reassess neurovascular status, monitoring closely for signs of compartment syndrome. Increasing pain after splinting is unusual and should prompt re-evaluation for potential compartment syndrome. Late findings such as pallor, pulselessness, and paresthesia are more challenging to assess in children.

Traumatic Injuries

Objectives

- Develop clear care protocols for individuals affected by fires and burn injuries
- Highlight the specific features of injuries resulting from explosions or blasts, along with their initial management
- Define crush syndrome, discuss its implications, and outline appropriate treatment options

Burn Injuries

Due to their distinct pathophysiology, burn injuries significantly elevate morbidity and mortality rates in trauma patients. Early intervention and resuscitation are crucial as they directly affect survival and the extent of long-term disability.

Pathophysiology

Burns result in both localized tissue damage and systemic changes, which vary according to the type and severity of the burn. The local response includes direct tissue coagulation and microvascular reactions in the adjacent dermis, leading to an increased area of injury. Some burns may continue to progress for up to 24 h even after irrigation, as harmful agents can penetrate deeply into the dermis (e.g., carbon-based agents like kerosene). The systemic response includes the release of vasoactive mediators, which can lead to interstitial edema throughout the body in cases of burns affecting more than 20% of total body surface area due to chemical mediators and hypoproteinemia. Securing the airway is the top priority during the initial evaluation. Inhalation injuries can occur when individuals are trapped in smoke-filled environments (e.g., inside a burning building) or during large-scale fires such as wildfires. However, facial burns are typically not linked to inhalation injuries if the heat source is smaller (e.g., a campfire or cooking fire) or not contained in an enclosed space.

Initial Therapy for Moderate to Severe Burns

- Remove all clothing.
- Assess the size and severity of the burn.
- Cool the affected areas with sterile water.
- Maintain the patient's warmth to prevent hypothermia.
- Conduct early rapid sequence intubation in cases of inhalational injury.
- Implement volume expansion according to the Parkland formula (see Appendix for additional options).
- Evaluate the necessity for escharotomy.
- Monitor for signs of rhabdomyolysis.
- Cover all burned areas with dry, sterile dressings.
- Transfer the patient to a burn center if necessary and transport resources are available.

Physical signs indicating inhalation injury include decreased mental status, respiratory distress, or upper airway obstruction, characterized by stridor or progressive gurgling and a hoarse voice. The presence of soot in the oropharynx may also signal exposure to harmful agents and possible inhalation injury.

The pathophysiological effects of inhalation injuries encompass upper airway edema from direct thermal damage, exacerbated by systemic capillary leak, bronchospasm due to aerosolized irritants, small airway blockage from sloughed endobronchial debris, and the loss of the ciliary clearance mechanism.

Additionally, complications may include increased dead space and intrapulmonary shunting due to alveolar flooding, along with decreased lung and chest wall compliance resulting from interstitial and alveolar edema. Infections of the tracheobronchial tree (tracheobronchitis) or pulmonary tissue (pneumonia) can occur (Sheridan, 2002).

For patients exhibiting significant inhalational injury symptoms, such as stridor, a worsening hoarse voice, or respiratory distress, consider emergency endotracheal intubation, as increasing edema may complicate later intubation. When intubating burn patients, a smaller endotracheal tube size than expected should be used, and tools for cricothyrotomy should be readily available for emergency intervention. Upper airway edema typically resolves within 2–3 days. Once intubation is performed, the patient will require mechanical or bag ventilation for several days, which may not be practical in resource-limited settings. If intubation is not viable, alternative treatments to reduce airway swelling, such as racemic nebulized epinephrine or corticosteroids, can be considered.

Other concerns related to smoke inhalation include exposure to toxic products released during combustion, such as carbon monoxide and hydrogen cyanide (from plastics), both of which impair the body's ability to utilize oxygen. In the field, initial ventilation support for burn patients should include administering 100% oxygen with a non-rebreather mask, if available. In cases of burn or smoke exposure in confined spaces or signs suggesting carbon monoxide exposure (e.g., altered mental status, loss of consciousness, headache, vomiting), administering 100% oxygen can reduce the half-life of carboxyhemoglobin from 4.5 h to 50 min. In this scenario, pulse oximetry readings may be misleading; thus, arterial blood gases are necessary for accurate oxygen saturation determination. If cyanide poisoning is suspected, especially following burn exposure in an enclosed area, cyanide antidote kits may be required. Administering newer cyanide antidotes (such as hydroxycobalamin) should be considered with a low threshold if cyanide exposure is suspected, without waiting for confirmatory tests.

Bronchospasm from inhaled particles and gases may respond to inhaled or intravenous bronchodilators, low-dose epinephrine infusions, or systemic steroids. Significant trunk burns may restrict the patient's ventilatory capacity due to compromised chest wall compliance, potentially necessitating escharotomies to facilitate chest expansion.

Circulation

Prompt fluid resuscitation is crucial to restore intravascular volume, especially for patients with burns covering more than 15–20% of total body surface area (Box 5.5). Research indicates that delays in initiating fluid resuscitation are a major factor contributing to mortality in patients with extensive burns. Most guidelines suggest delivering half of the calculated fluid volume within the first 8 h and the remaining half over the subsequent 16 h in a 24-h period. Typically, the initial 24-h fluids should consist of isotonic crystalloid solutions (normal saline or lactated Ringer's solution). The recommended resuscitation protocol aims to administer the minimum fluids necessary to achieve adequate tissue perfusion and maintain urine output of at least 1 mL/kg/h.

Box 5.5 Calculations of fluid needs for volume expansion for large burns
Recommended initial volume resuscitation for large burns (>20% BSA)

- Use isotonic fluids—lactated Ringer's solution (preferred) or 0.9% NS
- Treat shock with usual 20 cc/kg bolus if clinical signs of shock on initial presentation (max of 40 cc/kg or 2 L initially)
- Further fluid resuscitation

  - Adults—500 mL/h
  - Children—250 mL/h
  - Infants—125 mL/h

- Re-assess fluid needs within several hours to ensure urine production is adequate:

  - Adult—0.5 mL/kg/h
  - Child—1 mL/kg/h
  - Infant—1–2 mL/kg/h

Parkland fluid formula (more complicated but traditional)

1. Calculate maintenance rate for the patient as usual = MF rate
2. Calculate the BSA with 2nd/3rd (partial/full thickness burns) (do not include superficial burn area)
3. Additional fluid needed over 24 h = (2–4 mL/kg) × (weight in kg) × (% BSA) = AF

   (a) Give 1/2 the additional fluid needed over the first 8 h: initial extra fluid rate (mL/h) = (AF (mL)/2)/8 h
   (b) Give the remaining half over the next 16 h: subsequent extra fluid rate (mL/h) = (AF (mL)/2)/16 h

4. Total administered fluid rate:

   (a) First 8 h = Maintenance rate + initial extra fluid rate
   (b) Second 16 h = maintenance rate + subsequent extra fluid rate

5. Include dextrose containing fluids after initial 8 h

Several methods can be used to estimate initial fluid needs. Traditionally, the Parkland formula has been utilized, which calculates additional fluid requirements for the first 24 h as 2–4 mL/kg/% BSA. This volume is divided in half, with the first portion given over the initial 8 h and the second over the next 16 h. This volume is then added to the maintenance rate based on the patient's weight. However, if the rates are not adjusted after the first 8 h, it can lead to excessive fluid administration. A simplified approach suggests starting with an initial fluid rate tailored to large burns and adjusting it based on ongoing evaluations of the patient's needs and urine output. For adults, the starting rate is 500 mL/h; for children, it's 250 mL/h, and for infants, it's 125 mL/h. Following the initial resuscitation, precise calculations for ongoing fluid management can be determined based on the patient's condition, ensuring adequate urine output (0.5 mL/kg/h for adults, 1 mL/kg/h for children, and 1–2 mL/kg/h for infants).

Estimation of Burn Surface Area

Various charts can assist in calculating burn surface area. One common method is the Rule of Nines (Fig. 5.5), originally designed for adults (Fig. 5.5a) but adapted for children (Fig. 5.5b) and infants (Fig. 5.5c).

Burns can be classified based on their depth:

- Superficial burns are red, dry, and painful but do not penetrate the dermis (e.g., sunburn).
- Partial thickness burns appear red and moist, may develop blisters, and are very painful.
- Full thickness burns completely damage the dermis, injuring underlying capillaries and nerve endings. These burns are leathery, dry, and insensate, often appearing waxy, white, or charred. Deeper (fourth degree) burns may involve underlying tissues, tendons, and bones. Some sources continue to refer to burns using the first through fourth-degree classification, which is still present in current literature. When calculating the percentage of total body surface area burned, only partial and full thickness burn areas should be included, excluding superficial burns.

Oral Rehydration

While fluid resuscitation via the intravenous route is recommended for patients with total body surface area burns exceeding 15–20%, this may not be possible in disaster situations or areas with limited resources. Given the urgency of initiating fluids to reduce morbidity and mortality, several authors have proposed using oral rehydration solutions similar to lactated Ringer's, with added glucose or the World Health Organization's oral rehydration solution (with an osmolarity range of 260–330 mOsm/L), administered orally or via nasogastric tube. However, the

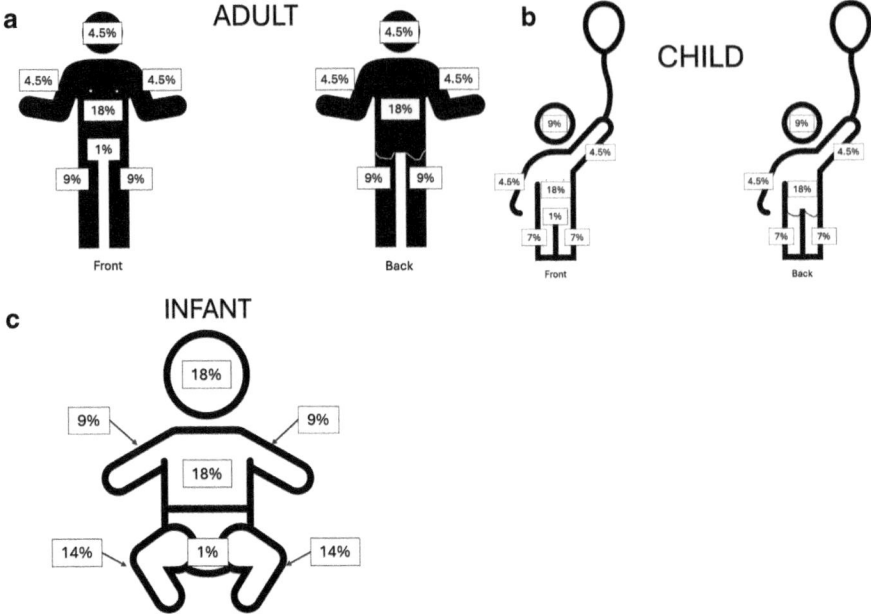

Fig. 5.5 (**a**) Rule of 9's body surface area calculation—adult. (**b**) Rule of 9's body surface area calculation—child. (**c**) Rule of 9's body surface area calculation—infant

challenge with oral rehydration in burn patients lies in the initially prolonged gastric absorption time compared to intravenous fluids and concerns about impaired gut function due to splanchnic under-perfusion.

Initial Wound Care for Burn Injuries

Initial treatment begins with halting the burning process. For children, rolling them in a blanket or rug (avoiding covering the face to prevent inhalation of fumes) is essential. Rinse chemical burns with ample clean water, remove clothing and jewelry, and avoid using cool or wet dressings. Instead, cover the burn with a clean, dry bandage or if a large burn area cover with a dry sheet.

Special Burn Situations

Chemical Injury

Irrigate chemical burns with copious amounts of clean water, and use isotonic crystalloid solutions for ocular injuries. Close monitoring of electrolytes is crucial. After thorough irrigation, treat chemical burns similarly to thermal burns. Hydrocarbon fuels pose a particular risk, as they can cause severe and prolonged chemical burns, along with the potential for thermal ignition.

Tar Injury

To manage tar injuries, begin by irrigating with water to cool the molten tar or asphalt and halt the burning process. After cooling, remove the tar using lipophilic solvents, such as Vaseline or petroleum jelly-based ointments, during the debridement process. Effective pain control is essential, and sedation may be required if available.

Electrical Injury

Low- and intermediate-voltage electrical exposures can lead to localized injuries and systemic complications, while high-voltage exposures may result in delayed neurological and ocular effects. It is essential to conduct serial examinations of the affected extremities to monitor for intra-compartmental edema, which may necessitate decompression. Electrical injuries can also result in rhabdomyolysis, leading to renal complications from myoglobinuria. To mitigate these risks, ensure adequate hydration with intravenous (IV) fluids if available, or increase oral or nasogastric (NG) fluid intake if resources are limited.

Summary of Burns

Overall, the prompt management of burn patients—with vigilant monitoring of the airway, fluids, electrolytes, and clinical status—significantly influences morbidity and mortality. The definitive management approach will depend on the severity of the injury, any concomitant injuries, and the resources available.

In disaster scenarios with numerous burn victims and limited resources, prioritize admitting children with:

- Burns covering more than 10% of total body surface area (BSA)
- Burns on the face, hands, feet, or perineum
- Burns that cross a joint
- Circumferential burn injuries
- Burns associated with other multisystem traumatic injuries

It is advisable to establish at least one IV access in patients with burns exceeding 10% BSA and initiate fluid replacement with crystalloid at a rate of 20 mL/kg. Burns that affect the airway require urgent onsite interventions, including airway protection and fluid administration.

Pain management should involve analgesics and sedatives, adjusting doses to achieve the desired effect. Transfer the patient as soon as possible, and if transportation is delayed, consult the Burn Department of the designated hospital to determine the appropriate rate of intravenous fluid replacement.

Blast Injury

Injuries from Bombs and Explosives

Bombs and explosives can inflict distinctive injuries due to the presence of a blast or shock wave, resulting in injuries not typically associated with other trauma types. Survivors of an explosion may experience a combination of blunt, penetrating, and shock-related tissue injuries, with blast lung emerging as the most common lethal injury among those who reach medical care. Patients with less severe injuries are typically the first to seek medical attention, as they are more capable of self-transport. The concept of the upside-down triage triangle illustrates this phenomenon: those who are less injured arrive at hospitals first, while more severely affected individuals—who may be trapped, closer to the explosion, or unable to move—arrive later and in smaller numbers after rescue.

Explosives are classified into high-order (HE) and low-order (LE) types. High-order explosives, such as TNT, C-4, nitroglycerin, and ammonium nitrate, produce a supersonic shock wave. In contrast, low-order explosives, like black powder and nitrocellulose, create a subsonic explosion that can still cause significant damage and shrapnel but lack a blast or shock wave. The blast wave generates an initial compression or over-pressurization wave, followed by a decompression or under-pressurization zone. This cycle of compression and expansion of gases and tissues leads to unique injury patterns.

Types of Injuries Associated with Blast Trauma

Primary injuries result from the excessive pressure produced by the blast wave, affecting all air- or fluid-filled cavities such as the lungs, ears, and gastrointestinal tract. This can lead to air embolism, potentially causing strokes or acute abdominal or spinal cord injuries. Areas at the interface of fluid, gas, and tissue are particularly vulnerable due to the rapid compression and decompression. Secondary injuries arise from flying debris acting as projectiles, causing penetrating or blunt trauma upon impact with the body; small objects can behave like ballistic projectiles, leading to wounds similar to gunshot injuries, accompanied by cavitation. Tertiary injuries occur when individuals are propelled by the blast wind, striking other objects or the ground, which can result in fractures, brain injuries, traumatic amputations, and other injuries. Quaternary injuries encompass a range of other trauma resulting from the blast, including burns from fires, crush injuries from collapsing structures, inhalation of dust and debris leading to respiratory injuries, and subsequent infections from wounds.

Blast Lung

Blast lung is the most prevalent primary blast injury among explosion victims, often manifesting up to 48 h post-explosion (Fig. 5.6). The acceleration-deceleration effect can tear the lung parenchyma from the stationary vascular tree, resulting in hemorrhage and air emboli. Additionally, smoke inhalation can contribute to lung injury, with symptoms that may include dyspnea, cough, hemoptysis, chest pain, and hypoxia. The initial triad of apnea, bradycardia, and hypotension may present, with pulmonary injuries ranging from petechiae to pulmonary hemorrhage. Primary blast lung injury typically manifests as pulmonary contusion, with respiratory symptoms and hypoxia developing either acutely or progressively over the first 48 h. Other potential complications may include bronchopleural fistula or arterial air embolism, which can arise due to low vascular pressures after hemorrhage or high airway pressures during resuscitation with positive pressure ventilation; arterial air embolism to the brain or heart can be a leading cause of immediate death from primary blast injuries or death upon initiating positive pressure ventilation.

For children suspected of having pulmonary primary blast injuries, immediate treatment with 100% oxygen is essential. In cases where patients present with asymmetrically reduced air entry and signs of shock, there is a need for urgent needle thoracentesis to decompress a possible tension pneumothorax, which is a life-threatening condition that may result from any combination of primary, secondary, tertiary, or other blast injuries. Furthermore, acute respiratory distress syndrome (ARDS) may develop within 24–48 h following the injury.

Fig. 5.6 Blast lung X-ray

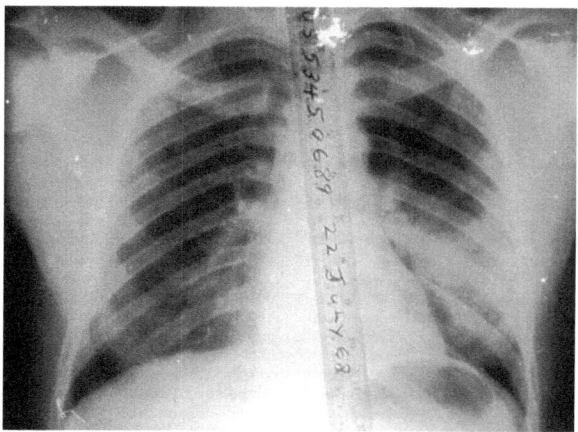

Head Injury

Blast fatalities related to head injuries are often due to subarachnoid and subdural hemorrhages. Among survivors, significant traumatic brain injuries are typically straightforward to identify; however, it is important to note that mild to moderate traumatic brain injuries are prevalent and can be easily overlooked. Despite a lack of external signs, these injuries may lead to considerable disruption and disability. Moreover, other concurrent injuries can distract medical providers, making the identification of subtle neurologic findings more challenging. Therefore, it is essential to consider subtle signs and symptoms indicative of potential mild traumatic brain injury, which may include memory problems, headaches, fainting, an uneven gait, blurred vision, irritability, and confusion.

Abdominal Injury

Primary intestinal blast injury is relatively rare and occurs primarily due to exposure to very high air pressure. Possible injuries include intestinal petechiae, hemorrhages, large intramural hematomas, intestinal lacerations, or bowel perforations. The colon, where gas accumulates, is the most frequently injured site. Ruptures can occur either acutely or several days post-explosion due to stretching, ischemia, and subsequent weakening of the bowel wall, and there is a possibility of developing a tension pneumoperitoneum. Additionally, mesenteric, retroperitoneal, or scrotal hemorrhages may occur as a result of the blast.

Eye Injury

Approximately 10% of all blast survivors experience eye injuries, which can manifest as perforations from high-velocity projectiles presenting as penetrating trauma. It is crucial to assess patients for altered vision, eye pain, foreign body sensation, decreased visual acuity, hyphema, or lacerations, as these symptoms can indicate significant ocular trauma.

Ear Injury

Blast injuries to the ear can often go unnoticed. The most common injury is tympanic membrane perforation, although injuries to the ossicular chain occur in about 33% of ear trauma cases. The rupture of the tympanic membrane serves as an early indicator that the patient has been subjected to the blast wave's pressurization and depressurization forces, necessitating careful evaluation for other associated injuries. Inner-ear sensorineural hearing loss may also result from such trauma. The local consequences of blast-related eardrum perforation can include infection, tinnitus, temporary or permanent hearing loss, and vertigo, so these patients require follow-up care from an otorhinolaryngologist.

Other Injuries

In addition to the aforementioned injuries, other complications associated with blast trauma may include compartment syndrome, rhabdomyolysis, acute renal failure, severe burns, and inhalation of toxic substances. If the explosion occurred in an enclosed space or was accompanied by fire, it is critical to conduct tests for carboxyhemoglobin and assess electrolytes, as well as evaluate acid-base status. Elevated lactate levels can indicate cyanide toxicity, necessitating prompt medical attention.

Crush Injuries

Building collapses are a common type of disaster, and the collapse of a multi-story structure may lead to crush injuries in up to 40% of the extricated survivors. For instance, during the 1995 Kobe, Japan earthquake, 372 patients with crush syndrome exhibited a mortality rate nearly twice that of other trauma patients. Unfortunately, there is limited information available regarding crush injuries in children. In studies conducted after the 1999 earthquake in Turkey, pediatric patients showed a pattern of injuries predominantly affecting the ankle (30%), thigh (28.6%), head (23.8%), and forearm (7%). Many of these children developed crush syndrome, and surgical amputations or multiple fasciotomies were necessary in 12.6% of cases. Additionally, acute renal insufficiency occurred in 27% of the pediatric population affected, underscoring the importance of modern disaster plans that anticipate such scenarios.

Even short periods of entrapment can lead to muscle compression injuries, potentially resulting in crush syndrome, also known as traumatic rhabdomyolysis. Crush syndrome (Box 5.6) manifests as a severe systemic reaction to trauma and ischemia affecting soft tissues, primarily skeletal muscle, due to prolonged and severe compression. This condition causes increased permeability of the cell membrane, leading to the release of potassium, enzymes, and myoglobin into the bloodstream. Consequently, ischemic renal dysfunction arises secondary to hypotension and reduced renal perfusion, resulting in acute tubular necrosis and uremia.

Box 5.6 Crush syndrome
Diagnostic criteria:

- Muscle mass involvement
- Prolonged compression (usually >4 h but can occur in as little as 1 h)
- Compromised local circulation

Clinical syndromes seen with crush:

- Extreme hypovolemic shock
- Hyperkalemia
- Hypocalcemia
- Metabolic acidosis
- Acute myoglobinuric renal failure
- Compartment syndrome

The clinical picture of crush syndrome and traumatic rhabdomyolysis includes muscle tissue destruction and the influx of myoglobin, potassium, and phosphorus into circulation, leading to hypovolemic shock and hyperkalemia. It is vital to initiate volume expansion as soon as possible, ideally starting intravenous (IV) fluid hydration even before extraction, if feasible. Crush syndrome can result in several serious medical conditions associated with significant morbidity and mortality.

Patients with rhabdomyolysis typically present with muscle weakness, malaise, and fever, but this clinical picture may understate the real danger posed by cardiovascular effects stemming from electrolyte imbalances and renal failure. Signs of skin trauma or local compression (such as erythema, ecchymosis, and abrasions) on the affected muscle mass should be assessed. The absence of a pulse or a weak pulse in the distal limbs may indicate muscle swelling or compromised circulation. Continuous assessment may reveal a pale, cool, diaphoretic limb, with compressed extremities eventually becoming tense and edematous due to inadequate vascular circulation. Secondary sensory and motor disturbances in the affected limbs are also common. If resources allow, laboratory evaluations for urine myoglobin, serum creatine phosphokinase, and serum electrolytes should be performed; urine test strips may also serve as a useful adjunct, as urine myoglobin can yield a positive result for blood on test strips.

Key therapeutic aspects focus on volume expansion through adequate fluid resuscitation, preferably via IV if resources permit, alongside ensuring alkalinized diuresis and early detection of metabolic abnormalities. A normal saline bolus of 20 mL/kg should be initiated at the disaster scene or as soon as possible. Once the patient stabilizes hemodynamically, intravenous fluids can be switched to 50% normal saline mixed with 40 mEq sodium bicarbonate for urine alkalinization, aiming for a urine pH between 6 and 7.

Diuresis can be promoted using either furosemide or mannitol. Furosemide is thought to assist by causing renal vasodilation, reducing renal oxygen demand, and increasing renal intratubular flow; if IV resources are limited, oral furosemide may be used. Mannitol acts as an osmotic diuretic and volume expander. It is also important to administer analgesics, such as opiates or ketamine, for pain management.

Severe hyperkalemia, defined as a serum potassium level greater than 7.0 mEq/L, is one of the leading causes of death from crush injuries. Hyperkalemia can lead to electrocardiographic (ECG) disturbances, including peaked T-waves, loss of P-waves, and widening of the QRS complex. To treat symptomatic hyperkalemia or hyperkalemia with ECG changes, calcium chloride 10% (0.2 mL/kg IV) or calcium gluconate 10% (0.5–1 mL/kg IV) should be administered to stabilize the cardiac membrane. However, intravenous calcium may be ineffective for hyperkalemia if the patient also presents with hyperphosphatemia, necessitating early dialysis if resources are available.

Additional treatment options include mobilizing potassium into the intracellular space through plasma alkalinization (sodium bicarbonate 1 mEq/kg IV) or glucose administration (0.5–1 g/kg, typically using 25% dextrose in water) combined with insulin (0.1 units/kg IV); albuterol aerosol may also serve as an adjunct therapy. In extreme cases, hemodialysis may become necessary.

Hypocalcemia is defined as a calcium concentration below 9 mg/dL and may present with symptoms such as weakness, paresthesias, and irritability, along with ECG findings including a prolonged QT interval, bradycardia, and arrhythmias. Treatment primarily involves calcium administration while closely monitoring ECG and serum calcium levels.

Intensive care support is often required for complications arising from crush syndrome, particularly for patients presenting with anuria or oliguria, who may need hemofiltration or dialysis. Aggressive treatment is critical to reduce mortality and morbidity; the focus during the acute phase of rhabdomyolysis is on maintaining adequate circulating volume and promoting sufficient diuresis to prevent renal, cardiac, and pulmonary complications.

Compartment syndrome may arise when there is increased pressure within a closed tissue compartment, typically affecting muscle tissue. This increased pressure can lead to ischemia, resulting in muscle necrosis and nerve damage (palsies). The anterior compartment of the lower leg is most commonly affected due to the presence of four susceptible compartments in this frequently injured area. In cases of severe trauma, the integrity of the compartment may be disrupted, preventing the achievement of high intra-compartment pressures. Clinicians should be vigilant for increasing and severe pain, particularly pain associated with passive extension of the affected compartment. While the classic teaching of the "five P's" may be less helpful for early detection, worsening pain despite splinting is often the first symptom noted. In small children, increased irritability may be the presenting symptom, followed later by pallor of the extremity, paralysis, paresthesias, and pulselessness.

Although confirmation of elevated compartment pressures can be obtained through direct measurement, the diagnosis of compartment syndrome ultimately relies on clinical evaluation, based on history and physical examination. In cases where compartment syndrome is confirmed, the definitive treatment is surgical release of the compartment connective tissue, or fasciotomy.

Always consider the possibility of compartment syndrome in patients suspected of having crush syndrome. The development of compartment syndrome in such injuries results from fluid uptake into damaged muscle tissue, which remains trapped within a restricted compartment. Once compartment pressure exceeds capillary perfusion pressure, typically around 30 to 40 mm Hg, ischemia occurs, and compartment syndrome develops. While traditional treatment involves fasciotomy, some evidence suggests that initial treatment with mannitol may help decompress the compartment, potentially avoiding the need for surgery.

The Role of Point-of-Care Ultrasound in Trauma

Point-of-care ultrasound (POCUS) can often be more readily available than CT scans and radiographs, particularly in disaster scenarios or mass casualty events. One of the significant advantages of using ultrasound in trauma settings is its ability to provide relatively quick diagnostic answers without exposing patients to radiation. Furthermore, its portability and low cost make it an invaluable tool for healthcare providers. POCUS is typically incorporated into the secondary survey during the trauma assessment process, as illustrated in Table 5.2.

Among the various applications of POCUS in major trauma cases, the extended focused assessment of sonography in trauma (E-FAST) stands out as one of the most widely utilized diagnostic approaches. Although the literature reports varying sensitivities for E-FAST, its specificity for positive findings in the appropriate clinical context is nearly 100%.

Section Summary

The prospect of facing a community-wide disaster can be overwhelming, even for well-prepared hospitals. No healthcare organization can be expected to function effectively during such an event without prior training and practice. The extent of relevant training and practice that a medical team or facility undergoes significantly impacts its ability to perform under crisis conditions.

Planning for the potential transfer of a large number of injured or traumatized children is crucial and requires advance preparation. It is essential to establish prior written transfer arrangements with other hospitals when anticipating mass disaster situations. In resource-limited contexts, delays in patient transport may occur, making it even more critical to have contingency plans in place.

Several factors must be carefully considered when preparing to transfer patients to other facilities. Most importantly, healthcare providers must ensure that patients are stable enough for transport. The medical team should confirm that the airway is secure, that breathing is not compromised by untreated conditions such as pneumothorax or hemothorax, and that any circulatory issues have been addressed and

Table 5.2 Uses of point-of-care ultrasound in trauma or disaster medicine

Study	Indications	Clinical use
e-FAST (evaluate 4 quadrants of abdomen, heart, and lungs)	Hemodynamic instability with concern for thoracic/abdominal injury	Determine need for urgent laparotomy or thoracotomy
Echocardiogram	Evaluate pericardial sac, cardiac function	Evaluate for cardiac injury, poor cardiac function Note—trace pericardial fluid can indicate significant cardiac injury in penetrating trauma as pericardium may not be intact
Extremity	Extremity injury if X-ray not available or if vascular injury is suspected	Evaluate for fracture, hematoma, significant fluid collections

controlled. Additionally, in the context of an ongoing disaster, safety along the route of travel must also be considered.

Essential interventions following a disaster include systematically sorting the injured into different categories, known as triage, and managing trauma through the stabilization of affected individuals. Familiarity with the common patterns of injuries is also vital for effective response and treatment.

Resources

1. Bendavid E, Boerma T, Akseer N, et al. The effects of armed conflict on the health of women and children. Lancet. 2021;397(10273):522–32. https://doi.org/10.1016/s0140-6736(21)00131-8.
2. Kadir A, Shenoda S, Goldhagen J, Pitterman S. The effects of armed conflict on children. Pediatrics. 2018;142(6) https://doi.org/10.1542/peds.2018-2586.
3. Kadir A, Shenoda S, Goldhagen J. Effects of armed conflict on child health and development: a systematic review. PLoS One. 2019;14(1):e0210071. https://doi.org/10.1371/journal.pone.0210071.
4. Umphrey L, Brown A, Hiffler L, et al. Delivering paediatric critical care in humanitarian settings. Lancet Child Adolesc Health. 2018;2(12):846–8. https://doi.org/10.1016/s2352-4642(18)30284-0.
5. Child Landmine Survivors: An Inclusive Approach to Policy and Practice. Save the Children. Accessed 12 September 2024. https://bettercarenetwork.org/sites/default/files/Child%20Landmine%20Survivors%20-%20An%20Inclusive%20Approach%20to%20Policy%20and%20Practice.PDF
6. Landmine and Cluster Munition Monitor. Landmine and Cluster Munition Monitor. 2024. Accessed 12 September 2024. https://www.the-monitor.org/
7. Political Declaration on Strengthening the Protection of Civilians from the Humanitarian Consequences arising from the use of Explosive Weapons in Populated Areas. Protecting Civilians in Urban Warfare, Department of Foreign Affairs of Ireland. 2022. Accessed 12 September 2024. https://www.gov.ie/en/publication/585c8-protecting-civilians-in-urban-warfare/#political-declaration-on-ewipa
8. Wild H, Reavley P, Mayhew E, Ameh EA, Celikkaya ME, Stewart B. Strengthening the emergency health response to children wounded by explosive weapons in conflict. World J Pediatr Surg. 2022;5(4):e000443. https://doi.org/10.1136/wjps-2022-000443.

9. Sarwer DB, Siminoff LA, Gardiner HM, Spitzer JC. The psychosocial burden of visible disfigurement following traumatic injury. Front Psychol. 2022;13:979574. https://doi.org/10.3389/fpsyg.2022.979574.

10. Fisher M. Pediatric burn reconstruction: focus on evidence. Clin Plast Surg. 2017;44(4):865–73. https://doi.org/10.1016/j.cps.2017.05.018.

11. Bhandari PS, Maurya S, Mukherjee MK. Reconstructive challenges in war wounds. Indian J Plast Surg. 2012;45(2):332–9. https://doi.org/10.4103/0970-0358.101316.

12. Aguirre AS, Rojas K, Torres AR. Pediatric traumatic brain injuries in war zones: a systematic literature review. Front Neurol. 2023;14:1253515. https://doi.org/10.3389/fneur.2023.1253515.

13. Kirollos M, Anning C, Fylkesnes GK, Denselow J. The War on Children: Time to end grave violations against children in conflict. Save the Children. 2018. Accessed 19 June, 2024. https://www.savethechildren.org.uk/content/dam/global/reports/education-and-child-protection/war_on_children-web.pdf

14. Children and armed conflict: Report of the Secretary-General 2024:1–49. https://documents.un.org/doc/undoc/gen/n24/095/07/pdf/n2409507.pdf.

15. Information Note: Disability and Inclusion in MHPSS. IASC Reference Group on Mental Health and Psychosocial Support in Emergency Settings. 2024. Accessed 12 September 2024. https://interagencystandingcommittee.org/sites/default/files/2024-01/IASC%20Information%20Note%20on%20Disability%20and%20Inclusion%20in%20MHPSS.pdf

16. Childhood in Rubble: The Humanitarian Consequences of Urban Warfare for Children. 2023:1–72. May 2023. file:///Users/lisaumphrey/Downloads/4703_002-ebook%20(1).pdf https://www.icrc.org>document>childhood-rubble: The humanitarian consequences of urban warfare for children. 2023:1-72 May 2023.

17. Haar RJ, Read R, Fast L, et al. Violence against healthcare in conflict: a systematic review of the literature and agenda for future research. Confl Heal. 2021;15(1):37. https://doi.org/10.1186/s13031-021-00372-7.

18. Fardousi N, Douedari Y, Howard N. Healthcare under siege: a qualitative study of health-worker responses to targeting and besiegement in Syria. BMJ Open. 2019;9(9):e029651. https://doi.org/10.1136/bmjopen-2019-029651.

19. Chung S, Baum CR, Nyquist AC. Chemical-biological terrorism and its impact on children. Pediatrics. 2020;145(2) https://doi.org/10.1542/peds.2019-3749.

20. Jawad M, Hone T, Vamos EP, Cetorelli V, Millett C. Implications of armed conflict for maternal and child health: a regression analysis of data from 181 countries for 2000–2019. PLoS Med. 2021;18(9):e1003810. https://doi.org/10.1371/journal.pmed.1003810.

21. Liu L, Villavicencio F, Yeung D, Perin J, Lopez G, Strong KL, Black RE. National, regional, and global causes of mortality in 5–19-year-olds from 2000 to 2019: a systematic analysis. Lancet Glob Health. 2022;10(3):e337–47.

Chapter 6
Pediatric Toxicologic Considerations in Disasters

Bryan Wilson, Shana Godfred-Cato, and Laurie Halmo

Introduction

Disasters that result in the widespread exposure of victims to toxicological substances present a distinct set of challenges and concerns for caring for children. Historically, natural disasters have exposed populations to toxic substances like smoke, poisonous gases, ash, and dust. The extensive industrialization of the twentieth century significantly elevated the risk of human-made disasters and introduced exposure to a broader array of potential toxicants. Additionally, the twentieth century saw the first large-scale production of chemical and biological weapons. The use of chemical, biological, and nuclear agents has since become a significant concern in the context of both warfare and acts of terrorism. Consequently, there is an increased focus on disaster preparedness involving chemical, biological, and radioactive agents, particularly related to the special care considerations required by children in case of these exposures. This module offers an overview and strategies for addressing the unique aspects of toxicological disasters, adaptable to various resource settings, and focusing on the unique physiology and needs of children.

B. Wilson
Southeast Texas Poison Center, University of Texas Medical Branch, Galveston, TX, USA

S. Godfred-Cato (✉)
Division of Pediatric Emergency Medicine, Department of Pediatrics, Spencer Fox Eccles School of Medicine at the University of Utah, Salt Lake City, UT, USA
e-mail: Shana.godfred-cato@hsc.utah.edu

L. Halmo
Department of Pediatrics, Section of Hospital Medicine, University of Colorado School of Medicine, Aurora, CO, USA
e-mail: laurie.halmo@childrenscolorado.org

© The Author(s), under exclusive license to Springer Nature   121
Switzerland AG 2025
L. Umphrey et al. (eds.), *Pediatric Considerations in Disaster Settings*,
https://doi.org/10.1007/978-3-031-85501-6_6

Vulnerability of Children

Objectives

- Acknowledge the heightened susceptibility of young children to various toxic substances.
- Examine the multiple factors that contribute to children's increased vulnerability to exposure to toxicants.

Children represent a particularly vulnerable group in disaster situations due to several anatomical, physiological, and developmental differences that, when compared to adults, present unique risks in the context of toxicologic exposure (Fig. 6.1). Although pediatric patients can be defined by various age cut-offs, prepubescent children, especially those under the age of 2, exhibit the most significant differences from a toxicological standpoint.

The most relevant physiological differences in children can be broadly summarized as generally reduced capacity for toxicant metabolism, increased minute ventilation, reduced cardiac reserve, greater penetration of certain drugs into the central nervous system, and lower glycogen reserves. Increased minute ventilation may lead to a higher relative dose of airborne exposures being absorbed. This dependence on high minute ventilation also makes children less capable of tolerating exposures that result in bradypnea or increase the work of breathing. Cardiovascularly, pediatric patients have a limited stroke volume reserve and rely primarily on heart

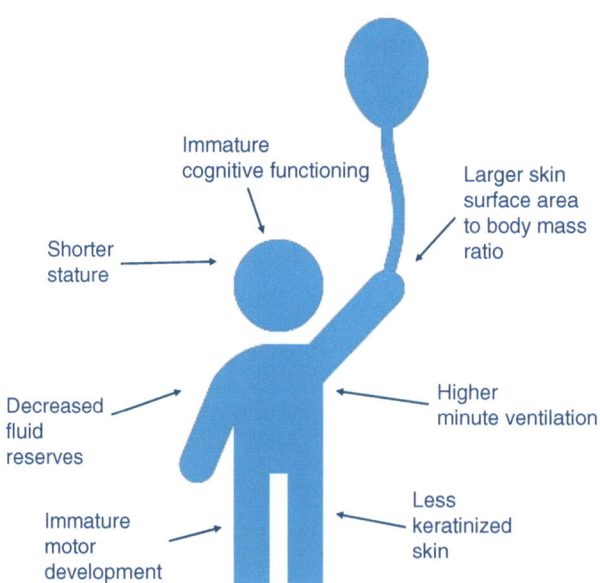

Fig. 6.1 Summary of key anatomic, physiologic, and developmental differences in children

rate to boost cardiac output. Consequently, toxicants that induce bradycardia are relatively less well tolerated in this population. Metabolically, due to their lower glycogen stores, toxicants such as alcohols that inhibit gluconeogenesis can lead to hypoglycemia in young children. Additionally, because of decreased active excretion from the central nervous system, certain toxicants that have minimal effects on adults can cause significant central nervous system symptoms in young children.

Anatomical considerations for children primarily focus on their small size and relatively high body surface area. Fundamentally, the small and variable sizes of pediatric patients necessitate a wider range of medical equipment and add complexity to many therapeutic interventions. Additionally, their shorter stature places children closer to the ground, which can increase their exposure to toxicants that are heavier than air or have settled on the ground. Despite their small size, children have a proportionately larger total body surface area, which, combined with their thinner subcutaneous fat, heightens their risk from dermally absorbed toxicants. This also makes them more susceptible to hypothermia, particularly during decontamination. Furthermore, children have a reduced fluid reserve compared to adults, making them more vulnerable to dehydration, especially in cases of repetitive vomiting or diarrhea caused by toxic exposures or food-borne illnesses.

From a developmental standpoint, children often rely on others to remove them from hazardous situations. Additionally, crawling on the floor and exploratory behaviors, such as ingesting unknown substances, can increase the risk of exposure to certain toxicants. Young children and those with developmental delays present additional challenges in the logistics of decontamination, treatment, and reunification with their caregivers.

Summary

- Children often struggle to avoid or extricate themselves from toxic exposures.
- Pediatric patients may exhibit reduced tolerance for bradypnea, bradycardia, and pulmonary injuries.
- There is an increased risk of hypoglycemia in pediatric patients.
- Pediatric patients are often exposed to relatively higher doses of airborne, dermally absorbed, and low-lying toxicants.
- The presence of pediatric patients complicates decontamination and treatment processes, adding logistical challenges.

Historical Context

Natural Disasters

Objective

- Detail the common toxic exposures that typically occur during natural disasters.
- Explore the relationship between natural disasters and the increased potential for exposure to hazardous materials.

In some cases, toxic exposure can be the most immediate consequence of a natural disaster. For example, in 2019, the eruption of the Whakaari/White Island volcano in New Zealand released volcanic gases and ash, posing health risks to nearby residents and tourists. Similarly, volcanic eruptions can emit harmful gases such as carbon dioxide, sulfur dioxide, and hydrogen sulfide, along with ash. Dust storms, like those that struck northern China in recent years, can also introduce irritating particulates and toxic pollutants into the atmosphere.

Typically, natural disasters are associated with physical injuries, displacement, insecurity, and the spread of infectious diseases, but they can also lead to secondary toxic exposures. For instance, the 2020 Beirut explosion in Lebanon resulted in the release of hazardous chemicals, including ammonium nitrate, which was involved in the blast. This explosion not only caused extensive physical damage but also contaminated the environment with toxic substances. Similarly, the 2017 Hurricane Maria in Puerto Rico led to widespread flooding and infrastructure damage, resulting in the release of pollutants from damaged industrial sites and untreated sewage.

Natural disasters that disturb soil or damage infrastructure can lead to toxic substance releases. For example, earthquakes can cause gas leaks, damage to sewer systems, electrical fires, and spills of household chemicals. The 2016 Kumamoto earthquake in Japan caused significant infrastructure damage and led to concerns about the release of hazardous materials. Additionally, fires often accompany natural disasters, either as a secondary effect or as the primary event, and present serious chemical hazards. For instance, the 2018 Paradise Fire in California released toxic smoke and particulate matter that posed health risks to affected communities. For more information on the hazards of combustion products like carbon monoxide and hydrogen cyanide, refer to section "Toxidromes."

The presence of significant toxic exposure may not be immediately evident amid the chaos of a disaster, especially when overshadowed by more visible injuries. Healthcare providers should be vigilant for clusters of symptoms, unusual odors or tastes, and direct reports of toxic exposures. Emergency planners should prepare for the types of natural disasters most likely to occur in their area and evaluate local sources of potential toxic exposure that could exacerbate these events.

Human-Made Disasters

Objectives

- Describe common toxic exposures associated with incidents resulting from human activities.
- Explore the connection between industrial activities and the risk of encountering hazardous materials.

Major toxicological disasters can occur independently of natural disasters. In the modern industrialized world, significant releases of hazardous chemicals can happen due to human errors or equipment failures. For instance, in 2021, the massive chemical fire at the Saint-Denis recycling plant in France led to the release of toxic fumes, resulting in evacuations and health concerns for nearby residents. This incident highlights the severe risks associated with industrial accidents.

Although less frequent, deliberate releases of chemical, biological, and nuclear agents as acts of terrorism remain a significant concern. The 2018 attack in the Syrian city of Douma, where chemical weapons were reportedly used, illustrates the continued threat of chemical warfare in conflict zones. Additionally, the 2019 Sri Lanka Easter bombings involved attacks that had indirect effects on public health and safety, though not through chemical means.

Accidental chemical releases generally reflect the types of industries and chemicals present in the area. For example, incidents involving respiratory exposure to irritants like chlorine, such as the 2018 chlorine gas leak in Syria, are common. Transportation routes, including trains, highways, and shipping lanes, can also pose risks from hazardous materials not typically associated with local industries. Terrorist acts, on the other hand, might introduce unexpected toxicants, including potent chemical warfare agents that pose significant risks beyond those of typical industrial or consumer chemicals.

The symptoms of chemical exposure usually appear quickly, helping to identify the source and timing of the exposure. Responders can aid treatment teams by gathering information about the toxicant, such as environmental clues, container labels, colors, odors, and the physical state of the substance (solid, liquid, or gas).

However, some chemical (and many biological or radioactive) exposures may present with delayed symptoms. In cases of terrorism, agents might be selected for their delayed effects to increase chaos and reduce the likelihood of the perpetrators being caught. This delay can complicate the identification of the exposure and its source. Therefore, healthcare workers and disaster responders should remain vigilant for unusual clusters of symptoms or illnesses, as these may provide essential initial clues about a toxic exposure.

Initial Response and Decontamination

Objectives

- Outline the primary objectives in the initial response to a toxicological disaster.
- Explain the zoning system used for organizing responses to toxicological disasters.
- Detail the various levels of personal protective equipment (PPE) utilized in hazardous materials response efforts.
- Discuss the steps involved in the decontamination sequence.

The initial response to a toxicological disaster focuses on securing the scene, preventing further exposures, evacuating and decontaminating patients, and minimizing additional casualties. Medical interventions beyond essential life-saving procedures are generally postponed until these primary concerns are addressed.

First responders, including emergency medical service (EMS) personnel, should base their planning on the following six key principles:

- *The potential influx of individuals with medical issues could be overwhelming.* Responders must be prepared for a surge in patients, which can strain available resources and facilities. Effective triage systems are crucial to manage the high volume of casualties and prioritize care based on the severity of injuries.
- *The number of "worried well" or "walking wounded" may exceed those with severe injuries.* This group includes individuals who are less critically injured but may still require medical attention or reassurance. Managing this population effectively helps ensure that resources are directed where they are most needed and that all individuals receive appropriate care.
- *A single incident may involve multiple toxic substances.* Complex scenarios may include a combination of chemicals, each with its own set of hazards. Responders must be equipped to identify and manage multiple toxic agents simultaneously, which requires comprehensive knowledge and resources.
- *Signs and symptoms of exposures may rapidly manifest, as occurs during attacks using the chemical Sarin.* In these cases, the onset of symptoms was swift and severe, necessitating immediate action from first responders. Recognizing these rapid manifestations is essential for timely intervention and treatment.
- *Signs and symptoms of exposures may also appear with a delay, as occurs during attacks with phosgene gas.* Some toxic exposures have delayed effects, which can complicate diagnosis and treatment. Awareness of such delays helps responders monitor affected individuals over time and adjust treatment protocols as necessary.
- *Emergency medical response personnel are vulnerable to becoming victims:* The safety of responders is paramount, and they must be equipped with proper protective gear and protocols to prevent secondary injuries or exposures. Planning for potential risks ensures that responders can effectively perform their duties without compromising their own safety.

Preparedness for Toxicological Disasters

As with any disaster, incidents involving hazardous materials depend heavily on pre-existing preparedness to mitigate impacts on victims, responders, and other emergency personnel. Additionally, it is crucial to implement measures that prevent toxic contamination in unaffected areas of the community. Promptly identifying the toxic substance is vital for refining the response strategy and enhancing its effectiveness. Box 6.1 illustrates the fundamental objectives of toxicological disaster preparedness.

Box 6.1 Essential preparedness for toxicological disasters

1. *Be Ready for Various Types of Disasters:* Prepare to manage different disaster scenarios that could involve toxicological hazards.
2. *Recognize Toxic Syndromes:* Develop the ability to identify signs and symptoms associated with toxic syndromes.
3. *Accessible Resources:* Ensure that resources for promptly identifying toxic syndromes are readily available.
4. *Treatment of Toxic Exposures:* Learn and practice the correct methods for treating injuries related to toxic exposures.
5. *Rescuer Safety:* Be prepared to respond in a way that sensibly and efficiently identifies and reduces risks that could endanger rescuers' safety.
6. *Proactive Community Education:* Offer education to the community on how to appropriately respond to various types of toxicological disasters.

Priorities in Response to a Toxic Disaster Scene

The primary objective in managing any disaster is to ensure the safety of medical and rescue personnel while maximizing the number of lives saved. To achieve this, several universal principles must guide disaster management. First, establishing a clear chain of command is crucial. An incident commander must oversee the scene and coordinate with nearby hospitals or healthcare facilities. In incidents involving hazardous materials (HAZMAT), it is essential to appoint a medical toxicologist, HAZMAT specialist, or another qualified expert as the medical coordinator at the command post (refer to Module 3). HAZMAT refers to any substance that poses a risk to people, property, or the environment. The selection of appropriate experts depends on available resources, so it is important to identify local and regional expertise during the planning phase.

The next step involves setting up appropriate zones for managing the disaster (see Fig. 6.2a–c). The type of disaster will dictate the specific zones required. The hot zone (Fig. 6.2a) is the most hazardous area on the disaster site, characterized by ongoing threats such as active fires, falling debris, or exposure to dangerous

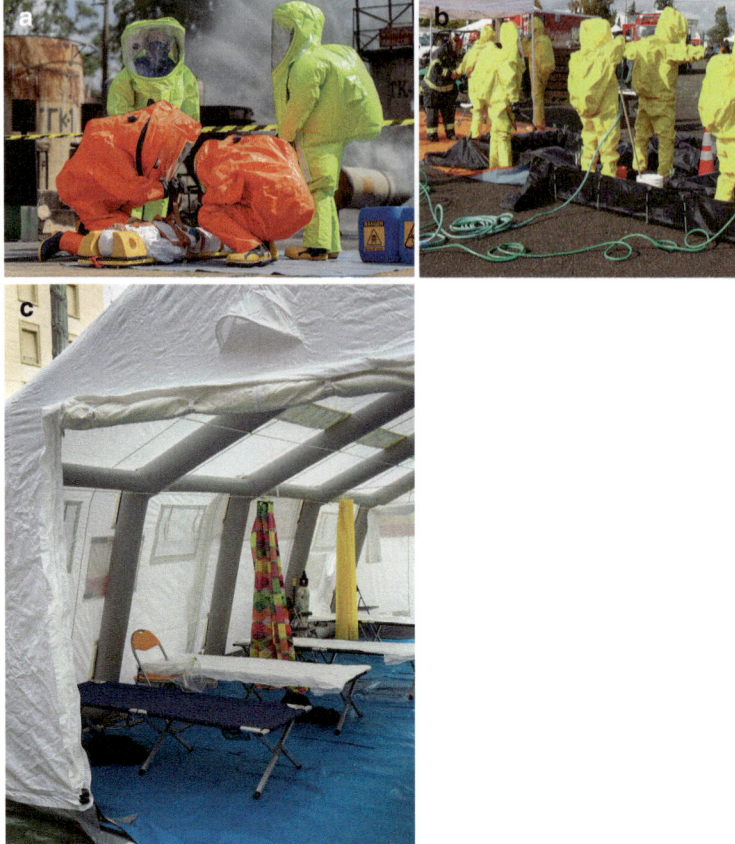

Fig. 6.2 (**a**) Disaster management zones, hot zone. (**b**) Disaster management zones, decontamination zone. (**c**) Disaster management zones, cold zone

materials. First responders should demarcate the perimeter of the hot zone using tape or rope if available. The incident commander will determine who is permitted entry into this zone. Generally, medical treatment should not be administered within the hot zone, although rapid, life-saving measures like the use of autoinjectors (devices that quickly deliver a fixed dose of medication with minimal training) or airway management may be necessary. Outside the hot zone, responders will establish a decontamination or warm zone, marking its perimeter with tape or rope. The decontamination zone (Fig. 6.2b) is where patients can be stabilized and cleaned of hazardous contaminants. Ideally, this zone should be situated upwind, uphill, and/or upstream from the hot zone to reduce further exposure.

The next area is the cold zone (Fig. 6.2c), also known as the support zone. This zone is situated beyond the decontamination area and is free from any risk of secondary contamination to equipment, victims, or personnel. It serves as the location for definitive patient treatment and triage. Typically, the incident command post is established within the support or cold zone. In some countries, specialized teams from the military or other government agencies may be deployed to assist with hazardous material responses.

A crucial aspect of managing a disaster scene is controlling unauthorized access between zones. No members of the general public or media should be permitted entry into any of the designated zones shown in Fig. 6.2. In the case of large-scale disasters, local authorities may struggle to secure or manage these zones effectively, necessitating additional support from police or military services, if available, to ensure proper security and control.

Levels of Protection for Personal Protective Equipment

HAZMAT incidents necessitate the use of personal protective equipment (PPE) to safeguard response workers from direct exposure and cross-contamination. The United States Environmental Protection Agency (EPA) and Occupational Safety and Health Administration (OSHA) have established four levels of protection for PPE (refer to Table 6.1). Other countries may have their own regulations, and the World Health Organization also offers guidance. It's important to recognize that not all countries will have access to the same resources, including PPE.

Level A provides the highest degree of protection, including respiratory, skin, and vapor protection. This level requires responders to wear a self-contained breathing apparatus (SCBA) beneath their suit. Level B offers the highest level of respiratory protection but less skin and no vapor protection. In terms of respiratory protection, the hierarchy follows: SCBA, powered air-purifying respirator (PAPR), and face masks with high-efficiency particulate air (HEPA) filters. Level C provides equivalent skin protection to Level B but with reduced respiratory protection. Level D is akin to a standard healthcare worker uniform and is generally insufficient for use in hot and warm zones.

Table 6.1 Different protection levels of rescuers personal protective equipment

Level	Degree of protection
A	Highest level of protection, used in environments with a high risk of exposure to harmful gases, vapors, or chemical splashes. It includes a fully encapsulated chemical-resistant suit, a self-contained breathing apparatus (SCBA), and gloves with multiple layers of chemical resistance.
B	Focuses primarily on respiratory protection. It uses the same SCBA as Level A but with less skin protection. This level is suitable for situations where respiratory hazards are high, but skin contact with contaminants is less likely.
C	Appropriate when the type and concentration of airborne contaminants are known and measurable. This level typically includes a full- or half-face air-purifying respirator and chemical-resistant gloves. It is used when there is a low risk of skin and eye exposure.
D	Minimum level of protection, used in environments where no respiratory hazards are present. It includes coveralls, safety boots, and goggles, providing basic protection against minimal risks.

While these US protection levels are applied internationally, the terminology may differ by region. It is crucial for responders to ensure they are familiar with and using the appropriate local terminology. Regardless of the specific terms used, these levels offer a valuable framework for determining the necessary PPE for a given situation.

Ultimately, the incident commander and medical coordinator will determine the appropriate level of PPE required for each zone. Typically, Level A and Level B PPE are used in the hot zone, where the risk of exposure is highest. Level C protection is generally suitable for the warm zone or for decontamination procedures at healthcare facilities. As a general guideline, responders should opt for the highest level of PPE when uncertain but may downgrade to a less restrictive level once the specific exposure is confirmed and the minimum necessary PPE is identified. In areas with no risk of secondary contamination, standard contact precautions such as gloves and face masks should be used.

Using PPE involves specialized training and presents unique logistical challenges for rescue workers and planners. PPE for HAZMAT incidents is often bulky and cumbersome, complicating patient handling and procedures such as venipuncture, especially on children. Responders in PPE are also at risk for heat-related illnesses, dehydration, and dermatitis. Additionally, Level A suits with SCBA provide ventilation for only about 20 minutes due to the limited air supply in each suit's oxygen tank, adding logistical complexity to the response. Adequate training is essential for understanding the risks and challenges associated with PPE and for ensuring its safe use. Rescue workers without proper training should not use PPE in a disaster scenario.

Although a comprehensive discussion of radiation emergency responses is beyond the scope of this chapter, a brief overview of PPE considerations is provided. To minimize radiation exposure, responders should reduce their time near the source, increase their distance from it, and use shielding effectively. In radiation disasters, PPE primarily prevents contamination from radioactive solids and liquids. Responders should stay uphill and upwind from the contaminated area, but be aware that wind directions can change, affecting previously established zones. Ideal respiratory protection includes a full-face mask with a HEPA filter; however, a wet cloth or handkerchief can offer some protection. Splash-proof clothing, gloves, and socks should be worn, with all seams (such as neck and arm cuffs) securely taped. A second pair of gloves that can be easily removed and replaced should be worn over the first, and waterproof shoe covers should be worn over shoes. If available, radiation dosimeters should be attached to the outside of clothing for easy reading. Radiation measurement equipment should be covered with plastic before entering contaminated zones. Rescuers should avoid smoking, eating, or drinking at the site and provide water only in closed containers.

After any HAZMAT exposure, first responders should clean all nondisposable gear with a 5% hypochlorite solution (1 part household bleach to 9 parts water). Protective clothing should be removed, bagged, and disposed of in a container labeled as "toxic waste." All personnel must then wash thoroughly with soap and water. Managing the tracking, collection, storage, and disposal of contaminated equipment and waste represents a significant logistical challenge in HAZMAT response.

Decontamination

Decontamination is essential in any disaster where toxic exposure is suspected. The primary aim of decontamination is to prevent further exposure to the patient and avoid contamination of the staff. All stable patients should be assessed for the need for decontamination before proceeding with further examination, triage, or treatment. Chemical and radioactive exposures typically require more stringent decontamination compared to biological exposures.

The decision to stabilize a patient before decontamination depends on the nature of the toxic exposure, the patient's condition, and the potential risk to personnel. Initial treatment prioritization for any victim, especially children, should follow the ABCs of Airway, Breathing, and Circulation.

Patients exposed only to gases or vapors, with no visible skin or eye irritation and no residual gas on their clothing, are less likely to cause secondary contamination. Such patients can often proceed directly to the support zone. For all other cases, decontamination should be carried out immediately after stabilization. Generally, critically ill patients should not be sent to the hospital before decontamination because they must undergo decontamination at the hospital anyway. Contaminated patients also pose a risk of secondary contamination to healthcare workers, emergency equipment, and transport vehicles. If transportation is necessary, protective clothing should be worn by transport personnel, and the vehicle's equipment should be safeguarded. Notify the receiving hospital in advance about the arriving patient requiring decontamination and ensure that a hospital-based decontamination area is prepared. Additionally, plan for patients who may arrive on foot or in private vehicles from the disaster scene without proper decontamination and will need to be decontaminated upon hospital entry.

In the decontamination zone, divide victims into two groups: those who can remove their own clothing and those who need assistance. Children, in particular, will generally need help, so ensure adequate staff is available. Remove and double bag all clothing and personal belongings, placing items carefully into small bags, especially when handling clothing contaminated with radioactive dust. Clearly label bags with the patient's name, address, and phone number. In cases where patients are considered crime victims, thorough documentation and evidence preservation are crucial.

The steps of decontamination are outlined in Box 6.2. It is important to consider that children are especially vulnerable to hypothermia during decontamination, so measures should be taken to keep them warm whenever possible. Infants may be difficult to decontaminate, so using an infant bath basin can be helpful. In scenarios with a large number of victims, communal decontamination showers may be used, with a focus on keeping children with their families. Lastly, in large-scale disasters or resource-limited settings, decontamination methods may need to be adapted to the situation.

Box 6.2 Sample decontamination sequence for children

 Remove all clothing: Place the clothes in double-bagged, labeled containers.

 Take out contact lenses: If present, ensure contact lenses are removed.

 Perform a full body rinse:
- Start from the head and work down to the toes, flushing the skin and hair with water for 3 to 5 minutes, while avoiding water entering the airways or eyes.
- Rinse irritated eyes with water or saline for at least 5 minutes.
- Wash all skin areas thoroughly, paying special attention to folds, underarms, and the genital area.
- Use mild soap to aid in removing oily contaminants.

 Protect children from thermal stress:
- If possible, use lukewarm water for decontaminating children.
- Dry them promptly.
- Swaddle them warmly to maintain body heat.

 Dispose of contaminated water properly: Whenever possible, collect water from decontamination areas in plastic containers marked as "toxic waste" for proper disposal.

In cases of unknown exposure or situations where the nature of the hazard is unclear, it is prudent to implement full PPE and decontamination procedures. However, it is important to periodically reassess the situation in consultation with toxicologists or other available experts if possible. As more information emerges, it might become unnecessary to maintain full decontamination measures, thereby allowing resources to be redirected to other urgent needs.

General Approach

Objectives

- Outline a systematic approach for delivering initial care to patients exposed to toxic substances.
- Acknowledge the critical role of effective supportive care as the foundation of high-quality toxicological management.

In disaster settings or mass exposure incidents, it may not be immediately clear if toxic exposure has occurred or which specific agent was involved. Fortunately, for most toxic exposures, specific treatments like antidotes or chelators are not required;

supportive and symptomatic care usually suffice. A fundamental principle is: treat the patient first, not the poison.

The management of any victim with toxic injury starts with a "Primary Survey" to evaluate the ABCs: Airway, Breathing, and Circulation. Ensuring a clear Airway is the initial step. Adequate breathing and ventilation must be secured, which may involve placing the patient in fresh air, providing supplemental oxygen, or administering positive pressure ventilation as needed. Circulation adequacy can be assessed by observing skin color, capillary refill, pulse, and blood pressure (refer to Module 4, Pediatric Trauma, for more details). Even in cases where serious toxicologic exposures are known, life-threatening traumatic injuries can lead to faster mortality than the toxic exposure itself. Therefore, after assessing and stabilizing the ABCs, address and stabilize any life-threatening traumatic injuries. Ideally, the airway, breathing, and circulation should be stabilized, and immediate life-threatening injuries should be managed before the patient undergoes decontamination (see sections "Levels of Protection for Personal Protective Equipment" and "Decontamination"). However, whether to stabilize a patient before decontamination depends on the toxic exposure, patient needs, and potential risks to personnel.

After stabilizing the patient's ABCs and completing decontamination, conduct a thorough physical examination. Special attention should be given to the patient's respiratory status, neurologic condition, and temperature, as abnormalities in these areas are both common and potentially life-threatening in toxicologic cases. Many patients exposed to gaseous or aerosolized toxins develop delayed respiratory symptoms, so even those with initially clear airways and adequate breathing should be reassessed carefully. Seizures, if present, should be treated promptly, as inadequate treatment can worsen toxic effects. It is crucial to prevent both hypothermia and hyperthermia; children are particularly susceptible to hypothermia, while hyperthermia, a pathophysiological state due to failed thermoregulation, can be fatal if not addressed. Unlike fever, which is a regulated increase in body temperature, hyperthermia requires immediate active cooling measures.

During the examination, noting whether the patient's symptoms align with a particular toxidrome can be useful. However, toxicological manifestations can vary widely; patients may show only partial toxidromes or a single symptom (e.g., respiratory distress or mydriasis) initially, with additional signs developing over time.

In the hospital setting, perform basic laboratory tests, such as arterial or venous blood gas analysis, electrolytes, blood urea nitrogen, creatinine, and lactate, as appropriate and available. Electrocardiography is particularly valuable, as it can detect life-threatening dysrhythmias common in critically ill toxicology patients and sometimes assist in identifying the toxicant, as some exposures are associated with specific ECG changes (e.g., cardiac glycosides, sodium channel blockers). Co-oximetry is also highly effective for diagnosing carbon monoxide poisoning, which is frequent among disaster victims (refer to the section "Carbon Monoxide" below).

Toxidromes

Objectives

- Define what constitutes a toxidrome.
- Describe the typical features of common toxidromes.

The term "toxidrome" is a blend of "toxic" and "syndrome" and refers to a specific set of symptoms linked to various types of toxic substances. In the initial stages of a disaster, the exact toxic agents involved may not be immediately known. In such cases, toxidromes can guide effective patient care by focusing on the observed signs and symptoms, even without knowing the precise exposure. This section provides an overview of several common toxidromes.

Anticholinergic

The anticholinergic toxidrome results from the inhibition of muscarinic acetylcholine receptors, leading to reduced parasympathetic nervous system activity and a relative increase in sympathetic activity. Clinically, this toxidrome is characterized by symptoms such as tachycardia, hypertension, flushed skin, dry mucous membranes, urinary retention, and reduced bowel motility. Delirium is also a common feature, attributable to the suppression of central nervous system acetylcholine receptors. Typical sources of anticholinergic exposure include antihistamines, antipsychotics, certain plant toxins, and some chemical warfare agents. Although antidotal treatment with an acetylcholinesterase inhibitor, like physostigmine, may occasionally be appropriate, the primary approach to management involves supportive care, including the use of benzodiazepines or other sedatives to address agitation.

Sympathomimetic

The sympathomimetic toxidrome arises from excessive stimulation of adrenergic receptors, leading to heightened sympathetic nervous system activity. Clinically, this manifests as tachycardia, hypertension, sweating, agitation, increased psychomotor activity, and hyperthermia. Severe cases of hyperthermia and heightened psychomotor activity can lead to serious complications, including rhabdomyolysis, kidney damage, electrolyte imbalances, and multisystem organ failure. There is no specific antidote for this toxidrome; treatment primarily involves sedation, active cooling, and supportive care. Common sources of sympathomimetic exposure include various recreational and prescription drugs, such as cocaine, amphetamines, phencyclidine hydrochloride (PCP), and lysergic acid diethylamide (LSD).

Cholinergic

The cholinergic toxidrome arises from the excessive activation of both nicotinic and muscarinic acetylcholine receptors, leading to overstimulation of the sympathetic and parasympathetic nervous systems, as well as neuromuscular junctions. Clinically, the presentation can be summarized using mnemonics that highlight symptoms such as excessive secretions, bradycardia, bronchospasm, constricted pupils, altered mental status, muscle fasciculations, and seizures. The primary treatment involves supportive care, with a focus on administering an anticholinergic agent like atropine to counteract bradycardia, excessive bronchial secretions, and bronchospasm. Management of seizures with benzodiazepines or other GABA agonists is also crucial. While some cholinergic agents might benefit from oximes, such as pralidoxime, addressing the critical cholinergic symptoms takes precedence. Cholinergic exposures typically stem from organophosphate or carbamate insecticides, but can also involve nerve agents used in chemical warfare.

Opioid and Sedative-Hypnotic

The opioid toxidrome results from agonism at mu opioid receptors and presents with the triad of a decreased level of alertness, decreased respiratory rate, and constricted pupils. The sedative-hypnotic toxidrome similarly presents with a decreased level of alertness but with a more variable presence of respiratory depression and constricted pupils. The primary purpose of differentiating these two toxidromes is to facilitate the administration of naloxone, or other opioid antagonists, as a reversal agent for patients with opioid toxicity. If in doubt, a trial of naloxone, as a test dose, can help differentiate the two toxidromes and guide further treatment. While opioid antagonists can be helpful, either toxidrome can be effectively treated with good supportive care emphasizing airway protection and respiratory support. Typical sources of opioid exposure are recreational drugs and prescribed analgesic medications. Of note, a mass casualty exposure to aerosolized opioids is believed to have occurred in 2012 in an attempt to subdue hostage-takers at a theater in Moscow. Sedative-hypnotic agents are typically found as recreational drugs or prescribed medications used for anxiety and muscle spasms.

Irritant Gases

Irritant gases, such as chlorine, ammonia, and phosgene, are among the most common hazardous material exposures. They typically cause pulmonary and airway irritation and inflammation. Highly soluble irritant gases lead to immediate symptoms by affecting the upper airway and oropharyngeal mucosa. In contrast, gases with lower solubility can penetrate deeper into the respiratory system before reacting with mucosal surfaces, often resulting in delayed symptoms and more severe pulmonary inflammation.

Treatment primarily involves administering supplemental oxygen and providing airway or respiratory support as needed. Bronchodilators and corticosteroids may also be beneficial in managing the symptoms.

Caustics

Caustic substances include a wide range of household and industrial chemicals with either acidic or alkaline pH levels. They can cause severe soft-tissue damage through direct chemical injury. The primary treatment for caustic exposure is rapid and thorough decontamination with water. Neutralizing an acidic exposure with an alkaline solution, or vice versa, is not recommended as it may cause further injury without providing additional benefit; water alone is the most effective method.

Special attention should be given to caustic injuries to the eyes, which require careful evaluation and decontamination to prevent serious damage.

Asphyxiants

Asphyxiants are substances that disrupt the body's ability to deliver and use oxygen effectively. Simple asphyxiants, such as carbon dioxide, nitrogen, methane, and propane, work by displacing oxygen in the environment. In contrast, chemical asphyxiants, including carbon monoxide and cyanide, interfere with the body's ability to use available oxygen. Exposure to asphyxiants typically leads to a rapid loss of consciousness and the onset of shock. While specific antidotes are available for some asphyxiants, such as cyanide, the primary treatment involves removing the individual from the exposure and administering supplemental oxygen. Asphyxiants also pose significant risks to rescuers, so it is crucial to take precautions to prevent further exposure in toxic or oxygen-depleted environments.

Carbon Monoxide

Carbon monoxide (CO) poisoning is commonly encountered after natural disasters. Faulty or inadequate exhaust systems in damaged furnaces, generators, camp stoves, or wood fires can pose significant hazards in the aftermath of an acute disaster. Even generators that are functioning properly but used indoors can lead to CO poisoning. The use of alternative heating and cooking sources in displacement camps or enclosed spaces further increases the risk of CO exposure. Since CO is both color-less and odorless, individuals often remain unaware of their exposure.

CO binds strongly to hemoglobin, forming carboxyhemoglobin, which impairs oxygen release compared to normal oxyhemoglobin. This results in reduced oxygen delivery to tissues and cellular hypoxia. Additionally, CO has direct cardiotoxic and neurotoxic effects. Symptoms of CO exposure can progress from fatigue, headache, and flu-like symptoms to confusion, ataxia, loss of consciousness, and even cardiac arrest as carboxyhemoglobin levels increase.

The most critical initial step in managing suspected CO poisoning is to remove the patient from the contaminated environment and ensure they breathe fresh air. If available, supplemental oxygen should be administered via a face mask. In a hospi-tal setting, laboratory tests such as measuring carboxyhemoglobin levels can con-firm the diagnosis. Hemoglobin/hematocrit tests can help identify underlying anemia, which may exacerbate the decreased oxygen-carrying capacity. It's impor-tant to note that peripheral saturation (pulse oximetry) may show normal or near-normal readings because carboxyhemoglobin's light absorption spectrum is similar to that of oxyhemoglobin.

In Depth: Cyanide

Cyanide can be released from the combustion of materials such as plastics, wool, silk, nylon, synthetic rubber, paper, and melamine resins. It is sometimes described as having a "bitter almond" odor, although this is not a reliable method for detecting cyanide exposure. Suspect cyanide poisoning if a fire involves synthetic materials, particularly if patients show symptoms like altered mental status, hypotension, or severe metabolic acidosis. Cyanide disrupts mitochondrial oxidative metabolism, affecting all tissues but especially those with high metabolic activity, such as the brain and heart. Initial symptoms may include tachypnea, hyperpnea, tachycardia, dizziness, headache, nausea, and vomiting. More severe exposure can lead to cen-tral nervous system depression, coma, seizures, and respiratory depression.

On-site management recommendations include decontaminating victims exposed to liquid cyanide by removing wet clothing and washing the skin. Administer 100% supplemental oxygen and provide additional respiratory support as needed. For seizures, use antiepileptic agents like benzodiazepines, and adminis-ter crystalloid fluids if the patient is hemodynamically unstable.

Upon hospital arrival, laboratory tests can be useful in managing cyanide poison-ing. Expected abnormalities include severe metabolic acidosis and hyperlactatemia. Although specific therapeutic measures for cyanide poisoning may not be available immediately, they are crucial for long-term care.

Hydroxocobalamin is the first-line antidote and should be administered intrave-nously. It is relatively safe but can cause temporary hypertension and turn bodily fluids deep red, potentially interfering with some laboratory tests and pulse oximetry. Hydroxocobalamin binds with cyanide to form cyanocobalamin, which is then excreted by the kidneys.

Older treatments include nitrites and sodium thiosulfate. Nitrites, such as amyl nitrite and sodium nitrite, induce methemoglobinemia, which helps detach cyanide from cytochrome oxidase. However, caution is needed as these agents can cause hypotension and excessive methemoglobinemia, which can impair oxygen transport, especially in patients with compromised conditions such as carbon monoxide toxicity. Sodium thiosulfate converts cyanide to thiocyanate, which is then excreted by the kidneys.

Recovery from cyanide poisoning can be rapid with prompt treatment, but without appropriate management, it can lead to swift death. Given that cyanide levels may not be immediately available, consider empirical treatment for suspected cyanide toxicity in patients with severe acidosis, hyperlactatemia, and hypotension who were exposed to a fire involving synthetic materials.

Fuels and Hydrocarbons

Hydrocarbons, including fuels and solvents, are common in both household and industrial settings. Prolonged skin contact with hydrocarbons can lead to irritation or even necrosis. Inhalation can cause respiratory irritation and, in severe cases, acute respiratory distress syndrome. Ingesting hydrocarbons may result in intoxication and altered mental status.

While each hydrocarbon may present unique toxicities, the primary focus in managing hydrocarbon exposures is diligent decontamination and supportive care. Additionally, hydrocarbons are often used as solvents in various chemicals, so exposure to hydrocarbons can be a concern in cases involving other chemical exposures or toxidromes.

Bioterrorism and Radiation

Objectives

- Compare the unique characteristics of bioterrorism with those of chemical terrorism.
- Describe the symptoms and impact of acute radiation syndrome.
- Summarize the triage methods for managing cases of acute radiation exposure.

An in-depth discussion of biological and radiation hazards in disaster scenarios extends beyond the scope of this module, but here are some key considerations. These considerations are vital for ensuring safety and effective response in the face of biological and radiation-related emergencies.

Biologic Exposures

Biological hazards encompass pathogens such as bacteria, viruses, and toxins that can lead to disease outbreaks. Essential considerations include the potential for rapid transmission, the necessity for suitable personal protective equipment (PPE), and the implementation of effective decontamination procedures. Prompt identification and isolation of affected individuals, along with timely vaccination and the use of antibiotics or antivirals, are vital for controlling such outbreaks.

In disaster and global health contexts, infectious diseases present a significant challenge. While naturally occurring illnesses are a common aspect of disaster response, there is also a considerable risk from intentional biological threats. The deliberate release of biological agents can potentially impact large populations. Unlike chemical threats, bioterrorism often involves more gradual and delayed symptom development, leading to patients presenting at various times and locations. Establishing a hot zone for bioterrorism is often challenging, if not impossible, due to the delayed onset of symptoms. Recognition of a biological event may be difficult, especially if unusual infections or symptoms appear in clusters. If a biological threat is suspected, it's crucial to alert local government and health authorities to initiate an investigation and implement appropriate infection control measures.

In the case of children, a bioterrorism event presents additional complications. Young children may struggle to describe their symptoms or their onset accurately. Infants or very young children may only exhibit general signs of distress, such as fussiness or clinginess, without clear symptoms. Furthermore, many treatments for biological threats have not been thoroughly studied in children, so dosing may need to be adjusted based on the child's size and age.

Radiation Exposures

Radiation exposure can result from nuclear accidents or the use of radioactive materials. Key management strategies include minimizing exposure time, increasing distance from the radiation source, and using shielding when feasible. Effective decontamination of affected individuals and equipment is crucial, and radiation detection instruments should be used to assess exposure levels. Treatment may involve specific antidotes or countermeasures to reduce the effects of radiation.

Radiation refers to the emission of energy as electromagnetic waves or subatomic particles, with ionizing radiation being the primary concern in disaster scenarios. Ionizing radiation can damage health by removing electrons from atoms or molecules in the body. This discussion focuses on ionizing radiation. Radiation comes from both natural and human-made sources. Natural sources account for about 80% of daily exposure and include sunlight (gamma radiation), radon gas (from decaying uranium in soil), and cosmic rays. The most common human-made source is in healthcare settings. Radiation exposure can be a primary disaster event or a complication of another disaster, occurring accidentally or intentionally.

Nuclear fission poses significant risks for disaster preparedness. Notable examples include the 2011 Fukushima Daiichi nuclear disaster in Japan, which was caused by a massive earthquake and subsequent tsunami, and the 2022 Zaporizhzhia nuclear plant incident in Ukraine amidst the ongoing conflict, which raised concerns about potential nuclear risks. Intentional sabotage of nuclear facilities is also a serious concern, including the potential detonation of nuclear weapons or improvised nuclear devices.

Accidental exposure from radiation in healthcare and industrial settings is another concern. For instance, in 2017, a radioactive source was inadvertently released during a cleanup operation at a healthcare facility in Mexico, leading to exposure of several individuals. Similar incidents involving unsecured or lost radioactive materials have been reported globally. There is also concern about malicious actors distributing radioactive materials to affect large populations.

Radiation exposure can cause public panic, potentially overwhelming healthcare systems with individuals seeking reassurance. Effective communication strategies are crucial to managing public perception and response during radiation disasters. Shelter-in-place and avoidance of contaminated food are often recommended actions.

It is important to differentiate between radiation exposure and contamination. Radiation exposure itself is harmful but typically does not make the patient radioactive or pose a risk to responders. However, patients contaminated with radioactive materials, such as fallout or powders, pose an ongoing risk. Decontamination involves removing contaminated clothing and using irrigation and scrubbing to remove residual contamination. Portable radiation detectors, like Geiger counters, can assist in identifying and locating contamination. Contaminated items should be tracked, contained, and stored for proper disposal.

Radiation exposure has two main health concerns: long-term risks of malignancy and chronic health effects, and immediate concerns related to high doses of radiation. Acute radiation syndrome (ARS) can range from mild bone marrow dysfunction to severe multiorgan failure and death, depending on the dose. ARS is categorized into four sub-syndromes: hematologic, gastrointestinal, neurovascular, and cutaneous. Symptom onset varies from hours to days, and various clinical and laboratory tools can help estimate exposure. For instance, the time to onset of vomiting can indicate the severity of exposure, with vomiting occurring within 1 h suggesting a need for extensive critical care.

Management of radiation exposure focuses on decontamination and supportive care, addressing challenges such as immune suppression, fluid and electrolyte balance, and sepsis. Specific chelating agents and antidotes, such as potassium iodide, Prussian blue, and diethylenetriamine pentaacetic acid (DTPA), may be used for certain radioactive isotopes but are adjuncts to decontamination and supportive care. Expert guidance is recommended for their use.

Table 6.2 provides an overview of acute radiation syndrome, including approximate timelines for each phase in cases of moderate to severe exposure. It's

Table 6.2 Acute radiation syndrome phases

Phase	Time until onset	Description
Prodrome	Hours	Nausea and vomiting
Latent	Days	Initial clinical symptoms resolve but biochemical injury progresses
Manifest illness	Weeks	Signs and symptoms of acute radiation syndrome sub-syndromes begin to develop and reach their peak severity. Rapidly dividing cells are most sensitive. *Hematopoietic syndrome*: Pancytopenia and immunodeficiency. Lymphocyte decline can be used as a sensitive marker for exposure and dosimetry. *Gastrointestinal syndrome*: Death of the mucosal lining leading to nausea, vomiting, bloody diarrhea, dehydration, electrolyte disturbances, and loss of the gut-blood barrier. Associated with critical illness and high risk of death. *Cerebrovascular syndrome*: Central nervous system dysfunction, seizures, shock. Associated with lethal exposures. *Cutaneous syndrome*: Vascular destruction leading to tissue death. Can occur in isolation with radiation exposure focused in a small anatomic area.
Death or recovery	Months	The patient either succumbs to their injuries or recovers from the acute illness but remains at risk for long-term impacts such as malignancy.

important to note that these timelines can shorten significantly with higher radiation doses, and not all phases or subsyndromes may be observed at lower levels of exposure.

Summary

Despite the many benefits of industrialization, our increasingly industrialized society has heightened the risk of disasters involving toxic exposures. This risk is further amplified by the growing focus on terrorism in disaster preparedness, making it essential to prepare for incidents involving chemical, biological, and radiation injuries. These types of exposures present distinct hazards and often cause significant emotional stress for both victims and responders. Effective preparedness and response should emphasize understanding the specific risks in the area, training to manage these unique hazards, and establishing communication plans to offer clear guidance to both victims and response teams. The following general principles offer a foundational framework for addressing these challenges:

- Identify local industries and other potential sources of toxic exposures.
- Consider the natural disasters more common in your region and how they might be exacerbated by toxic exposures.
- Determine the available local expertise for both planning and response efforts.

- Regardless of the type of exposure, prioritize limiting further exposure and contamination, decontaminating affected patients, and providing comprehensive supportive care.
- Use antidotal treatments as supplementary measures, without losing focus on the core principles of response and care.

Suggested Readings

Chung S, Shannon M. Hospital planning for acts of terrorism and other public health emergencies involving children. Arch Dis Child. 2005;90(12):1300–7.

Feldman RJ, Kazzi Z, Walter FG. Radiation injuries: acute radiation syndrome in children. Pediatr Ann. 2023;52(6):e231–7.

Ferguson B, Kaufman BJ. Hazardous materials incident response. In: Nelson LS, Howland MA, Lewin NA, Smith SW, Goldfrank LR, Hoffman RS, editors. Goldfrank's toxicologic emergencies. 11th ed. McGraw-Hill Education; 2019. p. 1806–13.

Hamele M, Poss WB, Sweney J. Disaster preparedness, pediatric considerations in primary blast injury, chemical, and biological terrorism. Pediatr Crit Care Med. 2014;3(1):15–23.

Linet MS, Kazzi Z, Paulson JA, Council on Environmental Health. Pediatric considerations before, during, and after radiological or nuclear emergencies. Pediatrics [Internet]. 2018;142(6) https://doi.org/10.1542/peds.2018-3001.

Maciulewicz TS, Kazzi Z, Navis IL, Nelsen GJ, Cieslak TJ, Newton C, et al. Pediatric medical countermeasures: antidotes and cytokines for radiological and nuclear incidents and terrorism. Disaster Med Public Health Prep. 2024;18:e76.

Markenson D, Reynolds S, American Academy of Pediatrics Committee on Pediatric Emergency Medicine, Task Force on Terrorism. The pediatrician and disaster preparedness. Pediatrics. 2006;117(2):e340–62.

Patt HA, Feigin RD. Diagnosis and management of suspected cases of bioterrorism: a pediatric perspective. Pediatrics. 2002;109(4):685–92.

Scalzo AJ, Lehman-Huskamp KL, Sinks GA, Keenan WJ. Disaster preparedness and toxic exposures in children. Clin Pediatr Emerg Med. 2008;9(1):47–60.

Chapter 7
Pediatric Considerations for Nutrition and Malnutrition in Disasters

Maureen Cunningham, Liliane Diab, and Douglas Taren

Introduction

Ensuring that children receive adequate nutrition to support their growth is essential in order to prevent an increase in malnutrition rates, which can lead to higher mortality during the recovery phase following a disaster. A child's nutritional health significantly affects their susceptibility to, and the severity of, infectious diseases in emergency situations. Frequent infections can result in heightened metabolism and related loss of appetite, exacerbating stress and the severity of malnutrition. Children who have been previously malnourished are especially at risk, as they lack the protective mechanisms that enable healthy individuals to cope with periods of food scarcity. Consequently, these children will experience further decline unless they receive prompt nutritional assistance. Conversely, proper nutrition fosters wound healing and enhances outcomes for both mothers and infants. In disaster contexts, providing sufficient food is vital to mitigate the risks associated with malnutrition. The World Health Organization (WHO) defines food security as a situation where everyone has consistent access to enough safe and nutritious food to meet their dietary needs and preferences, ensuring an active and healthy life.

Local healthcare providers, including doctors, nurses, nutrition experts, and epidemiologists, are invaluable for understanding the nutritional status of children prior to a disaster. Their participation in nutritional assessments and food resource planning is critical. Assessments may reveal significant disparities in pediatric nutritional health across a given area. Moreover, it is not uncommon to observe both malnutrition and obesity within the same household, particularly in low- and middle-income countries (LMICs) and among low-income populations.

M. Cunningham (✉) · L. Diab · D. Taren
University of Colorado, Department of Pediatrics, Aurora, CO, USA
e-mail: Maureen.cunningham@childrenscolorado.org; Lilian.diab@cuanschutz.edu;
Douglas.taren@cuanschutz.edu

143

Micronutrient deficiencies, particularly iron deficiency and anemia, can also be detected even in regions where the overall nutritional status appears satisfactory.

Nutritional Status Assessment

Objectives

- Acknowledge the significance of conducting an emergency food security assessment for communities affected by a disaster.
- Identify vulnerable population groups and specific risk factors in such situations.
- Outline various methods for anthropometric assessment of children.

Emergency Food Security Assessment

An emergency food security assessment (EFSA) evaluates how a disaster or humanitarian crisis affects the food security of communities and households in the impacted area. There are three types of EFSAs. The initial assessment provides quick, rough information. A rapid assessment gathers and analyzes data rigorously, though it often relies on assumptions, estimates, and approximations due to time and access limitations. The final type, an in-depth assessment, offers the most precise, quantifiable, and substantial information but is more time-consuming and challenging to conduct in the aftermath of sudden disasters. All EFSAs share similar objectives (see Box 7.1). Collaborating with multiple stakeholder organizations for EFSAs is beneficial when possible. Involving various stakeholders, including the affected community, ensures that:

- Different perspectives are taken into account.
- There is broad ownership of the assessments and recommendations.
- A diverse skill set is included.
- The process remains transparent.
- Multiple community assessments by different teams are avoided.

This approach helps identify nutritionally vulnerable groups (see Box 7.2) and assesses the quantity and quality of food supplies available to the affected population. The data collected through the EFSA, along with accurate demographic information about the impacted community, is essential for designing and implementing an effective food response after a disaster [1].

Box 7.1 Goals of Emergency Food Security Assessments
- Identify the prevalence of food insecurity and malnutrition within the affected area.
- Estimate how many people are affected.
- Determine where the affected people are located.
- Describe coping strategies used by different population groups and identify any that may have a negative impact on lives or livelihoods.
- Describe the food insecure and / or malnourished populations in terms of their individual and socio-economic characteristics -gender, ethnicity, etc.—and livelihoods.
- Establish the reasons why people are food insecure and / or malnourished by identifying factors associated with food insecurity or malnourishment.
- Determine whether food insecurity or malnutrition are chronic or transitory.
- Develop scenarios for the next 3, 6, or 12 months and use these to predict what will happen with the food security and nutrition of affected populations if no intervention is made.
- Evaluate the need for external assistance.
- Make recommendations for interventions including: What? How much? For Whom? How long?

Box 7.2 Vulnerable Populations
- Children under 5 years of age
- Children and adolescents separated from their families or communities, or those who have lost a parent
- Pregnant and lactating women
- Physically or emotionally disabled persons
- People with chronic disease
- Elderly people
- Families having lost their home or job as direct result of the disaster
- Families with women as head of household (depending on social and cultural norms)

Immediately following a disaster, a s uggested guideline for emergency rations is 2100 kcal per day per person. This figure can be adjusted based on readily available information that may influence the population's energy requirements, including:

- Temperature: Increase energy needs by 100 kcal for every 5 °C drop below 20 °C.
- Health and nutritional status: Increase needs by 100–200 kcal if the population is known to be in poor health or nutrition.

- Demographic distribution
- Activity levels

Additional immediate priorities should include ensuring that rations provide adequate protein, fat, and micronutrients for the population and meet the needs of all subgroups. It's important to outline strategies for gathering further information to adjust rations as needed, address food management issues and related conditions, and establish a monitoring system to verify that the rations remain sufficient [2].

Assessment During the Recovery Phase

During the recovery phase, as external resources increase and the local community becomes more organized, a key goal is to develop programs that ensure available food resources are effectively targeted to those in need. This requires a systematic assessment of the population's nutritional status. Such measures should continue until adequate nutrition resources are distributed efficiently and appropriately. Once the emergency situation stabilizes, planning priorities should shift to periodic reassessment to adjust reference ration figures based on factors influencing energy requirements specific to the context, as well as to establish a plan for long-term assistance and strategies for phasing down or out support.

Anthropometric Assessment in the Pediatric Population

Anthropometric methods provide insights into a person's height, weight, and body composition, particularly in assessing nutritional status in children. To interpret anthropometric data, individual measurements must be compared to reference standards for the relevant population. When anthropometric data are systematically collected, they can characterize the overall nutritional status of the community. Typically, data from children under 5 years old serve as an indicator of the community's health. In disaster scenarios, this information helps identify the global nutritional needs of the affected population and guides the efficient allocation of resources.

Anthropometric Indexes

Weight-for-Age Index (W/A)

The W/A index indicates a child's weight in relation to their age. It's important to consider factors like dehydration and edema, as these can affect weight measurements. For accurate assessment, a precision scale is necessary, and young children should wear minimal clothing during weighing.

Weight-for-Length (W/L) and Weight-for-Height Index (W/H) and Body Mass Index (BMI)

The W/L and W/H indices measure a child's weight in relation to their height. For children under 24 months, recumbent length is measured, while standing height is used for older children. The BMI is calculated as the ratio of weight to height for those older than 24 months. Both indices reflect the child's current nutritional status and are used to diagnose acute (wasting) or subacute malnutrition. Accurate measurements require a precision scale and a measuring board or tape, which are often not readily available in disaster situations and can take significant time to obtain. Additionally, W/H and BMI measurements can be influenced by dehydration and edema.

Length-for-Age (L/A) and Height-for-Age (H/A) Index

The L/A and H/A indices measure a child's height in relation to their age. These indices primarily reflect nutritional history, as children with chronic malnutrition—whether due to primary causes or underlying chronic diseases—often experience stunted growth.

Mid-Upper Arm Circumference (MUAC)

The MUAC (Mid-Upper Arm Circumference) measures the amount of fat and muscle in the upper arm. It is taken using a standard tape on the left arm, at the midpoint between the shoulder and the tip of the elbow. This measurement is used to screen large groups of children aged 6 months to 5 years for malnutrition.

Percentiles and Z-Scores

Percentiles are determined by an individual's measurement relative to reference values, indicating the percentage of values that are equal to or below the median. In the reference population, weight for a given height typically follows a normal distribution. The 50th percentile represents the weight that divides the population into two equal halves, with 50% above and 50% below. For example, if a child weighs more than 25% of the reference population, they are in the 25th percentile. Z-scores indicate how many standard deviations a measurement is from the median. A review of how these anthropometric tools can be used to assess an individual's nutritional status is presented in Table 7.1.

Table 7.1 Anthropometric indexes commonly used in the assessment of children

Nutritional status	MUAC	W/H z-score	Edema
Moderate Acute Malnutrition	110–125 mm	−2 to −3 SD	Not Present
Severe Acute Malnutrition	< 110 mm	<−3 SD	Present

Reference Tables

Measurements obtained from anthropometric parameters are only useful if the standards they are compared against accurately reflect the population being evaluated. Many countries have created their own growth tables and graphics, but some regions are still unrepresented. In 2006, the WHO published new growth reference charts based on data from Brazil, Ghana, India, Norway, Oman, and the United States. The selected children were exclusively breastfed, healthy, and had their basic needs met. Research shows that children up to age 5 grow similarly when their physiological needs are adequately addressed, making these reference charts applicable for assessing growth in children worldwide. More information can be found at www.who.int/childgrowth/en/.

Clinical Features of Malnutrition

Objectives

- Identify the key clinical findings of protein-energy malnutrition through physical examination, as well as signs indicating severe malnutrition.
- Recognize the characteristics and clinical and pathophysiological differences between marasmus and kwashiorkor.
- Describe the pathophysiology of refeeding syndrome.

Healthy, well-nourished individuals have some protection against acute malnutrition due to sufficient glycogen stores, protein reserves, and fat calories. Within the first three days without food, glycogen in the liver and muscles is depleted, prompting the liver to maintain blood sugar levels by converting mobilized amino acids into glucose (gluconeogenesis). Concurrently, fat breakdown (lipolysis) generates ketone bodies, providing an alternate fuel source for short-term survival. However, individuals who are malnourished at the onset of a disaster cannot activate these protective mechanisms, putting them at higher risk for acute nutritional decompensation.

Types of Acute Malnutrition

The term "Acute Malnutrition" has replaced the older designation of protein-energy malnutrition (PEM). Within this framework, Severe Acute Malnutrition (SAM) describes two primary forms: (1) severe wasting, or marasmus, and (2) kwashiorkor, also known as nutritional edema.

It is essential to highlight the multifactorial causes of severe malnutrition, including food scarcity, infections, and environmental factors, as well as their strong link to increased mortality rates. Additionally, various types of malnutrition often coexist in the same child over time, compounding the risk of mortality. For instance, many children with severe wasting or kwashiorkor also experience stunting. Those under 5 years of age are the most vulnerable, but other at-risk groups include pregnant women (which can affect fetal development), the elderly, and individuals with disabilities. Malnutrition in children typically arises from a combination of energy and protein deficiencies, often accompanied by micronutrient shortages. Frequent infections that reduce food intake play a significant role in this scenario.

Marasmus is the most prevalent form of PEM, characterized by significant energy and protein deprivation, resulting in a weight loss exceeding 20% of a child's initial body weight. This condition manifests as extreme wasting, fatigue, apathy, and irritability. An individual with a normal weight (10% to 12% body fat) could develop marasmus after about 60 days of total starvation. This form of malnutrition is most common in infants under 1 year, who may still express hunger despite their irritability.

Kwashiorkor often arises in malnourished individuals who then face additional catabolic stress due to infections (such as measles, tuberculosis, or pertussis), diarrhea, or trauma. Research indicates that there is little difference in the diets of children who develop marasmus compared to those who develop kwashiorkor. The production of free radicals and the depletion of antioxidants during inflammation seem to be linked to the edema seen in kwashiorkor. This nutritional edema is thought to be associated with increased secretion of an antidiuretic substance (likely antidiuretic hormone), which hinders the normal excretion of free water. Diets low in protein and calories may also influence the inactivation of this hormone.

Despite the extensive recognition of kwashiorkor, its underlying causes remain poorly understood. Many studies have not found significant differences in food group consumption between children who develop kwashiorkor and those who do not, or between those who experience wasting. Edema, the defining feature of kwashiorkor, is attributed to hypoalbuminemia. However, the correlation between the degree of hypoalbuminemia and recovery with nutritional support is weak concerning the severity of edema and its resolution.

Kwashiorkor presents with symptoms such as abdominal distension (often due to poor gut motility and sometimes malabsorption), bilateral peripheral edema, flaky skin lesions, hair discoloration, and hepatomegaly. Affected children frequently experience anorexia, complicating their management.

Some children with acute malnutrition may exhibit a form known as marasmic kwashiorkor, characterized by edema, significant loss of subcutaneous fat and muscle, stunting, and mild hepatomegaly. This subgroup faces high mortality rates, making cautious rehydration and careful refeeding essential.

Severe acute malnutrition is linked to various pathophysiological complications affecting every organ and system:

- Cardiac Function and Hemodynamic: Cardiac muscle atrophy and reduced cardiac output are observed, particularly in children with kwashiorkor.
- Enteropathy: Diarrhea is common in malnourished children, leading to poor clinical outcomes. Contributing factors include intestinal infections and inflammation. Malnutrition results in small intestinal villous blunting and malabsorption, especially of monosaccharides and disaccharides, which can further cause osmotic diarrhea.
- Hepatic Function: Severe malnutrition, particularly kwashiorkor, is associated with altered hepatic metabolic function and elevated liver enzymes. Hepatic steatosis (fatty liver) is notably linked with kwashiorkor.
- Brain Function: Severe malnutrition can lead to acute changes in brain function and behavior. Children with severe wasting often exhibit apathy, and the impact of malnutrition in early life on development is well documented. Stunting significantly affects cognitive development; for every 10% increase in stunting prevalence, there is an estimated 7.9% decrease in the proportion of children completing primary school.
- Infections: Children with severe malnutrition are highly vulnerable to life-threatening infections due to secondary immunodeficiency.
- Loss of Skin Integrity: Malnutrition can also compromise skin health, leading to increased risk of infections and complications [3].

Micronutrient Deficiencies

Objectives

- Identify specific micronutrient deficiencies, along with their risk factors and clinical signs.
- Explain the epidemiology, pathophysiology, and clinical presentation of deficiencies in vitamin A, iron, and zinc.
- Outline the general management strategies for preventing and treating micronutrient deficiencies in acute emergency situations.

Various dietary insufficiencies can result in specific micronutrient deficiencies, each with characteristic clinical manifestations. Table 7.2 highlights specific dietary risk factors for significant micronutrient deficiencies along with potential solutions.

Table 7.2 Micronutrient deficiencies: Risk factors and possible solutions

Micronutrient	Dietary risk factor	Possible solutions
Niacin (pellagra)	Maize-based diet	Foods rich in proteins and whole grain cereals; nixtamalization
Thiamin (beri-beri)	Polished rice-based diet	Whole or parboiled rice, legumes, beef, fish, eggs, milk; fortified cereal blends
Vitamin A	Diet with not enough fresh fruits or meat	Dark orange fruits and vegetables, yellow corn, fortified cereal, animal products, dark green leafy vegetables, vitamin A supplements, increase dietary fat with meals containing ß-carotene.
Vitamin C (scurvy)	Diet with not enough fresh fruits and extremely low-fat intake	Fresh raw fruits/vegetables, specifically citrus, liver
Iron (ferropenic anemia)	Diet lacking animal products	Animal products (liver, meat); dried fruits; consumption of vitamin C with meals; iron/folate supplements or fortified cereal blends. Avoid tea and coffee prior to taking supplements. From ages 6–24 months on, nearly all iron will need to come from complementary foods
Zinc	Diet lacking animal products	Animal products (liver, meat); fortified cereal, peanuts. From ages 6–24 months on, nearly all zinc intake is provided by supplementary foods
Riboflavin	Diet lacking animal products	Animal products (liver, eggs, fish); milk, leafy green vegetables. From ages 6–24 months on, nearly all riboflavin intake is provided by complimentary foods
Vitamin D (rickets)	Lack of exposure to sunlight	Fortified milk, liver, egg yolk
Calcium	Lack of milk; dark green leaves, or fish with bones	Milk, fish with bones (e.g., sardines), beans and green peas, dark green leaves, calcium carbonate (used in making tortillas)

Adapted from Savage, King, and Burgess, p. 430–431; and Médecins Sans Frontièrs [4], p. 27

Vitamin A Deficiency

Vitamin A is essential for vision and maintaining epithelial integrity. Additionally, vitamin A deficiency (VAD) is linked to issues in hematopoiesis and immune function. Treating VAD can have positive effects for patients with anemia and enhance recovery from infections, particularly measles. VAD often results from diets low in fresh fruits, vegetables, and animal products, including dairy and eggs. Globally, VAD significantly impacts health, affecting around 127 million preschool-aged children and 20 million women. It is estimated that undiagnosed VAD contributes to approximately two million infant deaths, especially due to increased morbidity and mortality associated with measles. VAD is the leading preventable cause of childhood blindness worldwide and is also prevalent among displaced populations.

The ocular manifestations of VAD are referred to as xerophthalmia. The stages of xerophthalmia include night blindness, conjunctival xerosis, and keratomalacia. Night blindness is the most common and initial sign of xerophthalmia. Since this symptom may occur before any visible physical signs, it is typically evaluated through careful history-taking and can also be assessed using various tests.

Conjunctival xerosis appears as a dry, non-wettable, rough, or granular surface, which can be observed with a handheld light. More advanced xerosis can lead to Bitot's spots, which are bubbly, foamy, or cheese-like patches on the conjunctival epithelium. Conjunctival xerosis may quickly progress to ulceration or, in severe cases, keratomalacia, characterized by necrosis of the cornea.

Supplementation

A diet that includes adequate amounts of vitamin A-rich foods is sufficient to prevent hypovitaminosis. If dietary sources are insufficient, supplementation should be considered. Research shows that vitamin A supplementation can reduce preschool child mortality by 25% to 35% and significantly decrease nutritional blindness in many low- and middle-income countries (LMICs). In acute humanitarian emergencies, if an adequate diet was not accessible and there was no existing vitamin A supplementation program prior to the disaster, all children aged 6 months to 5 years should receive vitamin A supplementation during their first contact with healthcare staff. This program can be integrated with immunization campaigns, including the measles vaccine. If dietary sources of vitamin A are inadequate, this supplementation should be repeated every 6 months. In areas with an existing vitamin A supplementation program, continue distributing supplements every 6 months, starting from the last administration. During the recovery phase, distribute fortified foods containing vitamin A and other essential micronutrients. Individuals showing symptoms of VAD should receive the recommended treatment. Table 7.3 outlines the preventive and treatment doses of vitamin A.

Table 7.3 Vitamin A treatment and prevention schedule

Age	Treatment[a]	Preventive dosage
<6 months	50,000 IU	50,000 IU every 4–6 months
6–12 months	100,000 IU	100,000 IU every 4–6 months
>1 year	200,000 IU	200,000 IU every 4–6 months
Women	200,000 IU[b]	200,000 IU < 8 weeks after delivery

Adapted from: West et al. [5]

[a]Treat all cases of xerophthalmia and measles with the same age-specific dosage the next day and again 1 to 4 weeks later

[b]For women of reproductive age, give 200,000 IU only for corneal xerophthalmia; for ocular eye signs (night blindness or Bitot's spots), give 5000–10,000 IU per day or <25,000 IU per week for >4 weeks

Low doses of vitamin A can be administered to pregnant women in their second and third trimesters, particularly those experiencing night blindness. Recommended doses include 10,000 IU per day or 25,000 IU per week. Additionally, vitamin A can be given to women postpartum to enhance the levels passed to their infants through breastfeeding.

The WHO advises providing high-dose vitamin A to severely malnourished children who are not already receiving Ready to Use Therapeutic Foods (RUTF), F-100, or F-75 for nutritional rehabilitation, or other multi-micronutrient supplements that contain adequate amounts of vitamin A (5000 IU per day). (Table 7.3).

Iron Deficiency

Iron deficiency (ID) is the most prevalent nutritional deficiency globally, particularly affecting women and children in developing countries. Risk factors for ID, aside from a diet low in animal products, include pregnancy, prematurity, low birthweight, early umbilical cord clamping, rapid growth, and feeding cow's milk (which can cause intestinal microhemorrhages). Additional factors that reduce iron absorption include high intake of phytates and tannins (found in coffee and tea), calcium (from cow's milk), and phosphates (from cola beverages), as well as menstruation and parasitic infections. ID is the leading cause of anemia, with the three primary causes of anemia in tropical regions being nutritional deficiencies, malaria, and intestinal parasites (such as hookworm, Trichuris, and schistosomiasis). The prevalence of anemia often serves as a proxy for ID prevalence in a population, with estimates suggesting that ID occurs 2 to 3 times more frequently than iron deficiency anemia (IDA).

Clinical signs of severe anemia include pallor of the skin, mucous membranes, and nail beds, along with dyspnea or tachypnea at rest. However, clinical examination alone is not a reliable method for diagnosing isolated iron deficiency or mild anemia. If laboratory tests are available, anemia can be confirmed through hemoglobin (Hb) or hematocrit measurements. Table 7.4 provides age-specific cutoff values for Hb and hematocrit according to WHO guidelines, which should be adjusted upward based on altitude (see Table 7.5). The decrease in tissue oxygen supply caused by anemia leads to various clinical manifestations and long-term effects associated with iron deficiency. Both iron deficiency and IDA can result in growth retardation, increased vulnerability to infections, and impaired cognitive and psychomotor development. Severe anemia (Hb <7 g/dL) is linked to higher mortality rates. While iron therapy can reverse some effects of ID, long-term studies indicate that iron deficiency anemia in early childhood may lead to irreversible developmental damage.

Table 7.4 Hemoglobin levels to define anemia at sea level (g/L)[a] in individuals and populations

		Anemia		
Population	Normal	Mild	Moderate	Severe
Children 6–59 months	≥110	100–109	70–99	<70
Children 5–11 years	≥115	110–114	80–109	<80
Children 12–14 years	≥120	110–119	80–109	<80
Non-pregnant Women 15–65 years	≥120	110–119	80–109	<80
Men 15–65 years	≥130	110–129	80–109	<80
Pregnancy	≥110	100–109	70–99	<70

From: World Health Organization [6]
WHO [7]
[a]Based on fifth percentile

Table 7.5 Altitude adjustments to measured hemoglobin levels

Altitude (meters above sea level)	Measured hemoglobin adjustment (g/L)
<1000	0
1000	−2
1500	−5
2000	−8
2500	−13
3000	−19
3500	−27
4000	−35
4500	−45

WHO [7]

Iron Supplementation for Prevention and Treatment of Anemia

The high bioavailability (approximately 50%) of lactoferrin-linked iron in human milk ensures that exclusive breastfeeding for the first 4 to 6 months provides a sufficient iron pool for healthy term infants.

Iron absorption can be improved by including animal protein in the diet. Adequate vitamin C intake and reducing dietary factors that inhibit iron absorption also enhance iron bioavailability. It is also important to ensure sufficient dietary intake of folic acid, as iron deficiency anemia (IDA) is often linked with folate deficiency. Preterm infants require early iron supplementation due to their insufficient iron stores at birth. Once solid foods are introduced around 6 months of age, supplementary feeding should focus on foods that offer high iron bioavailability.

Iron supplementation programs have proven effective in preventing ID. Starting preventive iron supplementation at 6 months of age is recommended, especially for those at risk, given the significant consequences of ID at this age. Table 7.6 provides guidelines for iron supplementation to prevent ID [9, 10].

The Integrated Management of Childhood Illness identifies palmar pallor as a sign of severe anemia and recommends hospitalization for children exhibiting severe palmar pallor. In some cases, if the child appears otherwise well,

Table 7.6 Iron supplements to prevent anemia in areas with high prevalence of anemia (>40%)

Age Group	Dosage (daily)	Duration
Children 6–23 months	10–12.5 mg elemental iron	3 consecutive months in a year
Children 24–59 months	30 mg elemental iron	3 consecutive months in a year
Children 5–12 years	30–60 mg elemental iron	3 consecutive months in a year
Adolescents and Adults	60 mg elemental iron	3 consecutive months in a year
Prevalence of anemia in pregnant women in the area		
<40%	30–60 mg elemental iron plus 400 µg. Folic. acid	Duration of pregnancy
>40%	60 mg elemental iron plus 400 µg. Folic. acid	Duration of pregnancy

From: World Bank [11]

Table 7.7 Iron and folic acid doses for treating severe anemia

Age	Iron and Folic Acid Doses	Duration[a]
Children <2 years	25 mg/day iron plus 100–400 µg/day folic acid	3 months
Children 2–12 years	60 mg/day iron plus 400 µg/day folic acid	3 months
Adolescents and Adults (including pregnant women)	120 mg/day iron plus 400 µg/day folic acid	3 months

From: World Bank [11]
[a]After completing 3 months of treatment children and pregnant women should continue on preventive supplementation

treatment may occur in an outpatient setting. Additional iron supplementation is not necessary if the child is already receiving nutritional rehabilitation with Ready to Use Therapeutic Foods (RUTF). Children with marasmus and kwashiorkor should be presumed to be severely anemic. Due to the risk of exacerbating underlying infections, oral iron supplementation should be delayed until the child is eating again and gaining weight. Table 7.7 outlines the management of severe anemia.

To ensure adequate iron status, it is crucial to implement public health programs aimed at controlling intestinal parasites, schistosomiasis, and other micronutrient deficiencies, in addition to providing sufficient dietary iron. In areas with endemic infections, routine administration of anthelmintic medication to individuals over 2 years of age is recommended, as helminthic infections, such as hookworm, can significantly affect iron status. Medications like albendazole are commonly used in community distribution programs for deworming children under 5 years old.

Zinc Deficiency

The exact global prevalence of zinc deficiency is not well-defined but is estimated to be similar to that of iron deficiency, highlighting it as an underrecognized public health issue. Zinc is crucial for the life, function, growth, differentiation, and replication of mammalian cells. It is one of the least visible micronutrient deficiencies. Zinc plays a vital role in maintaining health and immune function, as it is a component of over 200 enzymes and transcription proteins that regulate cell differentiation, nucleic acid synthesis, and the metabolism of proteins, lipids, and carbohydrates.

Zinc supplementation in children with deficiency has been shown to decrease the incidence, prevalence, and severity of diarrheal episodes and severe lower respiratory tract infections. Additionally, zinc supplementation reduces the frequency of malaria infections.

Reduced growth velocity or stunted growth is a common and early indicator of even mild zinc deficiency in infants, children, and adolescents. Table 7.8 presents

Table 7.8 Micronutrient deficiency signs and symptoms

Selected nutrients	Deficiency signs and symptoms
Vitamin A (retinol)	Night Blindness Various stages of xerophthalmia Hair Follicle blockage with permanent "goose bump" appearance, follicular hyperkeratosis Dry, itchy skin
Vitamin D (calciferol)	Rickets Osteomalacia and osteoporosis Epiphyseal swelling
Vitamin K (phylloquinone)	Small hemorrhages in the skin or mucous membranes (petechiae) Intraocular hemorrhage
Vitamin B1 (thiamine)	Beri Beri (cardiac and neurologic) Wernicke and Korsakov Syndromes (alcoholic confusion and paralysis) Sensory loss Blurred vision Dyspnea Muscular wasting Sometimes edema (wet beri beri) Malaise Ataxia Reduced muscle jerks (reflexes) Mental confusion Tense calf muscles Distended neck veins Jerky movements of eyes Staggering gait and difficulty walking Infants may develop cyanosis Round, swollen (moon) face Foot and wrist drop

(continued)

Table 7.8 (continued)

Selected nutrients	Deficiency signs and symptoms
Vitamin B2 (riboflavin)	Redness and scaling of nasolabial folds
	Diffuse depigmentation
	Non-specific: fatigue, eye changes, dermatitis, brain dysfunction, impaired iron absorption
	Tearing, burning, itching eyes
	Fissuring in the corners of the eyes
	Soreness and burning of the lips, mouth, tongue with fissuring and / or cracking of the lips or corners of the mouth
	Purple swollen tongue
	Seborrhea of the skin in the nasolabial folds, scrotum, or vulva
	Capillary overgrowth around the corneas
Vitamin B3 (niacin)	Pellagra identified by the four Ds: dermatitis, diarrhea, dementia, and death if not treated. The dermatitis from niacin deficiency has a classical presentation that is symmetric and occurs at pressure points (e.g. Buttocks) and on sun exposed skin
	Sensory loss
	Tremors
	Sore tongue
	Amblyopia
	Anorexia
	Indigestion
Vitamin B6 (pyridoxine)	Dermatitis
	Neurological Disorders, convulsions
	Anemia
	Inflammation of the lining of the mouth, tongue inflammation
	Fissures in the corners of the mouth
Vitamin B9 (folic acid)	Glossitis
	Neural Tube Defects
	Weakness, fatigue, and depression
	Pallor
	Dermatologic lesions
Vitamin B12 (cobalamin)	Lime-yellow tint to skin and eyes
	Smooth, red, thickened tongue
	Pallor
	Ataxia
Vitamin C (ascorbic acid)	Scurvy (fatigue, hemorrhages, low resistance to infection, anemia)
	Edema
	Swollen, bleeding, and/or retracted gums or tooth loss; mottled teeth; enamel erosion
	Painful subperiosteal hematoma
	Lethargy and fatigue
	Skin lesions
	Small red or purplish discolorations on skin and mucous membranes (petechiae)
	Intraocular hemorrhage
	Darkened skin around the hair follicles
	Corkscrew hairs and unmerged hairs
Calcium	Decreased bone mineralization, osteoporosis, rickets

(continued)

Table 7.8 (continued)

Selected nutrients	Deficiency signs and symptoms
Chromium	Corneal lesions
Copper	Hair and skin depigmentation
	Pallor
Fluoride	Increased dental decay, effects on bone health
Iodine	Goiter
	Developmental Delay
	Hypothyroidism
Iron	Fatigue
	Decreased cognitive function
	Headaches
	Glossitis
	Nail changes, koilonychias, thin concave nails with raised edges
	Skin pallor
	Pale conjunctiva
	Fatigue
Magnesium	Tremors, muscle spasms, tetany
	Personality changes
Selenium	Cutaneous changes including xerosis, erythematous scaly patches
Zinc	Dwarfism and hypogonadism
	Hepatosplenomegaly
	Hyperpigmentation
	Acrodermatitis enteropathica
	Alopecia
	Acral rash
	Skin and eye lesions
	Nasolabial seborrhea
	Decubitus ulcers

Taren and de Pee [12]

various clinical features associated with micronutrient deficiencies, including zinc deficiency.

Risk factors for zinc deficiency include insufficient dietary intake (particularly low-protein diets), high phytate and/or fiber content in the diet, diarrhea, and other malabsorption syndromes, intestinal parasitosis, hot and humid climates, and lack of breastfeeding.

In many developing countries, young children often do not get enough zinc in their diets, and data suggest that a significant number of women worldwide have zinc intakes that fall short of their pregnancy needs. Promoting exclusive breast-feeding for the first 6 months can help prevent zinc deficiency in infants. Fruits and vegetables are generally poor sources of zinc, as the zinc in plant proteins is less bioavailable compared to that in animal proteins.

Supplementation is the quickest method to improve zinc status, while fortification should be the primary long-term public health strategy to prevent deficiencies of this micronutrient. Box 7.3 provides the daily recommended intakes of zinc.

In the management of diarrhea, it is recommended to supplement with zinc alongside oral rehydration solutions.

Box 7.3 Zinc Daily Recommended Intake
- Infants: 5 mg
- Young Children: 10 mg
- Women: 12 mg
- Doses in diarrhea: 20 mg/day for 10–14 days

General Management for Micronutrient Deficiencies in Disasters

In disaster situations, two primary considerations are the prevention of protein-energy malnutrition and the provision of foods fortified with multiple micronutrients when feasible. Ensuring adequate micronutrient intake is crucial for reducing morbidity and mortality associated with deficiencies. Additionally, it is important to implement strategies aimed at decreasing micronutrient deficiencies during the early stages of the recovery phase.

An initial assessment of the affected population is essential to develop a management plan that addresses the identified needs. This plan should encompass the following elements:

1. Evaluate the pre-disaster prevalence of micronutrient deficiencies.
2. Review pre-disaster food sources to identify any existing deficiencies.
3. Assess current deficiency risks based on post-disaster food sources.

Table 7.9 outlines the classification of public health significance for selected micronutrient deficiencies.

Table 7.9 The classification of public health significance of selected micronutrient deficiencies

Micronutrient deficiency indicator	Recommended age group for prevalence surveys	Definition of a public health problem	
		Severity	Prevalence (%)
Vitamin A deficiency			
Night blindness (XN)	24–71 months	Mild	$0 \leq 1$
		Moderate	$1 \leq 5$
		Severe	5
Bitot's spots (X1B)	6–71 months	Not specified	>0.5
Corneal xerosis/ulceration/ keratomalacia (X2, X3A, X3B)	6–71 months	Not specified	>0.01
Corneal scars (XS)	6–71 months	Not specified	>0.05
Serum retinol (≤ 0.7 µmol/l)	6–71 months	Mild	$2 \leq 10$
		Moderate	$10 \leq 20$
		Severe	20

(continued)

Table 7.9 (continued)

Micronutrient deficiency indicator	Recommended age group for prevalence surveys	Definition of a public health problem	
		Severity	Prevalence (%)
Iodine deficiency			
Goitre (visible and palpable)	School-age children	Mild	5.0–19.9
		Moderate	20.0–29.9
		Severe	30.0
Median urinary iodine concentration (mg/l)	School-age children	Excessive intake	>300
		Adequate intake	100–199
		Mild deficiency	50–99
		Moderate deficiency	20–49
		Severe deficiency	<20
Iron deficiency			
Anemia (non-pregnant women hemoglobin <12.0 g/dl; children 6–59 months <11.0 g/dl)	Women, children 6–59 months	Low	5–20
		Medium	20–40
		High	40
Beriberi			
Clinical signs	Whole population	Mild	1 case and <1%
		Moderate	1–4
		Severe	5
Dietary intake (<0.33 mg/1000 kCal)	Whole population	Mild	5
		Moderate	5–19
		Severe	20–49
Infant mortality	Infants 2–5 months	Mild	No increase in rates
		Moderate	Slight peak in rates
		Severe	Marked peak in rates
Pellagra			
Clinical signs (dermatitis) in surveyed age group	Whole population or women >15 years	Mild	≥1 case and <1%
		Moderate	1–4
		Severe	5
Dietary intake of niacin equivalents <5 mg/day	Whole population or women >15 years	Mild	5–19
		Moderate	20–49
		Severe	50
Scurvy			
Clinical signs	Whole population	Mild	1 case and <1%
		Moderate	1–4
		Severe	5

From: The Sphere Handbook [13]

Nutritional Assessment and Management

Objectives

1. Evaluate and categorize the nutritional status of children using the Integrated Management of Childhood Illness (IMCI) and World Health Organization guidelines.
2. Develop appropriate management strategies based on the assessed nutritional status of children in alignment with IMCI and WHO recommendations.

Assessing the nutritional status of children and checking for anemia is a crucial component of the IMCI ask, look, and listen strategy. The risk of death from acute respiratory infections, diarrhea, malaria, and other serious viral and bacterial illnesses significantly increases when a child suffers from moderate or severe acute malnutrition or severe anemia. Consequently, children with medical issues such as severe pneumonia, who could typically be treated in an outpatient setting according to IMCI guidelines, require inpatient care if they also present with severe acute malnutrition.

The severity of malnutrition is evaluated by checking for bilateral edema of the feet and measuring the child's MUAC or W/H z score, as discussed earlier in this chapter. This information, along with the medical assessment for symptoms such as cough, diarrhea, fever, and HIV infection, allows for the classification of a child into categories: complicated severe acute malnutrition, uncomplicated severe acute malnutrition, moderate acute malnutrition, or no acute malnutrition. These classifications correspond to the red, yellow, and green zones in the IMCI chart for managing malnutrition, which can be found at: https://cdn.who.int/media/docs/default-source/mca-documents/child/imci-integrated-management-of-childhood-illness/imci-in-service-training/imci-chart-booklet.pdf?sfvrsn=f63af425_1.

Infants and children with complicated severe acute malnutrition should be urgently referred to a hospital, kept warm, and given the first dose of an appropriate antibiotic, along with a feed to prevent hypoglycemia. According to IMCI protocol, uncomplicated severe acute malnutrition and moderate acute malnutrition can be managed on an outpatient basis with oral antibiotics as necessary, ready-to-use therapeutic food, feeding assessments, and counseling.

In its 2023 guidelines, the WHO recommends that infants and children be triaged immediately upon entering a healthcare facility or meeting with a healthcare worker to identify and address any danger signs and to conduct a nutritional assessment. As a result, all infants and children who meet the criteria outlined below should be hospitalized. These recommendations align with the red zone on the IMCI chart for managing severe acute malnutrition.

For infants under 6 months:

- One or more IMCI danger signs
- Acute medical problems or conditions classified as severe per IMCI

- Nutritional edema
- Weight loss

For infants and children aged 6–59 months:

- One or more IMCI danger signs
- Acute medical problems
- Severe nutritional edema
- Poor appetite (failed the appetite test)

Infants under 6 months and infants and children aged 6–59 months who do not meet the above criteria but present with severe wasting or nutritional edema, along with any criteria listed in Box 7.4 and Box 7.5, should undergo an in-depth assessment to determine the need for hospitalization based on clinical judgment.

Box 7.4 Special Considerations Requiring In-Depth Assessment for Infants Less Than 6 Months
- Medical problems that do not need immediate inpatient care but do need further examination and investigation (for example, HIV related complications).
- Medical problems needing mid or long-term follow up care and with a significant association with nutritional status (for example, congenital heart disease, HIV, tuberculosis, cerebral palsy or other physical disabilities).
- Specific anthropometric criteria from the list of criteria used to identify infants at increased risk for poor growth and development WAZ < −2 SD, WLZ < −2 SD, MUAC <110 mm for infants between 6 weeks and less than 6 months of age, failure to gain weight on 2 consecutive measurements.
- Ineffective breastfeeding or perceived breastmilk insufficiency.
- Feeding concerns for non-breastfed infants (for example inappropriate or unsafe use of breastmilk substitutes for replacement feeding, milk refusal).
- Any maternal related or social issue needing more intensive support (for example, disability or depression of the caregiver, absent mother, adolescent mother or other adverse social circumstances [14].

> **Box 7.5 Special Considerations Requiring In-Depth Assessment for Infants and Children Aged 6–59 Months**
> - Medical problems that do not need immediate inpatient care but do need further examination and investigation (for example bloody diarrhea, hypoglycemia, HIV complications).
> - Medical problems needing mid or long-term follow up care and with a significant association with nutritional status (for example, congenital heart disease, cerebral palsy or other disability, HIV, tuberculosis).
> - Failure to gain weight or improve clinically in outpatient care.
> - Previous episode(s) of failure to gain weight and / or nutritional edema [14].

Infants under 6 months and infants and children aged 6–59 months can be managed on an outpatient basis if they meet the following criteria:

For infants under 6 months:

- No danger signs or conditions that require inpatient admission.
- No criteria needing in-depth assessment (Box 7.4), or if such criteria are present, an in-depth assessment has been conducted and determined that inpatient admission is unnecessary.

For infants and children aged 6–59 months:

- A good appetite (passed the appetite test).
- No danger signs or acute medical issues that necessitate inpatient admission.
- No criteria requiring in-depth assessment (Box 7.5), or if such criteria exist, an in-depth assessment has been completed confirming that inpatient admission is not needed.

These infants and children are classified in the yellow zone on the IMCI chart, and efforts should be prioritized to treat them in an ambulatory setting.

Appetite Test

The WHO recommends that children older than 6 months with uncomplicated severe acute malnutrition or moderate acute malnutrition undergo an appetite test to assess their ability to consume Ready to Use Therapeutic Food (RUTF). RUTF consists of soft or crushable foods that are designed for nutritional rehabilitation, being high-energy and fortified. Children who qualify for severe acute malnutrition but exhibit no medical complications and pass the appetite test are classified by IMCI as having uncomplicated severe acute malnutrition (yellow) and can be

Table 7.10 Minimum RUTF a child must eat in 30 min to pass the appetite test

	Number of 500 kcal, 92 g sachets a child should consume willingly during the test.	
Weight	Minimum	Maximum
<4 kg	1/8	1/4
4–6.9 kg	1/4	1/3
7–9.9 kg	1/3	1/2
10–14.9 kg	1/2	3/4
≥15 kg	3/4	1+

World Health Organization [15]

managed in an outpatient setting. If a child fails to consume the required amount of RUTF, they will need to be admitted for further care. Table 7.10 outlines the amount of RUTF that must be consumed to pass the appetite test.

To conduct an appetite test:

- Take the child and caregiver to a quiet area.
- Explain the purpose of the appetite test and the procedure to the caregiver.
- Ensure the caregiver washes their hands and sits comfortably with the child on their lap.
- Have the caregiver offer RUTF directly from the packet or place a small amount on their finger for the child to eat.
- Encourage the caregiver to offer RUTF gently and to continue encouraging the child without pressure. It's important that the child feels comfortable and is not forced to eat.
- Provide the child with plenty of clean water in a cup during the appetite test.

Nutritional Management

Community Based Management of Acute Malnutrition

Community-Based Management of Acute Malnutrition (CMAM) consists of four key components:

- Stabilization care for acute malnutrition with complications
- Outpatient therapeutic care for severe acute malnutrition without complications
- Supplementary feeding for moderate acute malnutrition
- Community mobilization

In a joint statement released in 2007, the World Health Organization, World Food Programme, United Nations System Standing Committee on Nutrition, and United Nations Children's Fund acknowledged CMAM as the preferred approach for early detection and treatment of severe acute malnutrition before life-threatening complications arise. CMAM utilizes Ready-to-Use Therapeutic Food (RUTF) for the nutritional rehabilitation of children with uncomplicated moderate and severe acute malnutrition who have successfully passed an appetite test. (Children must be at least 6 months old to receive RUTF; management of infants under 6 months is addressed separately [16]).

The WHO advises that all children aged 6–59 months with uncomplicated severe acute malnutrition should be administered a course of broad-spectrum antibiotics, such as amoxicillin, for five days. RUTF should be provided at home in adequate amounts to deliver 150–185 kcal/kg/day until the child is no longer severely wasted and edema has resolved. The RUTF quantity can then be reduced to 100–130 kcal/kg/day until anthropometric recovery is achieved. Weekly follow-up by a qualified home visitor, such as a nurse or trained community health worker, or regular visits to a health center, is recommended until recovery is confirmed.

For children aged 6–59 months with moderate acute malnutrition, a nutrient-dense diet high in vitamins, minerals, essential amino acids, and healthy fats is recommended. This diet should include animal products, beans, nuts, and various fruits and vegetables. Additionally, children with moderate wasting who meet specific criteria should receive Specially Formulated Foods (SFFs) and counseling, including those with:

- MUAC of 115–119 mm
- Weight-for-age z-score (WAZ) < −3 SD
- Age under 24 months
- Failure to recover from moderate wasting after other interventions
- History of severe wasting or severe acute malnutrition
- Comorbidities that require ongoing care associated with nutritional status

In high-risk contexts, such as humanitarian crises, children with moderate wasting should be prioritized for SFFs, counseling, and home food support for their families. SFFs should be provided in quantities sufficient to meet 40–60% of the daily energy requirement, aiming for 100–130 kcal/kg/day to facilitate recovery [14].

Box 7.6 Specially Formulated Foods (SFFs)
Designed for medical use to meet specific dietary needs.
  Types of SFFs:

- Lipid-based Nutrient Supplements (LNS):

  - Ready-to-Use Therapeutic Foods (RUTF)
  - Ready-to-Use Supplemental Foods (RUSP)
  - BP-100

- Fortified Blended Foods (FBF):

  - Super cereal with added sugar, oil, and/or milk

  Preference: LNS is preferred over FBF when available.

Patients may be discharged from outpatient therapy when the following criteria are satisfied:

- Weight-for-height z-score is greater than −2 and mid-upper arm circumference (MUAC) is greater than 125 mm during two consecutive visits/measurements.
- There is no nutritional edema recorded during two consecutive visits/measurements.
- Children with medical issues requiring mid- to long-term follow-up care, significantly affecting nutritional status, and/or additional social factors have been referred to appropriate support, or the limits of outpatient care have been reached [14].

Inpatient Care for Children with Complicated Severe Acute Malnutrition

Inpatient care for children with complicated severe acute malnutrition consists of two phases: Stabilization and Rehabilitation.

Stabilization Phase:

- Diagnosis and treatment of serious life-threatening complications.
- Feeding is gradually introduced, with a careful increase in caloric intake to prevent re-feeding syndrome.
- Duration: lasts a few days to a week, depending on the child's condition and associated morbidities, such as hypoglycemia, hypothermia, dehydration, infection, and electrolyte imbalances.

Rehabilitation Phase:

- Children are medically stable and can transition to outpatient care.
- Treatment follows the principles of Community-Based Management of Acute Malnutrition (CMAM).

A time frame for managing children with complicated severe acute malnutrition is provided in Table 7.11.

Similar to outpatient management, all infants and children hospitalized with severe acute malnutrition should receive a broad-spectrum antibiotic due to their high risk of severe infection. The WHO recommends the following treatment:

- Initial Antibiotic Therapy:

  - IV/IM benzylpenicillin: 50,000 U/kg every 8 h for 2 days
  - or IV/IM ampicillin: 50 mg/kg every 6 h for 2 days
  - Transition to oral amoxicillin: 25–40 mg/kg every 8 h for 5 days
  - PLUS IV/IM gentamicin: 7.5 mg/kg once daily for 5 days

Table 7.11 Time frame for the management of complicated severe acute malnutrition

	Stabilization		Rehabilitation
Hypoglycemia	███		
Hypothermia	███		
Dehydration	███		
Electrolytes	███	███	███
Infection	███	███	███
Micronutrients	███	███	Iron*
Initiating feeding	███	███	
Catch-up feeding			███
Sensory Stimulation		███	███
Follow up			███

Adapted from the World Health Organization [18]
Iron should not be introduced until Rehabilitation due to the risk of exacerbating an underlying infection

- For infants and children with complicated severe acute malnutrition and dehydration, intravenous fluids should be avoided for rehydration. Instead, they should be gradually rehydrated enterally using:
  - Oral rehydration solution for malnourished children (ReSoMal)
  - or ½ strength standard WHO low osmolarity rehydration solution with added glucose and potassium at a rate of 5–10 mL/kg/h for up to 12 h.

For additional guidance on managing medical complications related to complicated severe acute malnutrition, refer to the WHO Pocket Handbook of Hospital Care for Children, 2nd Edition. https://www.who.int/publications/i/item/978-92-4-154837-3 [17].

Special milk-based formulas F-75 (75 kcal and 0.9 g protein per 100 mL) and F-100 (100 kcal and 2.9 g protein per 100 mL) are recommended for initiating feeds and stabilization. Frequent small feeds, every 2–3 h, with F-75 are advised, aiming for a total of 130 mL/kg/day, which corresponds to 100 kcal/kg/day and 1–1.5 g protein/kg/day. The transition to F-100 should occur gradually over 2–3 days by replacing F-75 with equal amounts of F-100. After the child has transitioned to F-100, the feeding volume should be increased by 10 mL at each feed, targeting a total of 200 mL/kg/day, 150–185 kcal/kg/day, and 4–6 g protein/kg/day. Additionally, children can be transitioned directly from F-75 to Ready-to-Use Therapeutic Food (RUTF) in suitable amounts. For a sample feeding schedule for a child hospitalized with complicated severe acute malnutrition, refer to Table 7.12.

Table 7.12 Sample feeding schedule for a child with complicated severe acute malnutrition[a]

Day	Formula[a]	Frequency of Feed	Goal kcal/kg/day
1	F-75	2–3 h	100 kcal/kg/day
2	F-75	3–4 h	100 kcal/kg/day
3	F-75	4 h	100 kcal/kg/day
4	F-75 + F-100 / RUTF	4 h	130 kcal/kg/day
5	F-75 + F-100 / RUTF	4 h	130–140 kcal/kg/day
6	F-100 / RUTF	4 h	150–185 kcal/kg/day
≥7	F-100 / RUTF	4 h	150–185 kcal/kg/day

[a]*Duration of stabilization and transition to F-100 / RUTF will vary from patient to patient and is dependent on how well feeds are tolerated*

Children aged 6 to 59 months hospitalized with complicated severe acute malnutrition can be transferred to an outpatient program if they meet the following criteria:

- They do not exhibit any danger signs for 24–48 h prior to transfer.
- The medical problems that prompted their admission no longer require inpatient care.
- Children admitted with wasting and no nutritional edema do not show ongoing weight loss.
- Children admitted with nutritional edema no longer have severe edema (generalized to feet, legs, arms, and face) and edema is resolving.
- They have a good appetite.
- All efforts have been made to refer children with medical problems needing mid- to long-term follow-up care, which significantly affects nutritional status, to appropriate services, or the limits of inpatient care have been reached [14].

The Refeeding Syndrome

Refeeding syndrome is a serious condition that can occur when feeds are rapidly initiated in an undernourished patient. It can be fatal, so a slow reintroduction of feeding is essential to prevent its development and associated complications in patients hospitalized with complicated severe acute malnutrition.

Complications of refeeding syndrome include:

- Hypomagnesemia
- Hypoglycemia
- Hypokalemia
- Hypophosphatemia
- Thiamine deficiency

During refeeding, increased glucose levels lead to a rise in insulin and a decrease in glucagon secretion. Insulin facilitates the absorption of potassium into cells via the sodium-potassium ATPase symporter, which also transports glucose. This process, along with magnesium and phosphate uptake, results in decreased serum levels of these electrolytes, all of which are already depleted. The clinical manifestations of refeeding syndrome stem from the functional deficits of these electrolytes and water retention, potentially causing congestive heart failure, pulmonary edema, and cardiac arrhythmias.

Additionally, the refeeding process, particularly with carbohydrates, accelerates the use of thiamine, which is crucial for carbohydrate metabolism. This can lead to a "functional thiamine deficiency," particularly in patients with severe acute malnutrition who may already have low thiamine stores.

To prevent refeeding syndrome, the following recommendations are made:

1. Gradual advancement of feeding and avoidance of aggressive hydration.
2. Empiric thiamine supplementation.
3. Monitoring refeeding labs, including magnesium, potassium, and phosphorus levels [18].

Nutritional Management of Infants Less Than 6 Months

Assessing nutritional status and feeding issues in the first 6 months of life is crucial in health care. Early detection of feeding problems, along with prompt diagnosis and treatment for infants experiencing reduced weight gain or weight loss, can help prevent disease and mortality.

A newborn may lose up to 10% of body weight in the first week due to factors like edema reabsorption and fluid elimination. This weight loss is significantly influenced by gestational age, birth weight, feeding type and method, and other morbidity-related factors during the initial days of life.

The 2023 WHO guidelines for identifying and managing infants and children with wasting and nutritional edema recognize that infants exhibiting certain characteristics, as listed in Box 7.7, are at risk for poor growth and development.

Box 7.7 Infants Less Than 6 Months at Risk for Poor Growth and Development
Infants with poor growth based on sequential measures

- No weight gain or weight loss from one measurement to the next; or
- Downward crossing of the weight for age percentile lines; or
- Insufficient weight gain

Infants with poor anthropometry based on a single measure (if sequential measures aren't available)

- Weight for age z-score (WAZ) < −2.00
- Weight for length z-score (WLZ) < −2.00

- Nutritional edema; or
- Mid upper arm circumference (MUAC) <110 mm for infants 6 weeks to less than 6 months of age

Infants with known risk factors for poor growth and development

- Neurodevelopmental concerns; or
- Infant feeding concerns; or
- Maternal risk (physical or mental health problem(s) affecting infant care); or
- History of Hospitalization

Infants at risk due to poor birth outcomes

- Preterm birth; or
- Low birthweight; or
- Small for gestational age

Infants under 6 months who meet any of the criteria in Box 7.7, along with their mothers, should receive regular healthcare and monitoring to identify medical and psychological issues early and to prevent the infant from becoming severely underweight or wasted.

As previously mentioned, infants less than 6 months with wasting or nutritional edema can be managed on an outpatient basis if they:

- Show no danger signs or criteria necessitating inpatient admission.
- Do not meet criteria requiring in-depth assessment (Box 7.4), or if such criteria are present, a thorough assessment has been conducted and determined that inpatient care is not needed.

In-depth assessments must be carried out by a qualified healthcare worker and should include a comprehensive medical, feeding, and psychosocial evaluation of the infant and their mother or caregiver. Feeding assessments should specifically address the health status of both the infant and the caregiver, caregiver responsiveness to the infant's cues, and, for breastfeeding, aspects such as positioning, latching, sucking, and swallowing. Health workers should adhere to best practices for addressing breastfeeding and lactation challenges, as well as the underlying factors contributing to these issues. For more information on assessing and optimizing breastfeeding, please refer to the Global Health Media project: https://globalhealth-media.org/topic/breastfeeding/.

The decision to introduce supplementary formula alongside breastfeeding must be based on a thorough assessment of the infant's medical and nutritional needs, the physical and mental health of the mother or caregiver, and the availability of resources to safely provide formula. In emergency settings, resources such as clean water, suitable storage containers, and effective cleaning methods are often scarce, as is the availability of formula or milk. In such cases, if culturally appropriate, a wet nurse may serve as an alternative to human milk substitutes, pending appropriate testing for infectious diseases relevant to the context. Research indicates that it is generally safer and easier for HIV-positive mothers to continue breastfeeding with option B ART rather than switch to formula feeding. Always consult national guidelines regarding breastfeeding for HIV-positive mothers.

Infants under 6 months at risk for poor growth and development should be admitted for inpatient care if they meet any of the following criteria:

- One or more IMCI danger signs
- Acute medical problems classified as severe per IMCI
- Nutritional edema
- Weight loss

Inpatient care for these infants should prioritize breastfeeding, and caregivers should be encouraged and supported to breastfeed whenever possible. If breastfeeding is not feasible, support should be provided for the mother or female caregiver to relactate. If relactation is not possible, wet nursing should be promoted. Supplementary feeding should also be provided, focusing on supplementary suckling approaches. Acceptable supplementary feeds in the inpatient setting include expressed breast milk, commercial infant formula, F-75, or diluted F-100 (with an additional 30% water). Note that diluted F-100 should not be given to infants with nutritional edema. Clinically unstable infants with nutritional edema, dehydration, or diarrhea should not receive full-strength F-100 due to the increased renal solute load and risk of hypernatremic dehydration. If breastfeeding is not an option, infants should receive appropriate replacement feeds, such as infant formula, with caregivers instructed on safe preparation and usage.

Infants under 6 months can be transferred to outpatient care when they meet the following criteria:

- No danger signs have been present for at least 48 h prior to transfer.
- All acute medical problems are resolved.
- Nutritional edema is resolving.
- The infant shows a good appetite.
- There is documented weight gain for at least 2–3 days, satisfactory on exclusive breastfeeding or replacement feeding.
- All efforts have been made to refer children with medical problems requiring mid- to long-term follow-up care, with significant associations with nutritional status, to appropriate services, or the limits of inpatient care have been reached.
- The infant has received necessary immunizations and routine interventions or plans for follow-up have been established.
- The mother or caregiver has been linked with needed follow-up and support for any identified health, mental health, or social needs during the admission.

Infants can have reduced frequency of outpatient visits when they are effectively breastfeeding or feeding well with replacement feeds and have shown sustained weight gain for two consecutive weekly visits. Infants at risk of poor growth and development should be assessed at 6 months to determine if ongoing follow-up or referral to services is necessary based on their clinical and nutritional status.

Summary

Adequate nutrition is essential for everyone's health and well-being. Even in optimal conditions, there are numerous challenges to maintaining proper nutrition, which are significantly exacerbated in the aftermath of natural or man-made disasters. Understanding the local community and having reliable information about available resources are crucial for developing an effective recovery strategy. It's important to note that malnutrition increases morbidity and mortality rates, particularly among vulnerable groups such as children.

Assessing the nutritional status of the population through anthropometric measurements, identifying macro and micronutrient deficiencies, and implementing preventive and therapeutic strategies greatly enhance the chances of successful recovery in disaster-affected populations. In these situations, the WHO and IMCI primary health care strategy offers a practical framework to support this objective.

Resources

1. World Food Programme. Emergency food security assessment handbook. 2nd ed. Rome: World Food Programme; 2009.
2. Food and Nutrition Needs in Emergencies. Geneva: UNCHR, UNICEF, WFP, WHO; 2004. www.who.int/publications/i/item/food-and-nutrition-needs-in-emergencies.
3. Bhutta ZA, Berkley JA, Bandsma RHJ, Kerac M, Trehan I, Briend A. Severe childhood malnutrition. Nat Rev Dis Primers. 2017;3:17067. https://doi.org/10.1038/nrdp.2017.67. PMID: 28933421; PMCID: PMC7004825.
4. Médecins Sans Frontiers. Infant and young child feeding in emergencies: nutrition module for the interaction health training curriculum, academy for educational development, 1997; Updates from clinical guidelines – diagnosis and treatment manual, severe acute malnutition chapter, Medecins sans Frontieres / Doctors Without Borders, February 2024.
5. West K Jr, Caballero B, et al. Nutrition. In: Merson M, Black R, Mills A, editors. International public health: diseases, programs, systems, and policies. Gaithersburg: Aspen Publishers; 2001.
6. World Health Organization. Guideline on haemoglobin cutoffs to define anemia in individuals and populations. Geneva: World Health Organization; 2024. https://iris.who.int/bitstream/handle/10665/376196/9789240088542-eng.pdf?sequence=1.
7. WHO. Haemoglobin concentrations for the diagnosis of anaemia and assessment of severity. Vitamin and Mineral Nutrition Information System. Geneva: World Health Organization; 2011. http://www.who.int/vmnis/indicators/haemoglobin.pdf.
8. World Health Organization. Integrated management of childhood illness chart booklet. Geneva: World Health Organization; 2014.
9. World Health Organization. Guideline: daily iron supplementation in infants and children. Geneva: World Health Organization; 2016.
10. World Health Organization. WHO recommendations on antenatal care for a positive pregnancy experience. Geneva: World Health Organization; 2016.

11. World Bank. Anemia prevention and control what works part II: tools and resources. World Bank; 2003.
12. Taren D, de Pee S. The spectrum of malnutrition. In: De Pee, Taren, Bloem, editors. Nutrition and health in a developing world. 3rd ed. Humana Press; 2017.
13. The Sphere Handbook. Humanitarian charter and minimum standards in humanitarian response. https://handbook.spherestandards.org/en/sphere.
14. WHO Guideline on the prevention and management of wasting and nutritional oedema (acute malnutrition) in infants and children under 5 years. Geneva: World Health Organization; 2023. License: cc by-nc-sa 3.0 igo.
15. World Health Organization. Module 6 malnutrition and anaemia. Geneva: World Health Organization; 2014.
16. Community Based Management of Severe Acute Malnutrition Geneva: WHO, WFP, UN System, UNICEF, 2007. https://iris.who.int/bitstream/handle/10665/44295/9789280641479_eng.pdf?sequence=1.
17. World Health Organization. Pocket handbook of hospital care for children. 2nd ed. Geneva: World Health Organization; 2013.
18. Mehanna HM, Moledina J, Travis J. Refeeding syndrome: what it is, and how to prevent and treat it. BMJ. 2008;336(7659):1495–8. https://doi.org/10.1136/bmj.a301. PMID: 18583681; PMCID: PMC2440847.

Chapter 8
Management Strategies for Common Pediatric Infections in the Aftermath of Disasters

Hai Nguyen-Tran, Conrad W. Wanyama, Alemayehu Teklu Toni, and Stephen Berman

Introduction

Morbidity and mortality resulting from an acute humanitarian emergency in developing countries are related to the excessive childhood mortality that existed prior to the disaster. The main causes of mortality include neonatal issues (e.g., preterm birth complications, birth trauma), injury, and infectious diseases (e.g., pneumonia, diarrhea, malaria, measles) [1]. Malnutrition, as an underlying condition, increases the risk of dying from all of the above causes.

During acute humanitarian emergencies, mortality related to common childhood infections increases due to crowded living conditions; displacement to areas with higher disease prevalence; and compromised personal hygiene resulting from inadequate water supplies, contaminated water, and poor sanitation. The pre-existing nutritional status (particularly micronutrient and vitamin A deficiencies) and immunization rates of children, as well as the pre-existing primary care infrastructure and

H. Nguyen-Tran (✉)
University of Colorado School of Medicine I Department of Pediatrics Section of Infectious Diseases, Aurora, CO, USA
e-mail: hai.nguyen-tran@childrenscolorado.org

C. W. Wanyama
KEMRI Wellcome Trust Research Programme & University of Nairobi I Department of Nursing Sciences, Nairobi, Kenya

A. T. Toni
University of Gondar I Department of Pediatrics and Child Health, Gondar, Ethiopia

S. Berman
University of Colorado School of Medicine I Department of Pediatrics, Aurora, CO, USA

the degree of damage caused by the disaster, also affect childhood morbidity and mortality after a disaster.

Therefore, strategies to prevent and treat infections during an acute humanitarian emergency, such as utilization of the Integrated Management of Childhood Illness (IMCI) guidelines, must be employed quickly and effectively.

Integrated Management of Childhood Illness (IMCI)

Objectives

- Describe the rationale for the WHO evidence-based approach to case management as described in the IMCI.
- List the clinical illnesses included in the IMCI program and their relevance in situations associated with disasters.
- Assess and classify the condition of a child to determine its severity and establish the relationship between the classification and the subsequent management.
- List the danger signs that should be routinely checked in all children.

What Is Integrated Management of Childhood Illness (IMCI)?

The strategy for the IMCI was designed by WHO/UNICEF to enhance children's health and reduce mortality and morbidity caused by the most prevalent childhood diseases throughout the world, but especially in countries having the highest under 5 mortality rates [2–4]. Its strategy contains three major components: (1) improve clinical management skills of healthcare providers; (2) improve health systems; and (3) improve family and community health practices. The IMCI strategy addresses most, but not all, of the major reasons why a sick child needs medical attention. A child with a chronic condition or a less common illness may require additional special care; further, IMCI guidelines do not describe the management of trauma or other acute emergencies due to accidents or injuries.

This IMCI strategy seeks to integrate the acute care for children under 5 years of age across the continuum of clinical services: from community health worker encounters through first level referral health care facilities (e.g., camps, medical offices, and health care centers) and then in hospitals. The clinical decision-making approach involves using a limited number of symptoms and signs to classify the severity of illness, which determines the child's treatment and management. See Fig. 8.1.

IMCI management also includes guidelines for follow-up, counseling the parents, and instructions regarding when to return when additional care is needed. The IMCI approach focuses training and materials on the need to improve parental skills

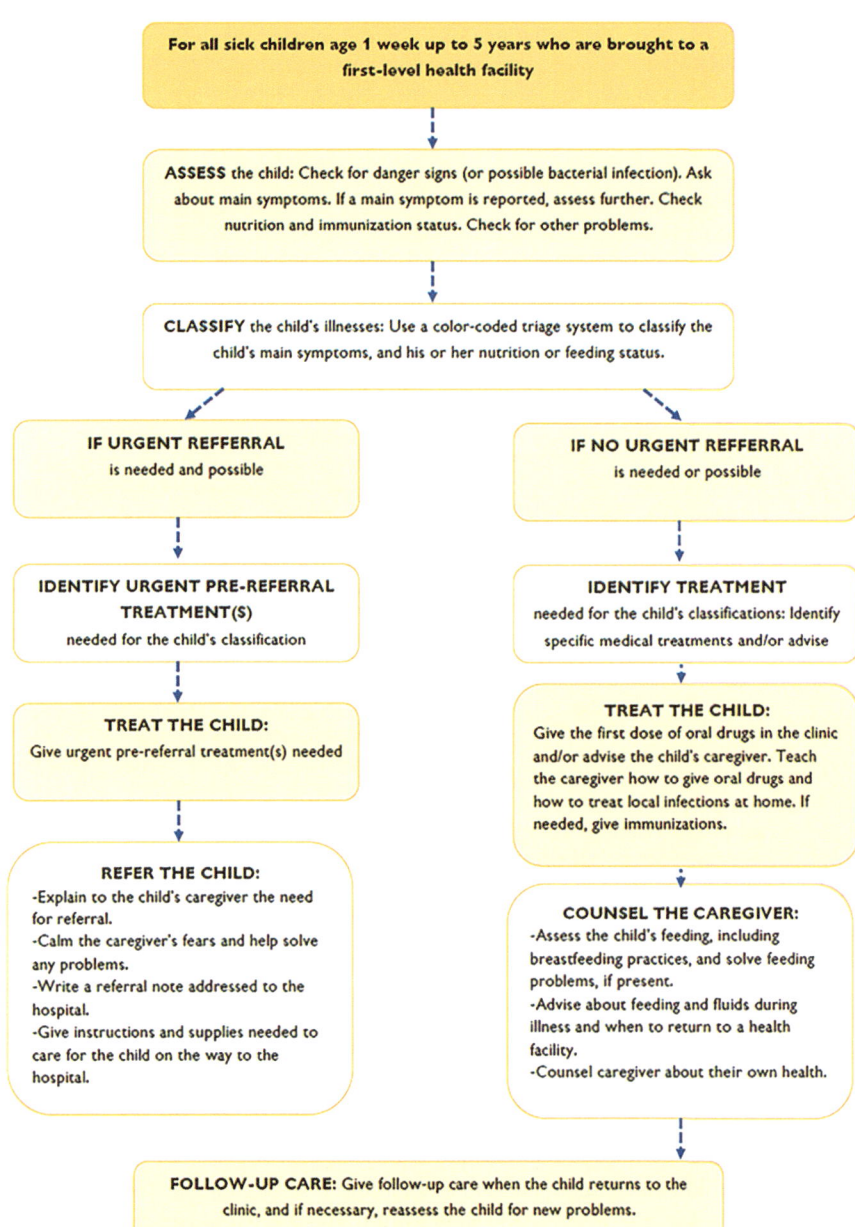

Fig. 8.1 Summary of the process of integrated care of children

and practices related to care seeking behaviors, the value of preventive services such as immunization and nutrition, and home care of children. The basic principles of IMCI are presented in Box 8.1. For full details and IMCI guidelines, please refer to the WHO website listed in the references.

Box 8.1: Principles of the Integrated Clinical Case Management

IMCI clinical guidelines are based on the following principles:

1. **Examining all sick children aged up to five years** of age for **general danger signs** and all young infants for signs of **very severe disease**. These signs indicate severe illness and the need for immediate referral or admission to hospital.
2. The children and infants are then assessed for main symptoms:
   - In older children the main symptoms include:
     — Cough or difficulty breathing,
     — Diarrhoea.
     — Fever, and
     — Ear infection.
   - In young infants, the main symptoms include:
     — Local bacterial infection,
     — Diarrhoea, and
     — Jaundice,
3. Then in addition, all sick children are **routinely checked** for:
   - Nutritional and immunization status,
   - HIV status in high HIV settings, and
   - Other potential problems.
4. Only a **limited number of clinical signs** are used, selected on the basis of their sensitivity and specificity to detect disease through classification.

A combination of individual signs leads to a **child's classification** within one or more symptom groups rather than a diagnosis. The classification of illness is based on a colour-coded triage system:
   - "PINK" indicates urgent hospital referral or admission,
   - "YELLOW" indicates initiation of specific outpatient treatment.
   - "GREEN" indicates supportive home care.
5. IMCI management procedures use a **limited number of essential drugs** and encourage active participation of caregivers in the treatment of their children.
6. An essential component of IMCI is the **counselling of caregivers** regarding home care:
   - Appropriate feeding and fluids,
   - When to return to the clinic immediately, and
   - When to return for follow-up

IMCI Guidelines

The IMCI strategy is divided into 2 components based on the child's age: (1) management of the sick child aged 2 months up to 5 years, and (2) management of the sick young infant aged up to 2 months.

The sick child management includes respiratory disease, diarrhea, febrile illness (malaria), measles, ear infections, malnutrition, anemia, HIV, and immunization status. See Fig. 8.2.

The sick young infant management includes severe disease (respiratory and sepsis), local bacterial infection, jaundice, diarrhea, HIV infection, weight gain, breastfeeding and other feeding problems, immunization status, and mother's health. See Fig. 8.3.

IMCI-related research involving traditional clinical history and physical examination data identified a limited number of clinical symptoms and signs that suggested the presence of certain diseases and their predicted mortality. Further, these clinical symptoms and signs were selected based on their sensitivity and specificity for diagnoses, in addition to a consideration of the available resources used to address them in first-level healthcare facilities worldwide.

Name: Age: Weight (kg):   Height/Length (cm):   Temperature (°C)

Ask: What are the child's problems?   Initial Visit?   Follow-up Visit?

ASSESS (Circle all signs present)	CLASSIFY
CHECK FOR GENERAL DANGER SIGN • NOT ABLE TO DRINK OR BREASTFEED • VOMITS EVERYTHING • CONVULSIONS • LETHARGIC OR UNCONSCIOUS • CONVULSING NOW	General danger sign present? Yes ___ No ___ **Remember to use Danger sign when selecting classifications**
DOES THE CHILD HAVE COUGH OR DIFFICULT BREATHING? • For how long? ___ Days • Count the breaths in one minute: ___ breaths per minute. Fast breathing? • Look for chest indrawing • Look and listen for stridor • Look and listen for wheezing	Yes ___ No ___

DOES THE CHILD HAVE DIARRHOEA?
• For how long? ___ Days
• Is there blood in the stool?
• Look at the childs general condition. Is the child:
  ▪ Lethargic or unconscious? Restless and irritable?
• Look for sunken eyes.
• Offer the child fluid. Is the child:
  ▪ Not able to drink or drinking poorly? Drinking eagerly, thirsty?
• Pinch the skin of the abdomen. Does it go back:
  ▪ Very slowly (longer then 2 seconds)? Slowly?
	Yes ___ No ___

DOES THE CHILD HAVE FEVER? (by history/feels hot/temperature 37.5°C or above)
Decide malaria risk: High ___ Low ___ No___
• For how long? ___ Days
• If more than 7 days, has fever been present every day?
• Has child had measles within the last 3 months?
Do a malaria test, if NO general danger sign in all cases in high malaria risk or NO obvious cause of fever in low malaria risk:
Test POSITIVE? P. falciparum P. vivax   *NEGATIVE?*
• Look or feel for stiff neck
• Look for runny nose
• Look for signs of MEASLES:
  ▪ Generalized rash and
  ▪ One of these: cough, runny nose, or red eyes
• Look for any other cause of fever.
	Yes ___ No ___

If the child has measles now or within the last 3 months:	• Look for mouth ulcers. If yes, are they deep and extensive? • Look for pus draining from the eye. • Look for clouding of the cornea.

Fig. 8.2 Assessment of the sick child aged 2 months up to 5 years. (Figure adapted from World Health Organization "Integrated Management of Childhood Illness Chartbook," 2014) [5]

ASSESS (Circle all signs present)	CLASSIFY
DOES THE CHILD HAVE AN EAR PROBLEM? • Is there ear pain? • Is there ear discharge? If Yes, for how long? ____ Days • Look for pus draining from the ear • Feel for tender swelling behind the ear	Yes ___ No ___
THEN CHECK FOR ACUTE MALNUTRITION AND ANAEMIA • Look for oedema of both feet. • Determine WFH/L z-score: • Less than -3? Between -3 and -2? -2 or more ? • Child 6 months or older measure MUAC _____ mm. • Look for palmar pallor. • Severe palmar pallor? Some palmar pallor? • If child has MUAC less than 115 mm or • WFH/L less than -3 Z scores: • Is there any medical complication: General danger sign? • Any severe classification? Pneumonia with chest indrawing? • Child 6 months or older: Offer RUTF to eat. Is the child: • Not able to finish? Able to finish? • Child less than 6 months: Is there a breastfeeding problem?	
CHECK FOR HIV INFECTION Note mother's and/or child's HIV status Mother's HIV test: NEGATIVE POSITIVE NOT DONE/KNOWN Child's virological test: NEGATIVE POSITIVE NOT DONE Child's serological test: NEGATIVE POSITIVE NOT DONE If mother is HIV-positive and NO positive virological test in child: Is the child breastfeeding now? Was the child breastfeeding at the time of test or 6 weeks before it? If breastfeeding: Is the mother and child on ARV prophylaxis?	

CHECK THE CHILD'S IMMUNIZATION STATUS (Circle immunizations needed today)
BCG   DPT+HIB-1   DPT+HIB-2   DPT+HIB-3   Measles 1   Measles 2   Vitamin A
OPV-0   OPV-1   OPV-2   OPV-3   Mebendazole
Hep B0   Hep B1   Hep B2   Hep B3
         RTV-1   RTV-2   RTV-3
         PCV-1   PCV-2   PCV-3
	Return for next immunization on:
	
	_____
	(Date)

ASSESS FEEDING if the child is less than 2 years old, has MODERATE ACUTE MALNUTRITION, ANAEMIA, or is HIV exposed or infected
• Do you breastfeed your child? Yes ___ No ___
  ■ If yes, how many times in 24 hours? ___ times. Do you breastfeed during the night? Yes ___ No ___
• Does the child take any other foods or fluids? Yes ___ No ___
  ■ If Yes, what food or fluids?
  ■ How many times per day? ___ times. What do you use to feed the child?
  ■ If MODERATE ACUTE MALNUTRITION: How large are servings?
  ■ Does the child receive his own serving? ___ Who feeds the child and how?
• During this illness, has the child's feeding changed? Yes ___ No ___
  ■ If Yes, how?
	FEEDING PROBLEMS

ASSESS OTHER PROBLEMS: Ask about mother's own health	

Fig. 8.2 (continued)

The presence of the IMCI symptoms and signs leads to a child's classification rather than a diagnosis. This classification indicates the severity of the condition, which then calls for specific actions based on whether the child: (a) needs to be urgently referred to a higher level of care, (b) requires specific treatments, or (c) can be safely managed at home. The classification is color-coded as: pink requires hospital referral or admission; yellow indicates the need to initiate treatment at home; and green indicates home supportive care management. See Fig. 8.4.

IMCI Recording Form: MANAGEMENT OF THE SICK YOUNG INFANT AGE BIRTH UP TO 2 MONTHS

Name:_____ Age:_____ Sex:_____ Weight:_____ Temperature:_____

ASK: What are the infant's problems?_____ Initial visit?_____ Follow-up Visit?_____

ASSESS (Circle all signs present)   CLASSIFY

CHECK FOR POSSIBLE SERIOUS BACTERIAL INFECTION OR VERY SEVERE DISEASE or PNEUMONIA or LOCAL BACTERIAL INFECTION • Is the infant having difficulty feeding? • Has the infant had convulsions?	• Count the breaths in one minute._____breaths per minute Repeat if (≥ 60) elevated_____Fast breathing? • Look for severe chest indrawing • Measure temperature High body temperature (temperature ≥ 38°C) or Low body temperature (below 35.5°C) • Look at young infant's movements. Does the infant move only when stimulated? Does the infant not move at all? • Look at umbilicus. Is it red or draining pus? • Look for skin pustules	
CHECK FOR JAUNDICE	• Is skin yellow? And infant is less than 24 hours of age? • Are the palms or soles yellow?	
DOES THE YOUNG INFANT HAVE DIARRHOEA? Yes_____No_____ If yes, ASK:	• Look at the young infant's general condition. Is the infant restless and irritable? Does the infant move only when stimulated? Does the infant not move at all? • Look for sunken eyes. Pinch the skin of the abdomen. Does it go back: Very slowly (longer than 2 seconds)? Slowly?	

CHECK FOR HIV INFECTION
ASK: HIV status of the mother?   Positive_____Negative_____Unknown_____
         HIV serological test of the infant? Positive_____Negative_____Unknown_____
         HIV virology test of the infant? Positive_____Negative_____Unknown_____		

THEN CHECK FOR FEEDING PROBLEM OR LOW WEIGHT FOR AGE

• Is the infant breastfed? Yes_____No_____ If Yes, how many times in 24 hrs?_____times • Does the infant receive any other foods or drinks? Yes_____No_____ If Yes, how often?_____times If yes, what do you use to feed the infant?	• Determine weight for age. Very low weight for age (<2 kg)_____ Low weight for age (< -2 Z score)_____ NOT low weight for age_____ • Look for ulcers or white patches in the mouth (thrush).	

If the infant has any difficulty feeding, is feeding < 8 times in 24 hours, is taking any other food or drinks, or is low weight for age, AND has no indications to refer urgently to hospital: ASSESS BREASTFEEDING:

• Has the infant breastfed in the previous hour?
• If infant has not fed in the previous hour, ask the mother to put her infant to the breast. Observe the breastfeed for 4 minutes.
• If the infant was fed during the last hour, ask the mother if she can wait and tell you when the infant is willing to feed again.
	• Is the infant able to attach? To check attachment, look for:
	  – More areola seen above than below the mouth Yes____No____
	  – Mouth wide open Yes_____No_____
	  – Lower lip turned outward Yes_____No_____
	  – Chin touching breast Yes_____No_____
	  Good attachment_____Poor attachment_____
	  No attachment at all_____
	• Is the infant suckling effectively (that is, slow deep sucks, sometimes pausing)?
	  Suckling effectively_____not suckling effectively_____
	  not suckling at all_____	

CHECK THE YOUNG INFANT'S IMMUNIZATION STATUS Circle immunizations needed today. <u>BCG</u> <u>Hep B0</u> <u>OPV0</u> <u>DPT1+Hib1+Hep B1</u> <u>OPV-1</u> <u>Rotavirus-1</u> <u>PCV-1</u>	Return for next immunization on:
ASSESS OTHER PROBLEMS:	
COUNSEL THE MOTHER ABOUT HER OWN HEALTH	

Fig. 8.3 Assessment of the sick infant aged up to 2 months. (Figure from World Health Organization "Integrated Management of Childhood Illness, Management of the Sick Young Infant Aged up to 2 months," 2019) [6]

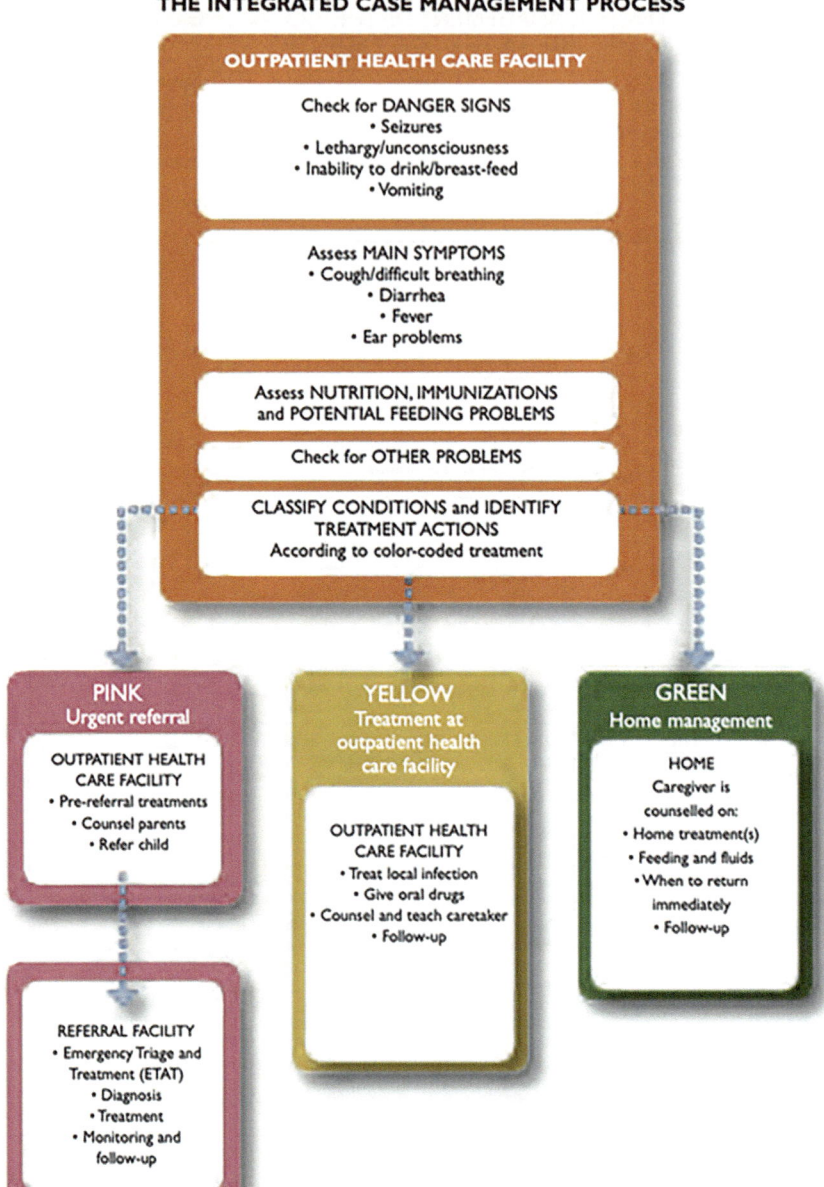

Fig. 8.4 IMCI strategy for case management in the outpatient health care facility, first-level referral service, and at home for the sick child from age 2 months to 5 years

Assessment of Sick Children 2 Months to 5 Years

The assessment procedure for this age group includes a number of important steps that must be taken by the health care provider: (1) take a history and talk with the caregiver about the child's problem; (2) check for general danger signs; (3) assess major symptoms; (4) evaluate nutritional status; (5) assess the child's feeding; (6) check immunization status; and (7) look for other problems.

Danger signs that should be routinely checked in all children:
1. Not able to drink or breastfeed
2. Vomits everything
3. Had convulsions
4. Lethargic or unconscious
5. Now convulsing

These general danger signs indicate the need for immediate referral to a hospital because they predict serious infections and conditions such as bacterial meningitis, cerebral malaria, and septic shock, which, if left untreated, often lead to death. To start treatment for severe illnesses without delay, quickly assess the child for the most important causes of serious illness and death, including acute respiratory infection (ARI), diarrhea and dehydration, sepsis, malaria, and measles.

Assessment of Sick Young Infant up to 2 Months

The assessment procedure for this age group includes a number of important steps that must be taken by the health care provider: (1) take a history and talk with the caregiver about the child's problem; (2) check for danger signs that may indicate a severe disease; (3) assess major symptoms; (4) evaluate nutritional status; (5) assess the child's feeding; (6) check immunization status; and (7) look for other problems.

Danger signs that may indicate severe disease in an infant:
1. Not feeding
2. Convulsions
3. Fast breathing (60 breaths per minute or more in infants less than 7 days old)
4. Severe chest indrawing
5. Fever (temperature 38 °C or more) or low temperature (temperature less than 35.5 °C)
6. Lack of movement

If a young infant has any of the above danger signs, they may have very severe disease and should be urgently referred to the hospital with a first antibiotic dose and treatment to prevent low blood sugar.

Summary

IMCI is family- and community-centered. This approach is essential for childhood health because it promotes healthy habits in the family, adequate care of children (e.g., feeding, clothing, stimulation, etc.), disease prevention, and prompt seeking of medical care when alarming signs and symptoms are noted. The IMCI strategy also helps healthcare professionals take advantage of opportunities for prevention, promote childhood development, and encourage the rational use of drugs and medications.

Outbreak Management

Objectives

- Gain familiarity with general concepts that relate to outbreaks.
- Be able to define what represents an outbreak, epidemic, and pandemic.
- Understand general strategies of outbreak management.

General Concepts

There have been numerous outbreaks and pandemics throughout history such as the 1817 Cholera pandemic, 1918 Influenza pandemic, 2014 Ebola Virus West African outbreak, and most recently the 2019 COVID-19 pandemic [7, 8]. These events have resulted in millions of deaths worldwide. Outbreaks can lead to and complicate current disaster and emergency situations, and one should be familiar with general concepts related to outbreaks to best prepare and respond.

Infectious Diseases

There are various infectious agents that can cause an infection. These include bacteria, viruses, fungi, parasites, and prions. Outbreaks can be caused by any of these infections but are more commonly caused by viruses and bacteria. It is important to know the infectious agent causing an outbreak or pandemic, as it has implications not only for treatment but also for prevention and public health measures. Influenza virus is one particular pathogen of importance given its potential to cause not only seasonal outbreaks but also epidemics and pandemics.

Modes of Transmission

Infections can be spread via various modes of transmission. These include:

- *Airborne*: Spread via very small particles that can remain in the air for a long period of time (e.g., measles, tuberculosis)
- *Droplet*: Spread via large droplets that do not remain suspended in air (e.g., influenza, meningococcus)
- *Contact:* Spread via direct contact with an infectious agent, for example, from skin-to skin or sexual transmission (e.g., herpes simplex virus)
- *Fecal-oral:* Spread via direct or indirect contact with infected stool, contaminated water, or food (e.g., hepatitis A, salmonella)
- *Vector-borne*: Spread via insects (e.g., malaria)

Definitions

There are several concepts within public health, epidemiology, and infectious diseases that are important to understand when discussing outbreaks. Familiarity with these terms is helpful for one to help prepare, recognize, and respond to outbreaks.

- *Active immunity*: Immune response and protection developed from natural infection or vaccination.
- *Close contact*: A person who was physically close to a person who was potentially infectious.
- *Communicable period*: Time when an infected person can transmit and spread an infectious agent.
- *Contact tracing*: Identification and monitoring of a person who has been exposed and possibly infected with an infectious agent.
- *Endemic*: A level of disease occurrence that is present constantly in a population.
- *Epidemic (outbreak)*: Occurrence of more cases of a disease than normally expected in a place/group of individuals over a given period of time.
- *Herd immunity*: Occurrence when a large portion of the population is immune to a disease and risk of spread is decreased.
- *Incubation period*: Time between exposure to infection and onset of symptoms.
- *Index case*: First person recognized in an outbreak to have a disease.
- *Isolation*: For those who have the disease and are attempting to separate from those who are not sick with the disease.
- *Latent period*: Time between exposure and onset of contagiousness.

- *Pandemic*: Epidemic/outbreak that has spread over several countries or continents.
- *Passive immunity*: Short-term protection against infection developed from the transfer of antibodies to a person.
- *Primary case*: Person who first has the disease in a population.
- *Quarantine*: For those who were exposed to the disease and attempting to separate from others and to monitor for illness.
- *Secondary case*: A person who acquires a disease from exposure to another person with the disease.
- *Surveillance*: Systematic collection, analysis, interpretation, and dissemination of health data for public health action.

Outbreak Management

Given the continued evolution of infectious agents, future outbreaks and pandemics are inevitable. While it is difficult to predict when the next outbreak or pandemic may occur, steps can be taken to prepare to help decrease the burden of disease, particularly in disaster settings. These include, but not limited to:

- Screening, surveillance, identification of cases, and contact tracing.
- Ensuring prevention strategies (e.g., quarantine, isolation, PPE).
- Preparing to work at surge capacity (e.g., creating disease-specific triage algorithms/admission criteria/treatment, utilizing alternative systems such as tents/transforming areas to accommodate additional medical beds) and ensuring adequate supply chains of tests, vaccines, medications, and healthcare supplies.
- Prevention through routine vaccination programs and implementing prioritization of high-risk groups for vaccinations.
- Supporting research for the development of tests, therapeutics, and preventative measures.
- Providing clear communication to the public.
- Commitment toward global collaboration and support.

Summary

Outbreaks can lead to and complicate disaster scenarios. They not only contribute to significant morbidity and mortality but can devastate healthcare systems and populations. Preparation, in addition to teamwork and clear communication, is key to outbreak management.

Acute Respiratory Infections

Objectives

- Be able to identify the key clinical signs used to assess a child with cough and/or difficult breathing.
- Diagnose and develop treatment plans (e.g., medications, supportive care, monitoring) using available resources for children with various acute respiratory infections.

Acute Respiratory Infections (ARI)

All types of respiratory infections are more common among people living in overcrowded conditions in low- and middle-income countries (LMIC). These include both upper respiratory tract infections (e.g., common colds) and lower respiratory tract infections (e.g., pneumonia). Most ARI cases are caused by viruses and do not warrant treatment with antibiotics. However, pneumonia remains a major cause of child mortality and morbidity and is the leading infectious cause of death in children worldwide. It is estimated that 7–13% of episodes are severe enough to be life-threatening and require hospitalization. Common causes of childhood pneumonia include *Streptococcus pneumoniae, Haemophilus influenzae*, and respiratory syncytial virus (RSV). Because of limited diagnostic capacities in resource-constrained settings, it is important to accurately identify and treat all ARIs.

IMCI Strategy for the Patient with Cough and/or Difficult Breathing

The IMCI strategy uses 4 key clinical signs to assess children with cough and/or difficult breathing as below. These are then used to help classify children into categories to guide treatment and management [9].

1. *Respiratory rate (RR):* Helps distinguish the presence or absence of pneumonia.
2. *Lower chest wall indrawing:* Represents increased work of breathing.
3. *Stridor:* Presence in a calm child indicates severe upper airway obstruction and the need for hospital admission.
4. *Wheezing:* Presence can indicate bronchiolitis or asthma.

Table 8.1 Respiratory rate
cutoffs for fast breathing
(tachypnea) in children

Child's age	General Cutoff rate for fast breathing (tachypnea)
2 weeks to <2 months	~60 breaths per minute or more
2 months to <12 months	~50 breaths per minute or more
12 months to <5 years	~40 breaths per minute or more
5 years to <12 years	~25 breaths per minute or more
12 years to ≤18 years	~20 breaths per minute or more

Respiratory Rate (RR)

No single clinical sign has a better combination of sensitivity and specificity to detect pneumonia in children under 5 years than RR, and counting respirations is an easier clinical skill to teach to different cadres of healthcare workers. Cutoff rates for fast breathing (tachypnea) depend on the child's age. Normal RR is higher in children aged 2 to 12 months than in children from 12 months to 5 years (Table 8.1).

Lower Chest Wall Indrawing

Lower chest indrawing occurs when a child employs accessory muscles of respiration to overcome trouble breathing, and this may be caused by any respiratory pathology from the lungs to the upper airway. Chest indrawing should only be considered present if it persists in a calm child; agitation, a blocked nose, or breastfeeding can all cause temporary chest indrawing.

Stridor

Look and listen for stridor in a calm child, which indicates severe upper airway obstruction and the need for hospital admission. Stridor is a harsh noise made when the child inhales. Children who present with stridor when calm are at substantial risk of upper airway obstruction. Some children with mild croup manifest stridor only when they are crying or agitated.

Wheezing

Sometimes a wheezing noise is audible on auscultation as a high-pitched noise. According to IMCI, a child with fast breathing is classified as having pneumonia. However, if wheezing is present, clinicians must also consider a diagnosis like asthma or viral bronchiolitis. The clinician may trial a bronchodilator and monitor the response for potential asthma diagnosis.

Classification of Children with Cough or Difficult Breathing

Based on a combination of the aforementioned clinical signs, children presenting with cough and/or difficult breathing can be classified into 3 categories:

1. pink (Severe pneumonia or very severe disease): Presence of general danger sign (not able to drink, persistent vomiting, convulsions, lethargic/unconscious), stridor in calm child, severe malnutrition
2. yellow (Pneumonia): Fast breathing and/or chest indrawing without danger signs
3. green (No pneumonia): Cough and cold

The group requiring referral for possible very severe disease includes children with any general danger sign, stridor when calm, or severe malnutrition. Children with very severe disease are more likely to have life-threatening invasive bacterial infections. A first dose of antibiotic should be given immediately via parenteral route if available prior to referral.

Give outpatient antibiotics to children with chest indrawing or fast RR for their age to treat bacterial pneumonia when they do not have additional danger signs. Fast breathing, as defined by WHO, detects about 80% of children with pneumonia who need antibiotic treatment. Treatment based on this classification has been shown to reduce mortality.

Patients with cough and no signs suggesting pneumonia or severe disease do not require antibiotics. A child with a cough will normally improve in 1 to 2 weeks. However, a child with chronic cough (more than 30 days) needs to be further assessed (and, if needed, referred) to rule out tuberculosis, asthma, whooping cough, or another respiratory problem.

Antibiotics

If a child is classified according to IMCI as just "pneumonia," the typical first-line treatment is an oral antibiotic. For severe pneumonia, parenteral antibiotics are the first-line treatment. For specific details about what antibiotic to use, clinicians should refer to IMCI or local guidelines.

Ear Problems

Ear problems can accompany or become a complication from an ARI and should also be assessed in children. Although otitis (inflammation of the ear) is rarely a cause of death, it is the main cause of deafness in low-income areas, which in turn can lead to learning problems.

Clinical Assessment

When otoscopy is not available, examine the child for the following clinical signs:

- *Tender swelling behind the ear:* The most serious complication of an ear infection is an infection in the mastoid bone (mastoiditis). It usually manifests with swelling behind one of the ears. In infants, this swelling may also be above the ear. When present, this sign is considered positive and should not be mistaken for swollen lymph nodes.
- *Ear pain:* In the early stages of acute otitis, a child may have ear pain, which usually causes the child to cry and become irritable.
- *Ear discharge:* This may be another sign of an ear infection.

Classification of Ear Problems

Based on the presence and duration of clinical signs (such as swelling behind the ear, ear pain, or ear discharge), the child's condition may be classified as mastoiditis, acute otitis, chronic otitis, or no ear infection.

- *Mastoiditis:*
  - Tender swelling behind the ear
  - Should be referred to a hospital for treatment and receive a dose of antibiotics and pain relief prior to referral

- *Acute Otitis:*
  - Ear pain and/or discharge <14 days
  - Treat with oral antibiotics for 5 days. Typically use first-line antibiotics similar to ones used for pneumonia

- *Chronic Otitis:*
  - Ear discharge >14 days
  - Treat with wicking or drying the ear
  - Antibiotics are NOT recommended

- *No Ear Infection:*
  - No ear pain or discharge
  - Do NOT require any specific treatment

Summary

Acute respiratory infections are a common cause of illness, morbidity, and mortality in children, especially in LMIC countries, and can be exacerbated in disaster settings. Though a majority of ARIs are caused by viruses, some are caused by bacteria, and it is important to distinguish the cause and severe disease to help guide management.

Important Infections in Disaster Settings: Acute Infections

Objectives

- Recognize the public health importance of acute infections in the context of disaster settings.
- Explain why measles infection can be so devastating in displaced populations and disaster settings and strategies to prepare for a measles outbreak.
- Be able to describe the epidemiology, manifestations, complications, treatment, and prevention of important acute infections in a disaster setting.

Introduction

There are numerous illnesses caused by infections. Some infections are endemic to certain areas of the world and further exacerbated in disaster settings. The following section reviews some acute infections with outbreak potential and the ability to cause severe disease, which is important to consider in a disaster setting: measles, vector-borne infections (specifically malaria and dengue), and meningitis. This is not an exhaustive list of infections, and knowledge of local epidemiology is important to understand other infections one should consider in the differential of a patient presenting with an acute infection in a disaster setting.

Measles

Measles is a virus, and a measles outbreak is potentially devastating in displaced populations and disaster settings because of how highly contagious it is compared to other infections [10]. Ensuring adequate administration of the measles vaccine is a high priority in a large displaced or refugee population because there may be enough susceptible children to cause an epidemic. Malnourished children living in crowded shelters following a disaster are especially vulnerable and at high risk for severe disease.

Clinical Presentation of Measles

Following an incubation period of 10 to 12 days from exposure, measles prodrome is characterized by 2 to 4 days of fever, cough, coryza, and conjunctivitis. During this period, Koplik spots can be seen as tiny blue-white spots on intensely reddened oral mucosa. These lesions disappear within 3 days. The maculopapular erythema or morbilliform rash of measles first appears after this prodrome on the hairline and forehead, then moves downward to involve the face, neck, and the rest of the body. Initially the lesions are discrete and then become confluent. The rash persists for 4 to 6 days. It becomes brownish in color for a few days before desquamating. If no complications occur, fever disappears within 2 to 3 days after the onset of rash. Many children may also have anorexia, conjunctivitis, diarrhea, and some have mild stomatitis.

Measles Complications

Measles is a highly catabolic disease, associated with reduced food intake, increased gastrointestinal losses, and rapid weight loss. Complications in developed countries like the United States occur in approximately 30% of cases, with complication rates even higher in developing countries. The most frequent acute complications are pneumonia, croup, otitis media, and diarrhea. Measles virus is immunosuppressive and can predispose individuals to secondary viral and bacterial infections. Major long-term sequelae in developing countries include measles-related blindness, malnutrition, and chronic lung disease.

Treatment of Measles

Vitamin A deficiency increases measles-associated morbidity and mortality. Moreover, measles infection increases the severity of the complications resulting from vitamin A deficiency. Children deficient in vitamin A who become infected with measles have higher corneal ulceration and fatality rates. Thus, vitamin A is part of the management of measles. Additional management depends on the classification of the individual as below. With all cases, ensuring adequate nutrition is also important, particularly in malnourished children.

- *Severe complicated measles* (pink): Any child with measles having a general danger sign, clouding of the cornea, or deep or extensive mouth ulcers.

  - Refer urgently to the hospital.
  - Prior to leaving for the hospital, the child should be given vitamin A, the first dose of an appropriate antibiotic (for potential bacterial superinfections), a dose of eye ointment if there is eye discharge or corneal clouding, and oral hygiene/medications (e.g., gentian violet) for mouth ulcers.

- *Measles with eye or mouth complications* (yellow): The presence of eye drainage and or mouth ulcers without other signs of serious illness.

  - Treatment includes vitamin A, eye ointment for eye discharge, and oral hygiene with salt water or gentian violet.
  - Follow up visit in 3 days.

- *Measles* (green): A child without complications

  - Needs only vitamin A.

Vitamin A Dosing in Measles

Give oral vitamin A once a day for 2 days at 50000 IU (for children aged <6 months old), 100,000 IU (for children 6–11 months old), or 200,000 IU (for children ≥12 months old). If the child has any eye signs of vitamin A deficiency, give a third dose 2–4 weeks after the second dose on follow-up.

Prevention and Mitigation of Measles Outbreaks in Disaster Settings

With measles outbreaks, unfortunately, isolation of patients is not an effective preventive measure since individuals are most contagious in the prodromal period before a diagnosis can be made. Ensuring the population is vaccinated and administration of measles vaccination is the highest priority early in disaster situations. One should not delay administration of vaccines until cases of measles have been reported. Consider vaccinating young children (6 months to 5 years) and high-risk populations first, such as those presenting with acute illness, malnourished children, and those with tuberculosis or HIV infection.

Additionally, one should develop a plan to administer prophylactic vitamin A in conjunction with a measles immunization program. When the measles vaccine is not yet available and a delay is anticipated, one should still administer vitamin A. This vitamin by itself reduces morbidity and mortality during measles outbreaks.

Vector-Borne Diseases

A vector-borne disease is one in which an infection causing illness is spread through a vector such as mosquitos, ticks, or fleas. Global temperatures are on the rise, rainfall patterns are changing, and there are more extreme weather events, which may favor the spread of the vectors, particularly in disaster settings such as flooding. Therefore, it is important to be aware of these vector-borne diseases in disaster settings. This section focuses on two acute vector-borne infections in particular (malaria and dengue) that are more commonly encountered and can cause severe fatal disease, but many other vector-borne diseases exist.

Malaria

Malaria is caused by a protozoan blood parasite (*Plasmodium*) and is transmitted through the bite of an infected *Anopheles* mosquito. Most *Anopheles* mosquitoes are not well adapted to urban environments or places about 3900 ft (1200 m) above sea level. However, with increasing global temperatures, this may change. Infection produces a clinical syndrome that ranges in severity depending on the species of the parasite and the immune status of the individual. There are four species that most commonly infect humans: *P. falciparum, P. malariae, P. ovale,* and *P. vivax.* There is a fifth species, *P. knowlesi*, that primarily infects non-human primates; however, it has been reported to cause infections in humans as well. *P. falciparum* is the most common species within Africa, and *P. vivax* is the most dominant species in other countries outside of sub-Saharan Africa. *P. falciparum* causes the most severe form of disease.

Clinical Presentation of Malaria

There are two distinct clinical malaria presentations:

- *Uncomplicated malaria:* Presents with fever, chills, headaches, myalgias, diarrhea, and anemia. Classic malaria fever has been described as paroxysms of fevers and shaking chills lasting 8 to 12 hours, every 2 to 3 days. During the afebrile period, fever disappears, and the patient feels relatively well (depending on the species).
- *Severe, complicated malaria:* Malaria is considered to be severe with any of the following features or complications: prostration (patient unable to sit or walk), multiple convulsions, failure to feed, impaired consciousness not attributable to another cause, abnormal bleeding, meningeal signs, jaundice, respiratory difficulty, and signs of shock. Hyperparasitemia (>5%) is considered very severe. According to IMCI, the presence of any danger sign or a stiff neck leads to a very

severe febrile disease classification. Cerebral malaria is associated with signs of acute encephalopathy, and mortality varies from 15% to 50%.

Malaria can cause non-specific signs and symptoms and thus may be hard to distinguish from other acute febrile illnesses. Therefore, the clinical diagnosis of malaria based on signs and symptoms tends to be highly inaccurate. While it is preferable to have rapid diagnostic tests or microscopy to rule out malaria in patients that present with febrile illnesses living in an area with malaria, in the absence of available diagnostic testing, one should consider treatment when the clinical history and presentation are highly consistent with malaria. However, it is also important to acknowledge that malaria can coexist with other conditions that cause fever as well as predispose to other intracellular pathogens. Thus, in the absence of specific diagnostic tests, empiric treatment of any serious febrile illness should include coverage for malaria, as well as other pathogens. It is also important to prevent any unnecessary treatment to prevent the development of resistance.

Treatment of Malaria

The treatment of malaria depends on the likelihood of a malaria infection, species, the risk of resistant strains, the severity of the infection, the setting, and the availability of drugs. One should refer to guidelines for specific regimens and dosing (e.g., WHO Guidelines for Malaria, local guidelines) [11].

In addition to antimalarial drugs, supportive management is also recommended and includes antipyretics, rehydration, and assessment and possible referral to a feeding program for malnutrition.

Surveillance and Prevention of Malaria

Surveillance measures are important to understand the epidemiology and burden of malaria. This can guide management not only in endemic areas but also in displaced populations and disaster settings to help guide management. Prevention of malaria is also important to help reduce the overall burden of disease. Various techniques and strategies have been implemented, including vector control, preventive chemotherapy, and vaccination.

Dengue

Dengue infections occur worldwide but are most prevalent in Southeast Asia, Pacific Islands, the Caribbeans, Central America, and South America. It is caused by an arbovirus, usually acquired by the bite of an *Aedes* mosquitoes. There are 4 closely related serotypes of dengue virus, all of which can cause severe disease.

Clinical Presentation of Dengue

A majority of infections are asymptomatic or mild. However, dengue infection can have severe clinical manifestations. WHO defines severe dengue by one or more of the following: (i) plasma leakage that may lead to shock (dengue shock) and/or fluid accumulation, with or without respiratory distress, and/or (ii) severe bleeding, and/ or (iii) severe organ impairment. After the incubation period (~4–10 days), the illness begins abruptly and is followed by the three phases: febrile, critical, and recovery.

- *Febrile phase:* The acute febrile phase, lasting 2–7 days, usually has a sudden onset of high fever associated with facial flushing, skin erythema, generalized body ache, myalgia, arthralgia, and headache. Anorexia, nausea, and vomiting are also common. It is hard to distinguish dengue from other febrile illnesses during this period. However, several tests are helpful, including a positive tourniquet test, a progressive decrease in the total white cell count, and a falling platelet count.
- *Critical phase:* The critical phase begins during a 24–48-hour period when there is an increase in capillary permeability, which is associated with increasing hematocrit levels. This usually occurs after the fever decreases or resolves. Most patients recover without developing conditions caused by an increase in capillary permeability. In others, the severity of the plasma leakage is quite variable, in which hemoconcentration is a good indicator of the severity of plasma leakage. During this period, shock, progressive organ failure, metabolic acidosis, and disseminated intravascular coagulation (DIC) may occur.
- *Recovery phase:* The capillary permeability gradually improves after the 24–48-hour critical phase so that patients begin to stabilize who received appropriate fluid management. There is a reabsorption of fluid and a diuresis. However, bradycardia and electrocardiographic changes are common during this stage. During this phase, a patient's rash may start to desquamate or be pruritic.

Treatment of Dengue

In an area where dengue is endemic all patients who have a clinical presentation consistent with the febrile phase of dengue should, if feasible, have an initial CBC to identify leukopenia and decreased platelets and possibly a tourniquet test and followed to evaluate for signs of severe dengue (e.g., decreasing platelet, increasing hematocrit). Warning signs for developing severe dengue include any of the IMCI danger signs, presence of ascites or pleural effusions, increasing hematocrit, signs of shock (narrowed pulse, poor capillary perfusion/delayed capillary refill, cold extremities, and rapid pulse), severe bleeding, or organ impairment. Make sure that the family understands the importance of returning to the clinic immediately if any of the IMCI danger signs or bleeding develop. Patients who appear to be entering the critical 24–48 phase of dengue with any warning signs should be hospitalized.

Treatment of dengue is supportive. Fevers should be treated with paracetamol. Do not give acetylsalicylic acid (aspirin), ibuprofen, or other non-steroidal anti-inflammatory agents (NSAIDs) as these drugs may aggravate gastritis or bleeding. All patients with warning signs or severe dengue should be admitted to a hospital with access to intensive care facilities and blood transfusion. There should be prompt attention to fluid resuscitation for treatment of shock. Further specifics for treatment can be found in the WHO Dengue Handbook[12].

Surveillance and Prevention of Dengue

Mosquito population control and personal protection from mosquito bites are methods to prevent dengue. Active surveillance of dengue and mosquitoes is also important for the implementation of control measures. There is also a licensed vaccine (licensed in 2015) that has shown to be efficacious and safe in the prevention of dengue in individuals with a previous dengue virus infection.

Meningitis (Meningococcal Meningitis)

Meningitis is the inflammation of the membranes (meninges) that surround the brain and spinal cord. Encephalitis is the inflammation of the cerebral cortex. Meningoencephalitis involves both the meninges and the cerebral cortex. Meningitis affects individuals of all ages, but young children are at increased risk, and thus is important to recognize in disaster settings.

A majority of infections are caused by viruses, but some are caused by other pathogens such as bacteria. While many infectious agents can cause meningitis, in a disaster *N. meningitidis* is a pathogen of importance given its epidemic potential particularly in crowded settings (also causes meningococcemia, which is dissemination of the bacteria into the bloodstream).

Clinical Manifestations of Meningitis

When assessing a child for meningitis, evaluate for fever and look for changes in mental status and level of activity, including irritability, changes in feeding and sleeping patterns, unresponsiveness, and seizures. One should check for signs of meningeal irritation: nuchal rigidity, bulging fontanelle, paradoxical irritability, and Brudzinski and Kernig signs. It is also important to evaluate hydration status and signs of shock.

Signs associated with central nervous system complications include focal neurologic findings, prolonged seizures, persistent changes in mental status, enlarging head circumferences, or ataxia. Complications include subdural effusion or empyema, cerebral edema, cerebral abscess, cerebral infarction, or hydrocephalus.

Treatment of Meningitis

Ultimate treatment of meningitis depends on the pathogen identified and susceptibility pattern of the child's isolate. Parenteral antibiotics are used to treat bacterial meningitis. Until pathogen identification is made, initial antibiotic therapy should be directed towards the most common bacteria suspected. Refer to local guidelines for specific recommendations for agent, dosing, and duration.

Prevention and Mitigation of Meningitis Outbreaks in Disaster Settings

There are available vaccines to prevent certain pathogens that have been associated with meningitis, including *N. meningitidis*, *Haemophilus influenzae,* and *Streptococcus pneumoniae*. Routine childhood vaccinations for children are important to prevent infection.

Identification of *N. meningitidis* is particularly important because of its outbreak potential. Steps to mitigate outbreaks include steps such as ensuring adequate surveillance, case detection, and appropriate treatment of cases; identification of at-risk populations; and prevention and chemoprophylaxis. During confirmed *N. meningitidis* outbreaks, implement vaccination and chemoprophylaxis of high-risk close contacts. The goal of chemoprophylaxis is to eradicate *N. meningitidis* carriers and prevent the occurrence of secondary cases. Rifampin is the first-line agent for chemoprophylaxis in children, but there are alternatives.

Summary

During disaster settings and in displaced populations, it is important to recognize and distinguish between acute infections, as treatment and management between them differ. Understanding the local epidemiology of various pathogens is important to understanding what infections are most common and which are important not to miss. It is important to utilize any available resources in these settings including WHO guidelines, national guidelines, and knowledge from local community providers.

Other Infectious Considerations in Disaster Settings

Objectives

- Recognize and distinguish other infections that may be present during disaster settings, including chronic infections and diarrheal infections.

- Be able to triage and manage other clinical entities requiring attention in disaster settings.

Children may have other infections, including chronic infections, that one should consider during disaster settings. Though long-term management of these chronic infections are not the immediate goal at the time of a disaster, recognition of these infections is still important as they can become worse during a disaster setting if children are not receiving their typical management or even make them more susceptible to other infections. Infections discussed include tuberculosis and HIV. Infectious diarrhea is also common during disasters, which is briefly discussed here.

Tuberculosis

Tuberculosis (TB) is caused by *Mycobacterium tuberculosis* and is the leading infectious cause of death in some parts of the developing world. TB treatment and control programs are not part of an emergency relief response. TB is a chronic infection, and effective treatment is very resource intensive. Treatment programs need to include resources to identify and monitor true cases by sputum smear exam, a stable population for at least 6 months (to complete therapy), enough available drugs to treat all cases, and enough personnel to supervise therapy in the first couple of months. Administration of anti-TB drugs to persons who will not adhere to or complete treatment is likely to contribute to drug resistance in the community. Though initiation of TB treatment and control programs may not be part of disaster responses, it is important to recognize that individuals in displaced populations may have TB and it is important to consider when managing these patients for any concurrent infections.

Human Immunodeficiency Virus

Human immunodeficiency virus (HIV) is a virus that affects the immune system. HIV causes significant morbidity and mortality worldwide. Keys to caring for children with HIV include: (1) recognizing children and risk for HIV infection and diagnosing them early; (2) treating all individuals with HIV; (3) managing co-infections and opportunistic infections (OIs); and (4) ensuring excellent adherence by avoiding missed doses and treatment interruptions. Children exposed to and living with HIV are generally at higher risk of common childhood infections, important acute infections in a disaster setting as mentioned in section "Important Infections in Disaster Settings: Acute Infection", and opportunistic infections. Recognition of these infections is important in order to provide prompt treatment.

In a disaster setting, initial management of HIV-infected children should include documentation of the last CD4 and viral load if known and an antiretroviral therapy (ART) regimen if a child is taking ART. Children who had their ART and/or prophylaxis or treatment for OIs interrupted by disaster-related displacement should restart these medications as soon as possible. There is no need to start ART immediately in those HIV-infected patients who were not receiving antiretroviral medications before the disaster, but eventually they should start as soon as they are able. IMCI guidelines provide a simplified approach to starting ART in children; however, whenever possible, refer to in-country guidelines [13].

Diarrheal Infections

Diarrheal infections are common causes of illness in children, particularly during disaster scenarios. Infections can be caused by multiple pathogens. Specific antimicrobial treatment depends on the pathogen, but in all cases, ensuring and maintaining adequate hydration is crucial. Further discussions about diarrheal illnesses are discussed in other chapters.

Summary

TB, HIV, and diarrheal infections are other additional conditions one should be able to recognize during disaster settings.

Vaccination in Disaster Settings

Objectives

- Acknowledge the importance of routine and catch-up immunizations in disaster settings.
- Describe outbreak situations that require the use of certain vaccines and prophylaxis in a disaster.

Immunization During Disasters

Programs to ensure adequate baseline population immunization are important for the prevention of many devastating infections in children [14, 15]. In disaster settings, particularly those involving populations in flight, both outbreaks requiring urgent immunization campaigns and the implementation of routine and catch-up immunization programs for all children are critical for the health of a population both during and in the wake of a disaster.

Strategies for Immunization Programs and Catch-Up Vaccinations

In disaster scenarios, the only vaccine that must be routinely administered during immediate emergency relief efforts is measles (see the "Measles" section for details). A routine immunization program for other vaccines should be considered if the population affected by a disaster is displaced and expected to stay in an area away from their homes for longer than 3 months. Routine immunization programs in these settings also rely on the ability to keep appropriate records for a population and on the expectation that vaccination efforts should not disrupt or compromise other assistance efforts. This type of vaccination activity would be more commonly found in internally displaced persons camps or among refugee populations. It is important to also note that routine childhood vaccination programs vary between countries and should refer to local guidelines if you are in a situation where you are implementing a routine vaccination program.

According to the WHO framework, "Vaccination in Acute Humanitarian Emergencies," there are three steps one should take in deciding to implement a vaccine in a disaster setting for a vaccine-preventable disease:

1. Assess the epidemiologic risk of the vaccine preventable disease
2. Assess the vaccines availability, characteristics, and deliverability
3. Assess for any contextual constraints and/or competing needs to delivery of vaccine

Implementation of a routine immunization program requires concerted efforts. For further specific details and guidance on the implementation of such a program, refer to local guidance and WHO resources ("Vaccination in Acute Humanitarian Emergencies" and "Vaccination in Acute Humanitarian Emergencies: Implementation Guide") [16, 17].

Catch-up vaccination is another consideration for populations in a disaster setting. Elements for catch-up vaccination strategies according to the WHO's "Leave no one behind: guidance for planning and implementing catch-up vaccination" include [18]:

• Developing a policy and schedule for catch-up vaccination
• Ensuring vaccine and supply availability
• Establish data systems for recording and reporting
• Build community engagement through effective communication
• Enhance health worker knowledge and practice of catch-up vaccinations
• Identify strategies to determine those in need of catch-up vaccinations

Refer to local guidelines or the WHO's recommendations for specifics of timing and doses for catch-up vaccines.

Disease Specific Situations Requiring Prophylaxis

While routine immunization is not an immediate priority for childhood vaccine preventable diseases in a disaster setting, there are specific diseases in which prophylaxis with either a vaccine or medication (chemoprophylaxis) is recommended, if available, to prevent infection as described within this section.

Diphtheria

Diphtheria infection is caused by *Corynebacterium diphtheriae* and causes a respiratory infection as well as a cutaneous infection. When cases of diphtheria are suspected, mass vaccination is indicated, taking into account the rates of incidence by age groups. Asymptomatic contacts whose immunization regimen is complete and who have received their last dose more than 5 years ago must receive a booster. Close asymptomatic contacts whose immunization regimen is incomplete (<3 doses of diphtheric toxoid) or whose immunization status is unknown must receive a dose and complete the schedule. Whatever their immunization status, close contacts must be kept under surveillance for 7 days to detect any evidence of the disease, have cultures taken for *Corynebacterium diphtheriae* (if able), and receive antimicrobial prophylaxis (if available).

Haemophilus Influenzae Type b (HiB) Disease

Prior to the vaccine era, Hib was a major contributor to childhood pneumonia and meningitis in young children, though infection still occurs, particularly in unimmunized areas. Vaccines are key to reducing the incidence of Hib disease. Outbreaks can occur and risk of invasive Hib disease is increased in unimmunized individuals. Unimmunized or those incompletely immunized should receive a dose if available and complete their vaccine series. Chemoprophylaxis is indicated for those individuals who meet the criteria for close contacts. This generally includes prophylaxis for household contacts if the household has a young child/infant who is unimmunized, incompletely immunized, or is immunocompromised. Generally, rifampin is used, but ceftriaxone is an alternative.

Hepatitis A

Hepatitis A causes a self-limited acute illness with symptoms including fever, nausea, vomiting, and abdominal pain. Given its transmission via the fecal-oral route, with the breakdown of infrastructures during disasters including access to clean water, outbreaks of Hepatitis A are possible. If available, hepatitis A vaccination or immune globulin (depending on age, underlying history, and vaccination status) should be administered within 14 days of exposure.

Measles

See "Measles" portion in section "Important Infections in Disaster Settings: Acute Infections."

Meningococcal Disease

See "Meningitis" portion in section "Important Infections in Disaster Settings: Acute Infections."

Pertussis

Pertussis is caused by *Bordetella pertussis* and primarily causes a respiratory illness characterized by prolonged cough. In an outbreak, household contacts and other close contacts of patients may require booster vaccinations depending on the number of previous doses and timing of the last dose. For those that are not yet immunized, they should start their series if the vaccine is available. All household contacts and other close contacts, regardless of their age or immune status, should receive chemoprophylaxis within 21 days of onset of symptoms of the index patient because immunity after vaccination is not total and infection may not be prevented. Options depending on availability and age include: erythromycin, clarithromycin, azithromycin, and trimethoprim-sulfamethoxazole.

Tetanus

Tetanus is caused by a toxin produced by the bacterium *Clostridium tetani*. This can cause both generalized or local tetanus, which manifests as muscle spasms. There is also a form of neonatal tetanus that can occur in infants. Tetanus vaccine can be given prophylactically to individuals who have tetanus-prone wounds if the time of the last tetanus immunization is unknown or greater than 5 years, or when the child has not received the primary 3-dose vaccination series. If available, tetanus immune globulin should also be given to those that have not received their primary 3-dose vaccine series. The characteristics of tetanus-prone wounds are a wound that was first cleaned more than 6 hours after its occurrence; irregular wounds; wounds from bullets, crushing, burns, or frostbite; and the presence of devitalized tissue or wound contaminants.

Varicella-Zoster Virus

Varicella infection causes a generalized pruritic and vesicular rash that has varying stages of development and resolution. Complications can occur, including superimposed bacterial infections. In outbreaks, those exposed without prior evidence of immunity should receive a varicella vaccine if available up to 5 days after exposures. In certain circumstances and if available, varicella zoster immune globulin may be used.

Summary

Routine childhood vaccination programs are generally not the first priority in a disaster scenario, though programs ensuring baseline population immunization are important for the prevention of many infections. There are certain vaccine-preventable infections that are extremely contagious and do require prompt attention in emergency scenarios to prevent massive outbreaks (e.g., measles).

Acknowledgments Acknowledgment for contribution in this chapter: George Paasi, MBChB, MPH, Mbale Clinical Research Institute, Mbale, Uganda.

References

1. World Health Organization. Child mortality and causes of death. Accessed 12 May 2024. Available at https://www.who.int/data/gho/data/themes/topics/topic-details/GHO/child-mortality-and-causes-of-death.
2. World Health Organization. Handbook: IMCI integrated management of childhood illness. Geneva: World Health Organization; 2005. https://iris.who.int/bitstream/handle/10665/42939/9241546441.pdf;jsessionid=AAB6F3988A78398A9705766FE273890E?sequence=1.
3. World Health Organization. Manual for the health of care of children in humanitarian emergencies. Geneva: World Health Organization; 2008. https://iris.who.int/bitstream/handle/10665/43926/9789241596879_eng.pdf?sequence=1.
4. World Health Organization. Pocket book of hospital care for children. 2013. https://iris.who.int/bitstream/handle/10665/81170/9789241548373_eng.pdf?sequence=1.
5. World Health Organization. Integrated management of childhood illness chart booklet. Geneva: World Health organization; 2014. https://cdn.who.int/media/docs/default-source/mca-documents/9789241506823_chartbook_eng.pdf?sfvrsn=cccea3a6_1&download=true.
6. World Health Organization. Management of the sick young infant aged up to 2 months. Geneva: World Health Organization; 2019. https://iris.who.int/bitstream/handle/10665/326448/9789241516365-eng.pdf?sequence=1.
7. Piret J, Boivin G. Pandemics throughout history. Front Microbiol. 2021;11:631736. PMID: 33584597.
8. World Health Organization. Ebola virus disease. Accessed 12 May 2024. Available at https://www.who.int/en/news-room/fact-sheets/detail/ebola-virus-disease.
9. World Health Organization. Revised WHO classification and treatment of childhood pneumonia at health facilities. Geneva: World Health Organization; 2014. https://iris.who.int/bitstream/handle/10665/137319/9789241507813_eng.pdf?sequence=1.
10. Centers for Disease Control and Prevention. Measles (Rubeola). Accessed 12 May 2024. Available at https://www.cdc.gov/measles/index.html.

11. World Health Organization. WHO Guidelines for malaria. Geneva: World Health Organization; 2023. https://iris.who.int/bitstream/handle/10665/373339/WHO-UCN-GMP-2023.01-Rev.1-eng.pdf?sequence=1.
12. World Health Organization. Dengue guidelines, for diagnosis, treatment, prevention and control. Geneva: World Health Organization; 2009.
13. World Health Organization. HIV and AIDS. Accessed 12 May 2024. Available at https://www.who.int/news-room/fact-sheets/detail/hiv-aids.
14. World Health Organization. Essential Programme on Immunization. Accessed 12 May 2024. Available at: https://www.who.int/teams/immunization-vaccines-and-biologicals/essential-programme-on-immunization/implementation.
15. World Health Organization. Vaccines and immunization. Accessed 12 May 2024. Available at https://www.who.int/health-topics/vaccines-and-immunization#tab=tab_1.
16. World Health Organization. Vaccination in acute humanitarian emergencies: a framework for decision making. Geneva: World Health Organization; 2017. License: CC BY-NC-SA 3.0 IGO.
17. World Health Organization. Vaccination in humanitarian emergencies: implementation guide. Geneva: World Health Organization; 2017. License: CC BY-NC-SA 3.0 IGO.
18. World Health Organization. Leave no one behind: guidance for planning and implementing catch-up vaccination. Geneva: World Health Organization; 2021. License: CC BY-NC-SA 3.0 IGO.

Chapter 9
Pediatric Considerations for Diarrhea and Dehydration in Disaster Settings

Rosemarie Gachie-Lopokoiyit and Lisa Umphrey

Introduction

Diarrheal diseases pose a significant threat to the health and well-being of children, contributing to both illness and mortality rates. In areas affected by disasters, inadequate sanitation, contaminated water sources, and poor hygiene practices exacerbate the risk of diarrheal infections. The repercussions extend beyond immediate health concerns, impacting the nutritional status of affected children and escalating morbidity and mortality rates. Malnutrition, often exacerbated by diarrheal illness, further increases susceptibility to such infections. Timely diagnosis and treatment are crucial in alleviating these adverse effects. Moreover, prompt identification of cases enables the implementation of preventive measures essential for curtailing outbreaks among displaced populations. The Integrated Management of Childhood Illness (IMCI) strategy emerges as a valuable resource in resource-limited settings, including disaster areas, facilitating early detection and management of various diarrheal illnesses.

Diarrheal Illnesses

Objectives
- Define acute diarrhea and identify its defining characteristics.
- Discuss the management of acute diarrhea.

R. Gachie-Lopokoiyit (✉)
The Pediatric Clinic Karen, Nairobi, Kenya

L. Umphrey
Center for Global Health, Aurora, CO, USA
e-mail: Lisa.umphrey@childrenscolorado.org

© The Author(s), under exclusive license to Springer Nature Switzerland AG 2025
L. Umphrey et al. (eds.), *Pediatric Considerations in Disaster Settings*,
https://doi.org/10.1007/978-3-031-85501-6_9

- Examine the symptoms and strategies for managing epidemic cholera outbreaks.
- Outline the clinical manifestations of dysentery, including predominant causative agents and appropriate antibiotic interventions.

Definition of Diarrhea

Diarrhea is characterized by the passage of loose or watery stools at least three times within a 24-h timeframe. However, it's the consistency of the stools rather than the frequency that holds greater significance. Various infectious agents, including viruses, bacteria, and parasites, can trigger acute diarrhea. Rotavirus and Escherichia coli rank among the most prevalent pathogens causing moderate to severe diarrhea in low- and middle-income countries (LMICs). Shigella stands out as a notable cause of bloody diarrhea. Treatment of diarrhea is typically guided by the clinical presentation of the illness, which can be readily established during the initial examination of a child. Laboratory tests are usually unnecessary.

In disaster settings, where overcrowded living conditions, insufficient clean water supply, and inadequate stool disposal are prevalent, diarrhea emerges as a foremost cause of morbidity and mortality, especially among children. Early detection and prompt treatment are indispensable components of public health interventions, essential not only for managing individual cases but also for averting disease transmission within the population at large. Implementing effective hygiene measures significantly diminishes the incidence of diarrheal illnesses.

Types of Diarrhea

In disaster situations, a child with diarrhea might exhibit three potentially serious or extremely severe clinical conditions: (1) acute watery diarrhea, including cholera, lasting for hours or days, leading to dehydration; (2) acute bloody diarrhea or dysentery, which can result in intestinal harm, sepsis, malnutrition, and dehydration; and (3) persistent diarrhea, lasting beyond 14 days.

Assessment of all children with diarrhea is imperative to ascertain the duration of diarrhea, presence of blood in stools, and the occurrence of dehydration. Acute watery diarrhea predominantly results from infections by rotavirus, norovirus, enterovirus, enterotoxigenic Escherichia coli (ETEC), Vibrio cholerae, Salmonella, Giardia, and cryptosporidia. Shigella and Entamoeba histolytica are the primary pathogens associated with acute bloody diarrhea, although Campylobacter sp., invasive Escherichia coli, Salmonella, Clostridium difficile, and Yersinia sp. can also induce bloody diarrhea.

Management of Acute Watery Diarrhea

Dehydration represents the most prevalent complication of acute watery diarrhea in children. The assessment and management of this complication are detailed below.

Acute watery diarrhea caused by pathogens other than Vibrio cholerae typically resolves spontaneously and does not necessitate antibiotic therapy. Notably, antibiotics have the potential to prolong intestinal dysbiosis and impede the restoration of normal bowel flora. Consequently, the Integrated Management of Childhood Illness (IMCI) advises oral antimicrobial use solely for children with bloody diarrhea (amoebic or bacterial dysentery), cholera, and giardiasis, with treatment protocols addressed later in this section.

While antidiarrheal and many antiemetic medications are discouraged for acute diarrhea management due to their potential to diminish intestinal motility, thereby prolonging illness duration and exacerbating systemic symptoms, a single dose of oral ondansetron, where available, may be beneficial in reducing vomiting and facilitating oral rehydration [1].

Nutrition plays a crucial role in managing diarrhea in children. It is widely acknowledged that fasting does not influence the outcome or severity of diarrheal illness. Hence, in children with diarrhea and normal hydration status, continuation of breastfeeding (or bottle feeding with regular milk or formula if breastfeeding is not feasible), along with age-appropriate food consumption, is recommended. A lactose-reduced or lactose-free diet offers no advantage to children with acute diarrhea.

Feeding should resume in dehydrated children once normal hydration is restored through appropriate rehydration therapy tailored to dehydration severity. Notably, malnourished children face an elevated risk of diarrhea due to intestinal mucosal alterations, which can prolong illness duration owing to reduced enterocyte turnover. Hence, diminished food intake exacerbates preexisting malnutrition before acute diarrhea onset. Children with diarrhea lacking signs of dehydration typically exhibit a fluid deficit of less than 5% of their body weight. Despite the absence of overt dehydration signs, these children should receive increased fluid intake compared to usual to preempt dehydration development. Table 9.1 outlines the classification of diarrhea without dehydration or blood in stools, as per the IMCI approach.

Table 9.1 Classification of children with diarrhea without dehydration or blood in stools

Assess signs	Classify	Treatment
(Green) Not enough signs to classify as dehydration	(Green) No dehydration	(Green) Give food and fluids for treatment at home (see Plan A, Table 9.4) Tell the mother which signs require immediate medical attention If diarrhea persists, follow-up in 5 days

Management of Acute Bloody Diarrhea

Bacterial Dysentery

In pediatric cases, dysentery is diagnosed when a caregiver observes blood in the child's stools, signaling an invasive enteric infection that poses a significant risk of severe morbidity and mortality. Although dysenteric episodes comprise approximately 10% of all diarrhea incidents in children under 5 years old, they contribute to up to 15% of all diarrheal fatalities. Infants and undernourished children or those who develop dehydration during illness are particularly vulnerable to severe dysentery. Episodes of diarrhea that commence with dysentery are more prone to persistence compared to those lacking blood in stools initially. Dysentery treatment aims at clinical amelioration and curtailing fecal pathogen shedding to curb transmission. After assessing children with acute bloody diarrhea, administering appropriate fluids to prevent or treat dehydration and providing sustenance is imperative. Furthermore, initiating a 5-day course of oral antimicrobial active against Shigella, which accounts for the majority (up to 60%) of dysentery cases in children, is recommended [2].

Given the prevalence of antimicrobial resistance, knowing the sensitivity of local Shigella strains is crucial. In the absence of such data, information from neighboring regions or previous outbreaks may be utilized. Certain antimicrobials commonly employed for dysentery management, such as amoxicillin and trimethoprim-sulfamethoxazole (TMP/SMX), may prove ineffective against shigellosis regardless of local strain sensitivity and should be avoided. Ciprofloxacin is the preferred treatment for dysentery across all age groups. Ideally, stool culture should be conducted to pinpoint the causative organism and tailor treatment based on antimicrobial susceptibility. Hospital referral is advisable for malnourished children or those with preexisting conditions that could complicate diarrheal illness.

In regions like parts of Latin America, such as Argentina, where hemolytic uremic syndrome (HUS) is prevalent, induced by Shigella and Shiga toxin-producing strains of E. coli, which can lead to acute renal failure, antibiotic therapy might exacerbate renal failure. Hence, before initiating empirical antibiotic treatment, stool sampling for culture, yielding results within 48 h, is warranted.

Signs of improvement in bloody diarrhea include reduced fever, diminished blood in stools, less frequent bowel movements, enhanced appetite, and a return to normal activity. If minimal or no improvement is observed after 2 days, hospital referral for further evaluation and treatment is advised. Considerations for differentials, such as intussusception and cow milk allergy, should be contemplated if the child's condition does not ameliorate. If referral is unfeasible, perform stool culture to identify the organism and adjust antibiotic therapy accordingly. If the child demonstrates improvement, continue the antimicrobial regimen for 5 days.

Amoebic Dysentery

Amoebic dysentery, caused by the protozoan parasite Entamoeba histolytica, manifests as bloody diarrhea. Transmission typically occurs via the fecal-oral route, primarily through contaminated water and food sources. The most severe cases often afflict infants, pregnant women, and malnourished children. Similar to dysentery associated with Shigella, stools in amoebic dysentery frequently contain visible blood, accompanied by fever and abdominal pain. Hepatomegaly may also be evident.

Complications of amoebic dysentery encompass fulminant colitis, toxic megacolon, bowel perforation, and liver abscess formation. Metronidazole administration for 5–10 days is warranted when microscopic examination reveals amoebic trophozoites or cysts or when patients with bloody diarrhea fail to respond to two distinct antibiotic regimens.

Epidemic Cholera

Cholera, triggered by the toxin produced by Vibrio cholerae, is endemic in numerous global regions, particularly tropical and subtropical areas. In disaster scenarios, cholera transmission primarily occurs through contaminated water and heightened fecal-oral spread due to environmental factors. Vibrio cholerae can endure in water for 7–10 days, while contaminated food can also incite outbreaks. Early outbreak detection and preventive actions are crucial due to cholera's status as a public health emergency. Initial suspected cases require confirmation through culture, prompting immediate notification to public health authorities.

Upon confirming the diagnosis via a qualified laboratory, determining antibiotic susceptibility becomes paramount. Subsequent case identifications in cholera-affected areas often rely on clinical assessments. Given the prevalence of severe dehydration-related diarrheal illnesses in children, cholera's initial detection usually hinges on identifying adult cases. Suspect cholera in adults displaying severe, profuse, watery diarrhea and marked dehydration, especially if fatalities result from the illness. Controlling outbreaks necessitates identifying even milder cases among individuals who might not seek medical attention. Community interventions should emphasize enhancing sanitation, educating on personal hygiene and food safety, and ensuring access to uncontaminated water. Occasionally, household water chlorination or boiling may be necessary. Clinical signs of cholera encompass painless diarrhea without fever, with stool volume varying significantly. In severe cases, stools resemble rice water, with patients potentially losing between half a liter to one liter of fluid per hour. Such severe fluid loss can induce shock within the first 4–12 h if left untreated. Additional manifestations include anxiety, muscle cramps, weakness (attributed to electrolyte imbalances and hypoglycemia), and altered mental status.

Management of Cholera

Administering oral rehydration solution (ORS) alone has been shown to lower the case fatality rate (CFR) to below 1%. However, supplementing with appropriate antibiotics alongside ORS treatment can decrease the volume and duration of diarrhea, shorten hospital stays, and reduce the duration of bacteria shedding in stool, thereby aiding in transmission control. Antibiotic options include macrolides, tetracyclines, and fluoroquinolones. Zinc serves as an adjunctive therapy for children under 5, not only reducing diarrhea duration but also decreasing recurrence in subsequent months. Address mental status alterations with glucose to correct potential hypoglycemia. In areas where cholera is confirmed, monitoring CFR is crucial for assessing the adequacy and availability of rehydration therapy.

Assessment and Management of Dehydration Dehydration

Objectives
- Discuss dehydration, including definition and classification.
- Implement the Integrated Management of Childhood Illness (IMCI) guidelines for management of dehydration.
- Define the physiological mechanisms of oral rehydration therapy (ORT) and its application in dehydration management.
- Describe the inputs necessary for establishing an oral rehydration therapy (ORT) unit at disaster sites.

Dehydration stemming from acute diarrheal illness represents a major contributor to morbidity and mortality among populations displaced by disasters. During the early phases of humanitarian emergencies, it can be responsible for over 50% of deaths. However, the implementation of oral rehydration therapy (ORT) has significantly diminished both the morbidity and mortality linked to dehydration induced by diarrheal illness, irrespective of its cause.

Classification of Dehydration

Dehydration is a physiological state characterized by insufficient fluid levels in the body to sustain normal bodily functions. This condition arises when fluid losses surpass intake, leading to an overall reduction in body water content. In clinical contexts, dehydration may be categorized as hypotonic, isotonic, or hypertonic, with isotonic dehydration being the most prevalent. However, in disaster scenarios where access to laboratory resources is limited, dehydration severity is often assessed based on clinical presentation. While the most accurate method to gauge dehydration severity is by calculating weight loss percentage, it's often impractical due to the lack of pre-episode weight measurements in children. Hence, clinical signs become crucial for diagnosis. Table 9.2 outlines clinical signs corresponding to various dehydration degrees. Although precise dehydration assessment may be challenging, clinical signs can guide the diagnosis of mild (fluid loss <5% of body weight), moderate, or severe (fluid loss >10%, often with significant hemodynamic disturbance) dehydration. These classifications align with the Integrated Management of Childhood Illness (IMCI), which categorizes dehydration and guides treatment based on clinical observations (see Table 9.2). It's noteworthy that reduced skin turgor (skin pinch) may not always indicate dehydration, particularly in malnourished children. The IMCI approach relies on clinical findings for dehydration classification and treatment determination (see Table 9.3).

Shock

Dehydration-induced shock in children poses a life-threatening risk, often stemming from severe fluid depletion due to conditions like diarrhea and vomiting. The FEAST (Fluid expansion as supportive therapy) trial, a pivotal multicenter randomized controlled study, sought to determine the most effective treatment strategy for shock in febrile pediatric patients in resource-limited areas. Results from the trial indicated increased mortality associated with multiple fluid boluses. Consequently, current practice limits the administration to a maximum of two boluses of normal saline at 20 mls/kg before proceeding with step 2 of Plan C. It's important to acknowledge that these trial findings may not be directly applicable in settings where comprehensive intensive care is readily available [3–9].

Table 9.2 Clinical signs according to degrees or dehydration

Sign	Mild (No Dehydration)	Moderate (Some Dehydration)	Severe
Enophthalmos	+/−	++/+++	+++++
Mucus membranes	Partially moist	Dry	Very dry
Tears	+	−	−
Fontanelle	Normal	Sunken	Sunken
Skin temperature and color	Pink or slightly pale	Pale and cold	Very cold
Heart rate	Normal	Increased/mildly weak	Increased/ thready
Blood pressure	Normal	Mild or orthostatic hypotension	Markedly decreased/ shock
Sensorial status	Normal	Drowsy	Lethargic/coma
Capillary refill	<2 s	3–5 s	>5 s
Urine output	Reduced	Oliguria	Oligoanuria
Skin turgor (skin pinch)	No or slight delay	Delay = 2.5 s	Delay >5 s

Table 9.3 Classification of dehydration

Assess clinical signs	Classify as	Identify treatment

All four of:
  Weak/absent pulse;
  AVPU<A;
  Cold hands+ temp gradient
  Capillary refill<3 secs
PLUS Sunken eyes and slow skin pinch
	SHOCK
	(Note: this is not included in IMCI Classification)
		Normal saline 20 mls/kg bolus IV/IO
		A second bolus may be given if required before proceeding to step 2 of Plan C
		Treat for hypoglycemia

(Pink)
Two of the following signs:
  Lethargy/ unconsciousness
Sunken eyes
  Drinks poorly or unable to drink
  Skin turgor: skin pinch goes back very slowly to normal
	(Pink)
	Severe dehydration
		(Pink)
		  If the child does not have another severe classification: give fluid for severe dehydration (Plan C, see Table 9.6)
		  If the child has another severe classification: urgently refer to a hospital with the mother giving frequent sips of ORS during the trip
		  Advise the mother to continue breastfeeding if the child's state of consciousness allows it
		  If any case of cholera has been detected in the area, administer an antibiotic for this disease

(Yellow)
Two of the following signs:
  Restless, irritable
  Sunken eyes
  Drinks avidly, shows thirst
  Skin turgor: skin pinch goes back slowly to normal
	(Yellow)
	Some dehydration
		(Yellow)
		  If there is some degree of dehydration, administer fluids and food (Plan B, see Table 9.5)
		  If the child has another severe classification: urgently refer to a hospital with the mother giving frequent sips of ORS during the trip
		  Advise the mother to continue breastfeeding if the child's state of consciousness allows it
		  Tell the mother which signs require immediate medical attention
		  If diarrhea persists: schedule a follow-up visit in 24–48 h

(Green)
Not enough signs to classify as dehydration
	(Green)
	No dehydration
		(Green)
		  Give food and fluids adequate to treat diarrhea at home (Plan A, see Table 9.4)
		  Tell the mother which signs require immediate medical attention
		  If diarrhea persists, schedule a follow-up visit in 5 days

Management of Dehydration

Oral Rehydration Therapy (ORT)

The effectiveness and safety of ORT have been established globally. The discovery of the sodium-glucose cotransport system in the intestinal mucosa in 1964 paved the way for various oral dehydration treatment solutions. A significant drop in mortality rates from diarrheal illnesses, from 25% to 3%, was observed during the 1961–1975 cholera pandemic in Bangladesh when ORT replaced IV therapy. ORT is highly effective in preventing and treating dehydration associated with diarrheal illnesses in the majority of patients during disasters.

Physiologic Basis of ORT

Under normal physiological circumstances, water absorption transpires within the small intestine through tight junctions among epithelial cells, facilitated by a sodium gradient upheld by two mechanisms of sodium absorption within the brush border membrane of the luminal cell: passive sodium/potassium diffusion and active cotransport of sodium alongside monosaccharides such as glucose. Consequently, intracellular sodium undergoes active transportation into the intercellular space via ATPase carrier enzymes, establishing an osmotic gradient between the intercellular and luminal compartments, facilitating the unimpeded diffusion of water (see Fig. 9.1).

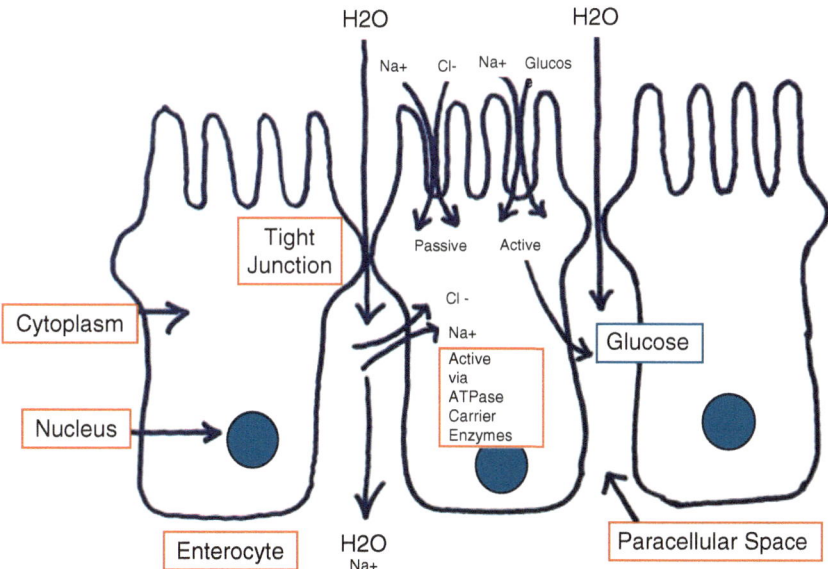

Fig. 9.1 Water absorption in the intestinal mucosa

During diarrheal illness, the passive absorption of sodium and chloride is compromised, while glucose absorption generally remains unaffected. This preservation allows for the absorption of adequate water and sodium to counterbalance fluid losses akin to those observed in cholera. The osmotic gradient within the intercellular space sustains the absorption of potassium and bicarbonate, thereby mitigating the metabolic acidosis typically associated with dehydration without the risk of excessive correction.

Advantages of Oral Rehydration Therapy

Oral rehydration therapy (ORT) presents several advantages over parenteral rehydration (Box 9.1). Utilizing the normal physiological mechanisms of intestinal absorption, ORT carries no risk of complications like water overload or electrolyte and acid-base imbalances associated with dehydration overcorrection. Consequently, ORT can be administered to any dehydrated child, irrespective of dehydration type. Furthermore, routine laboratory tests are typically unnecessary for patient evaluation. Normal hydration can usually be restored in children undergoing ORT within 4–6 h, facilitating early refeeding and reducing the risk of malnutrition linked to diarrheal diseases.

The costs of ORT are minimal compared to IV therapy expenses. Additionally, its primary components (salt, water, and sugar or starchy foods like rice) are often readily available within communities when pre-mixed oral rehydration solutions (ORS) are not accessible. ORT is straightforward and can be administered by trained health assistants, promoting family involvement in the child's health through caregiver participation. With minimal requirements, ORT can be administered at disaster sites, alleviating pressure on hospital-based medical personnel and enabling patients to remain close to their families (Box 9.2). Moreover, complications associated with invasive procedures, notably infections linked to IV therapy, are entirely circumvented.

Box 9.1: Advantages of ORT
- Use of normal physiologic mechanisms
- Early refeeding
- 90%–95% effective
- Effective for all types of dehydration
- No need for laboratory tests
- Low economic and social cost
- Availability
- No infectious, metabolic, or electrolytic complications

Box 9.2: Requirements for ORT
- Oral rehydration salt packets
- Drinking water
- Refrigerator
- Watch
- Pencil and paper
- Scale
- Containers (glasses, pitchers)
- Nasogastric tubes
- Trained staff

Composition of Oral Rehydration Solution

The World Health Organization (WHO) formulation stands as the most widely employed oral rehydration solution (ORS). A paramount aspect of this solution is the inclusion of equimolar quantities of sodium and glucose, which augments the intestinal absorption of both molecules. Additionally, the solution incorporates a source of bases (bicarbonate or citrate) and potassium. Despite initial apprehensions regarding hypernatremia linked to the WHO solution, particularly in hypertonic dehydration cases, the ORS has demonstrated efficacy and safety, irrespective of the patient's serum sodium levels.

The updated WHO ORS formulation, reducing osmolarity from 311 mOsm/l to 245 mOsm/l, has shown promise in diminishing stool output by 20% and vomiting by 30% in children experiencing acute non-cholera diarrhea, without significantly compromising effectiveness in cholera patients. Consequently, the WHO advocates for the adoption of a hypo-osmolar solution, particularly for children with acute, non-cholera diarrhea.

In scenarios where prepackaged ORS is unavailable, rehydration can be achieved with various extemporaneous solutions. The simplest method involves rice, water, and salt. One hundred grams of rice is boiled in 1 l of water for 10 min or until the rice pops. The water is then drained from the rice into a container, and any residual water is extracted from the rice using a spoon. Once all water is extracted, additional water is added to bring the total volume to 1 l, along with a pinch of salt.

It is imperative to utilize only drinking water when preparing rehydration solutions. Other beverages, such as mineral water or carbonated drinks, will alter the concentrations of various components, thereby diminishing efficacy. Ideally, prepared solutions should be refrigerated, and any unused solution should be discarded 24 h after preparation.

Contraindications for ORT

Contraindications to oral rehydration therapy (ORT) are outlined in Box 9.3. Additionally, the presence of other severe diseases, such as sepsis or meningitis, serves as a contraindication to ORT. However, vomiting before or during ORT does not necessarily preclude its use; only untreatable vomiting necessitates parenteral therapy.

Severe hemodynamic disturbances warrant immediate intravenous (IV) fluid replacement. Nonetheless, in the absence of supplies, ORT should be initiated until IV treatment becomes feasible. Before commencing ORT, it is essential to auscultate the abdomen to assess for bowel sounds and exclude diarrhea-related ileus, particularly with severe hypokalemia.

Box 9.3: Contraindications for ORT
- Shock
- Patient younger than 1 month of age
- Ileus
- Significantly altered sensorium
- Severe difficulty breathing
- Painful abdominal distension

Dehydration Management with the IMCI Guidelines

The Integrated Management of Childhood Illness (IMCI) guidelines delineate three plans for managing dehydration in children with diarrhea. Plan A is administered to children experiencing diarrhea without dehydration or those who have already been adequately rehydrated. Plan B is tailored for children exhibiting some degree of dehydration, while Plan C is designated for cases of severe dehydration.

Organization of ORT Units in Disaster Settings

Morbidity and mortality linked to diarrhea can be markedly mitigated through early hydration. Hence, it is imperative to establish oral rehydration therapy (ORT) units promptly in nearly every disaster relief scenario. The setup requires minimal supplies, and training auxiliary personnel in the Integrated Management of Childhood Illness (IMCI) approach to ORT is straightforward. Necessary supplies for establishing an ORT unit encompass a sufficient quantity of ORS packets, an ample supply of potable water, and other aforementioned items. Staff overseeing the unit should maintain patient treatment records and possess the ability to recognize cases of severe dehydration and suspected cholera cases. These records are indispensable for surveillance purposes, aiding in enhancing public health interventions during disaster scenarios (Tables 9.4, 9.5 and 9.6).

Table 9.4 Plan A, treating diarrhea

Plan A[a]: Oral treatment for diarrhea	
What	Oral rehydration with ORS Early future treatment of diarrhea to prevent dehydration
Where	At home
Who	Children able to drink on their own Children who are recovering from Plan B or Plan C but have ongoing diarrhea Children who cannot visit a health worker
How	Child should drink more fluid than normal, as much as they will take Keep up regular nutrition (food or breastfeeding) Teach the mother how to mix ORS appropriately and with clean water
Amount of ORS to give after each episode of diarrhea	**< 2 years-old** = 50–100 mL **2-9 Years** = 100–200 mL **> 10 years old** = as much as the child wants
What to do next	Child should see a health worker if: Diarrhea does not stop within 3 days There is fever There are many watery stools Child will not drink well There is repeated vomiting Child is very thirsty Stools are bloody

[a]See IMCI for full treatment details and algorithms

Table 9.5 Plan B, treating moderate dehydration

Plan B[a]: Oral treatment for moderate dehydration	
What	Oral rehydration with ORS
Where	At a health center
Who	Children who are dehydrated but are not in shock
How	Calculate the correct amount of ORS required over first 4-h of treatment Total fluid amount mL = body weight (kg) x 50–100 mL The child may have more if they want If no body weight is known, give ORS until the child will not take anymore **If the child is < 12 months-old:** Give one teaspoonful (= 5 ml) by mouth continuously **If the child is > 12 months-old:** Give frequent sips from a cup
Monitoring	Check on the child every hour while receiving Plan B
What to do next	Assess the child after 4 h, then decide if they need Plan A, B, or C If no dehydration: go to Plan A If some dehydration: continue Plan B for 2 more hours If severe dehydration: go to Plan C If the child is not improved by 6-h, switch to Plan C for IV hydration

[a]See IMCI for full treatment details and algorithms

Table 9.6 Plan C, treating severe dehydration

Plan C[a]: Intravenous (IV) or nasogastric (NG) treatment for severe dehydration	
What	Rapid hydration for severe dehydration
Where	At a health center
Who	Children with severe dehydration
When	If IV fluids are available now: start IV fluids urgently (ALSO give ORS orally)
	If IV fluids are available at a health center within 30-min away: send the child to the health center urgently (ALSO give ORS on the way)
	If no IV fluids are available: start NG, if available, or refer to another hospital (ALSO give ORS on the way)
How: IV rehydration	Give only isotonic fluids (like normal saline) by IV
	First dose is 30 mL/kg of IV isotonic fluid:
	For children < 12 months/old: give fluid over 1 h
	For children 12 months-old to 4 years-old: give fluid over 30 min
	Second dose is 70 mL/kg of IV isotonic fluid:
	For children < 12 months/old: give fluid over 5 h
	For children 12 months-old to 4 years-old: give fluid over 2.5 h
How: NG rehydration	Give ORS by NG
	Dose is 20 mL/kg/h continuously
	Refer urgently to another health center with IV therapy available, if possible
Monitoring	Reassess the child every 30 min
What to do next	If the child is not improving, give IV infusion more rapidly
	As soon as the child can drink, ALSO give ORS at a rate of 5 mL/kg/h)
	After 3-h, decide if the child needs Plan A, B, or C
	Observe the child for 6-h after resolution of dehydration

[a]See IMCI for full treatment details and algorithms

Diarrhea in Special Populations

Objectives
- Discuss the various types of diarrhea in newborns.
- Outline treatment strategies for infants aged 0–2 months experiencing diarrhea.
- Identify the diverse causes and approaches to managing persistent diarrhea.
- Explain the unique considerations for managing diarrhea in children with concurrent malnutrition.

Diarrhea in Infants 0 to 2 Months of Age

Within this age range, diarrheal illness presents specific characteristics. Stool consistency typically exhibits elevated water content compared to usual. It's important to note that frequent passage of normal stools does not constitute diarrhea, as bowel movements can vary based on dietary factors and age. For instance, loose stools in breastfed infants aged 5–10 days are considered normal. However, if the newborn is in good health overall, exhibiting no signs of

Table 9.7 Classification of diarrhea in infants younger than 2 months

Signs	Classify as	Treatment

(Pink)
Two of the following signs:
  Movement only when stimulated or no movement at all
  Sunken eyes
  Skin pinch goes back very slowly
	(Pink)
	Severe dehydration
		(Pink)
		If infant has no other severe classification
		  Give fluid for severe dehydration (Plan C)
		OR
		  If infant also has another severe classification
		    Refer URGENTLY to hospital with the mother giving frequent sips of oral rehydration salts (ORS) on the way
		    Advise the mother to continue breastfeeding
		    Advise the mother how to keep the infant warm on the way to the hospital

(Yellow)
Two of the following signs:
  Restless, irritable
  Sunken eyes
  Skin pinch goes back slowly
	(Yellow)
	Some dehydration
		(Yellow)
		  Give fluid and breast milk for some dehydration (Plan B)
		OR
		  If the infant also has another severe classification:
		    Refer URGENTLY to hospital with the mother giving frequent sips of ORS on the way
		  Advise the mother to continue breastfeeding
		  Advise the mother when to return immediately
		  Follow-up in 2 days if no improvement

(Green)
  Not enough signs to classify as some or severe dehydration
	(Green)
	No dehydration
		(Green)
		  Give fluids and breastmilk to treat diarrhea at home (Plan A)
		  Advise mother when to return immediately
		  Follow-up in 2 days if no improvement

illness, and feeding appropriately, these stools are likely transitional and typically do not necessitate treatment. Subsequently, breastfed infants may continue to have loose stools without mucus or blood. Parents usually identify diarrhea in infants by notable deviations in stool consistency or frequency from the norm. However, it's crucial to regard diarrhea in infants under 2 months as a serious infection and treat it accordingly (refer to Table 9.7) [10].

Persistent Diarrhea in Newborns

Consider infants from 0 to 2 months of age with persistent (7 days or more) diarrhea severely ill and refer them to a hospital whenever possible. These patients require special care to prevent fluid loss. It might also be necessary to make dietary changes and to perform laboratory tests to identify the cause of diarrhea.

Bloody Diarrhea in Newborns

Bloody diarrhea is a concerning issue in newborns. Common causes in neonates include hemorrhagic disease (linked to vitamin K deficiency), allergic colitis, necrotizing enterocolitis, or coagulation disorders like disseminated intravascular coagulation due to sepsis. In infants older than 15 days, blood in stools may stem from anal fissures, cow's milk allergy, or surgical conditions such as intussusception. While bacterial dysentery is rare, particularly in exclusively breastfed infants, suspicion should lead to consideration of Shigella and appropriate therapy. Amoebic dysentery is uncommon in very young infants. It's crucial to view bloody diarrhea in this age group as a severe condition necessitating urgent hospital referral (refer to Table 9.8).

Identifying the causative agent in infants under 2 months with diarrhea is challenging. Infection can occur either at birth, with organisms from the mother's feces, or afterward, through various organisms from infected children or contaminated hands. Poor hygiene practices with feeding bottles can elevate the risk of such infections. Common infecting agents in infants under 2 months often include Escherichia coli, Salmonella, echovirus, and rotavirus. Symptoms may start abruptly, with poor feeding and/or vomiting. Stool consistency may change from yellow and loose to greenish and watery, with an increase in evacuation frequency. The most critical aspect is acute fluid loss, leading to dehydration and electrolyte imbalances. Proper hand hygiene, exclusive breastfeeding, and cautious feeding practices can mitigate dehydration risks and potential fatalities.

Management of Persistent Diarrhea

Persistent diarrhea, lasting at least 14 days, is a significant concern, accounting for a substantial portion of diarrhea cases and a higher percentage of fatalities. It often coincides with weight loss and can be associated with severe non-intestinal infections. Many affected children are malnourished, elevating the risk of mortality. However, persistent diarrhea is rare among infants exclusively breastfed. Children with diarrhea persisting for 14 days or more should be categorized based on dehydration status (refer to Table 9.9).

Table 9.8 Classification of bloody diarrhea in infants less than 2 months

Assess signs	Classify as	Treatment
(Red) Blood in stools	(Red) Bloody diarrhea	URGENT referral to a hospital Counsel the mother to continue breastfeeding if tolerated by the infant Give a dose of intramuscular vitamin K Give the first dose of the recommended antibiotics

Table 9.9 Classification of children with persistent diarrhea

Has the child had diarrhea for 14 days or more?		
Assess signs	Classify	Treatment
With dehydration	Severe persistent diarrhea	Treat dehydration before and during the child's transfer, unless the child has another severe condition Refer to hospital
Without dehydration	Persistent diarrhea	Teach the mother how to feed the child with persistent diarrhea[a] Tell the mother which signs require immediate medical attention Follow-up in 5 days

[a]Advise the mother to temporarily decrease the intake of animal milk if it's already part of the child's regular diet, while continuing breastfeeding. For children older than 6 months, introduce suitable complementary foods in small, frequent portions, at least 6 times daily

For children with severe persistent diarrhea and any level of dehydration, specialized treatment is necessary, necessitating hospital referral rather than outpatient management. Dehydration treatment typically takes precedence unless another severe condition is present. Children with persistent diarrhea but no dehydration signs can usually be managed initially in an outpatient setting. Effective feeding practices are paramount in managing persistent diarrhea.

Nutritional therapy aims to:

(a) temporarily reduce animal milk (or lactose) intake
(b) ensure sufficient intake of energy, protein, vitamins, and minerals to aid gut mucosa repair and improve nutritional status
(c) avoid exacerbating foods or drinks and
(d) ensure adequate food intake during recovery to address any malnutrition

Routine antimicrobial treatment for persistent diarrhea is generally ineffective. However, some children may have specific infections, intestinal or otherwise, requiring targeted antimicrobial therapy. Persistent diarrhea in such cases will not resolve until these infections are diagnosed and treated.

Management of Giardiasis

Giardiasis, an intestinal infection caused by a protozoan parasite, can lead to non-bloody diarrhea with a distinct foul odor, often accompanied by chronic malabsorption. Symptoms may include abdominal cramps, epigastric pain, and flatulence, while fever is rare. Transmission typically occurs through the fecal-oral route via contaminated water sources (especially surface water), person-to-person contact, or contaminated objects. Even minimal exposure can lead to infection. Consider treatment with metronidazole for children with chronic malabsorptive non-bloody diarrhea and no fever, as well as for those with identified cysts or trophozoites in a microscopic stool examination.

Management of Diarrhea in Children with Malnutrition

Diarrhea is both a consequence and a contributor to malnutrition. Malnourished children are more susceptible to diarrhea, and each bout of diarrhea exacerbates malnutrition. Children in disaster situations face heightened risks of both conditions. Initial management of acute diarrhea in these cases should prioritize addressing fluid and electrolyte imbalances.

In cases of severe acute malnutrition, children are at risk of hypokalemia, leading to the recommendation of ResoMal over the standard WHO ORS formulation by WHO. ResoMal has a higher potassium and lower sodium concentration compared to standard ORS, and its administration rate is slower due to the risk of fluid overload. Early resumption of feeding is crucial and should only be interrupted for management of severe dehydration or shock. Additionally, adjunctive treatment with zinc has been found to be beneficial.

Malnutrition is covered elsewhere in this book and will not be reviewed further here.

Conclusions

- Acute diarrhea is characterized by the sudden onset of loose stools and may be accompanied by symptoms such as abdominal cramping, nausea, and vomiting.
- Clinical criteria for antibiotic treatment in acute emergency situations include severe dehydration, bloody stools, high fever, and signs of systemic infection.
- Dysentery presents with bloody diarrhea and abdominal pain, often caused by bacteria such as Shigella or Entamoeba histolytica, requiring appropriate antibiotic therapy.
- Epidemic cholera outbreaks demand swift action with strategies including oral rehydration therapy (ORT) and antibiotic treatment for severe cases to manage symptoms and prevent further transmission.
- Dehydration can be classified into no dehydration, some dehydration and severe dehydration based on clinical signs such as thirst, skin turgor, and capillary refill time.
- The Integrated Management of Childhood Illness (IMCI) guidelines provide a framework for classifying dehydration severity and guiding appropriate treatment interventions.
- Oral rehydration therapy (ORT) utilizes a solution of salt and glucose to replace lost fluids and electrolytes, addressing dehydration through physiological mechanisms such as sodium-glucose co-transport.
- Establishing ORT units at disaster sites involves planning for equipment, personnel, and supply chains to ensure timely administration of rehydration therapy to affected populations.

- Diarrhea in newborns may stem from infectious, allergic, or metabolic causes, requiring tailored treatment approaches such as breastfeeding promotion and fluid replacement.
- Treatment strategies for infants aged 0–2 months with diarrhea focus on supportive care, including fluid replacement and monitoring for signs of dehydration or complications.
- Persistent diarrhea necessitates thorough investigation into underlying causes such as infections, malabsorption disorders, or immune deficiencies, with management tailored to specific etiologies.
- Children with concurrent malnutrition and diarrhea require integrated care addressing both conditions, including nutritional rehabilitation, infection control measures, and micronutrient supplementation.

References

1. Freedman SB, et al. Oral Ondansetron for gastroenteritis in a pediatric emergency department. N Engl J Med. 2006;354:1698–705. https://doi.org/10.1056/NEJMoa055119.
2. World Health Organization. Guidelines for the control of shigellosis, including epidemics due to Shigella dysenteriae 1. World Health Organization; 2005. ISBN 92 4 159233 0
3. George EC, Walker AS, Kiguli S, Olupot-Olupot P, Opoka RO, Engoru C, Akech SO, Nyeko R, Mtove G, Reyburn H, Berkley JA, Mpoya A, Levin M, Crawley J, Gibb DM, Maitland K, Babiker AG. Predicting mortality in sick African children: the FEAST Paediatric Emergency Triage (PET) Score. BMC Med. 2015;13:174. https://doi.org/10.1186/s12916-015-0407-3. PMID: 26228245; PMCID: PMC4521500.
4. George EC, Kiguli S, Olupot PO, Opoka RO, Engoru C, Akech SO, Nyeko R, Mtove G, Mpoya A, Thomason MJ, Crawley J, Evans JA, Gibb DM, Babiker AG, Maitland K, Walker AS. Mortality risk over time after early fluid resuscitation in African children. Crit Care. 2019;23(1):377. https://doi.org/10.1186/s13054-019-2619-y. PMID: 31775837; PMCID: PMC6882199.
5. Kiguli S, Akech SO, Mtove G, Opoka RO, Engoru C, Olupot-Olupot P, Nyeko R, Evans J, Crawley J, Prevatt N, Reyburn H, Levin M, George EC, South A, Babiker AG, Gibb DM, Maitland K. WHO guidelines on fluid resuscitation in children: missing the FEAST data. BMJ. 2014;348:f7003. https://doi.org/10.1136/bmj.f7003. PMID: 24423891; PMCID: PMC5693317.
6. Maitland K, et al and the FEAST Trial Group. Mortality after fluid bolus in African children with severe infection. N Engl J Med. 2011; PMID:21615299.
7. Maitland K, George EC, Evans JA, Kiguli S, Olupot-Olupot P, Akech SO, Opoka RO, Engoru C, Nyeko R, Mtove G, Reyburn H, Brent B, Nteziyaremye J, Mpoya A, Prevatt N, Dambisya CM, Semakula D, Ddungu A, Okuuny V, Wokulira R, Timbwa M, Otii B, Levin M, Crawley J, Babiker AG, Gibb DM, FEAST trial group. Exploring mechanisms of excess mortality with early fluid resuscitation: insights from the FEAST trial. BMC Med. 2013;11:68. https://doi.org/10.1186/1741-7015-11-68. PMID: 23496872; PMCID: PMC3599745
8. Nteziyaremye J, Paasi G, Burgoine K, Sadiq Balyejjusa J, Tegu C, Olupot-Olupot P. Perspectives on aetiology, pathophysiology and management of shock in African children. Afr J Emerg Med. 2017;7(Suppl):S20–6. https://doi.org/10.1016/j.afjem.2017.10.002. Epub 2017 Nov 21. PMID: 30505670; PMCID: PMC6246868.

9. Obonyo NG, Olupot-Olupot P, Mpoya A, Nteziyaremye J, Chebet M, Uyoga S, Muhindo R, Fanning JP, Shiino K, Chan J, Fraser JF, Maitland K. A clinical and physiological prospective observational study on the management of pediatric shock in the post-fluid expansion as supportive therapy trial era. Pediatr Crit Care Med. 2022;23(7):502–13. https://doi.org/10.1097/PCC.0000000000002968. Epub 2022 Apr 21. PMID: 35446796; PMCID: PMC7613033

10. World Health Organization. Integrated Management of Childhood Illness: management of the sick young infant aged up to 2 months. IMCI chart booklet. Geneva: World Health Organization; 2019. License: CC BY-NC-SA 3.0 IGO

Chapter 10
Disaster Considerations for Newborn Delivery and Postnatal Care

Gabrielle Coleman, Yo Nishihara, Celia Wanda Kariuki, Caren Ito Emadau, and Lisa Umphrey

Introduction

This chapter centers on the initial care of the newborn, closely aligning with the World Health Organization's Essential Newborn Care guidelines.

In 2021, out of the 6.5 million children who died, nearly 70% were under the age of five. Of these, 47% passed away within their first 28 days of life, equating to 2.3 million neonatal deaths each year or approximately 6400 deaths per day. Although there has been steady progress in reducing the neonatal mortality rate, this improvement has lagged behind the under-5 mortality rate, indicating an ongoing need to address the specific and underlying causes of morbidity and mortality in newborns.

This situation starkly contrasts with high-income countries, where the infant mortality rate is currently at its lowest in history. According to WHO, neonatal deaths per 1000 live births range from 2 to 6 in the wealthiest nations, compared to 27 deaths per 1000 live births in Sub-Saharan Africa and 21 per 1000 in Southern

G. Coleman
University of Colorado, School of Medicine, Aurora, CO, USA
e-mail: gabrielle.coleman@cuanschutz.edu

Y. Nishihara (✉)
University of Colorado, School of Medicine, Department of Pediatrics, Aurora, CO, USA
e-mail: yo.nishihara@cuanschutz.edu

C. W. Kariuki
Mama Lucy Kibaki Hospital- Embakasi, Nairobi County, Kenya

C. I. Emadau
Child Health and Paediatrics (Moi Uni), Pumwani Maternity & Referral Hospital, Nairobi County, Kenya

L. Umphrey
Center for Global Health, Aurora, CO, USA
e-mail: Lisa.umphrey@childrenscolorado.org

© The Author(s), under exclusive license to Springer Nature Switzerland AG 2025
L. Umphrey et al. (eds.), *Pediatric Considerations in Disaster Settings*, https://doi.org/10.1007/978-3-031-85501-6_10

227

Asia. The United Nations estimates that a baby born in a developed country has only one-tenth the risk of dying in the first 28 days compared to a baby born in a developing nation. Ten countries, primarily in Africa and East Asia, account for nearly 60% of all under-five deaths globally, with more than 80% of these occurring in Sub-Saharan Africa and South Asia. These statistics highlight the profound impact that a baby's geographic location at birth has on their survival chances.

While various public health initiatives, such as vaccinations and access to clean water, have improved overall child mortality, these measures do not fully address the unique needs of newborns. Nearly 80% of neonatal deaths are attributed to pre-term birth, complications during or shortly after delivery, congenital abnormalities, and infections. Most of these causes are preventable, as evidenced by the ability of wealthier nations to make neonatal mortality exceedingly rare.

Despite the significant need for more medical supplies, knowledge, and personnel in lower-income countries, the interventions required to save newborn lives are primarily low-cost but highly impactful. This chapter emphasizes the importance of actions taken during delivery and the immediate postpartum period, including recognizing risk factors and taking supportive steps to ensure positive outcomes for both mother and baby.

Newborn Care in Disaster Settings

Neonatal resuscitation and newborn care are critically important in disaster settings due to the heightened vulnerability of infants in these environments. Disasters, whether natural or man-made, often disrupt healthcare infrastructure, deplete resources, and lead to overcrowded conditions, all of which significantly increase risks to newborns. Infants are especially prone to life-threatening conditions such as hypothermia, respiratory distress, and infections, which can be exacerbated by the chaotic circumstances of a disaster. Effective neonatal resuscitation and immediate care are essential to address these risks promptly and prevent potentially fatal outcomes.

In disaster settings, prioritizing the unique needs of neonates is crucial for their survival and long-term health. Newborns require prompt and specialized care to stabilize their condition, which includes resuscitation for birth asphyxia, careful management of their thermoregulation to prevent hypothermia, and vigilant monitoring for signs of infection or complications; Fig. 10.1 summarizes the necessary steps for neonatal resuscitation in the first minutes of life. The scarcity of medical supplies and trained personnel in these environments underscores the need for well-defined protocols and training to guide healthcare workers in providing effective newborn care. Without these measures, even minor health issues can quickly escalate into life-threatening conditions for vulnerable infants.

Neonatal care in disaster settings presents unique challenges due to both the extreme vulnerability of newborns and the severe disruption of healthcare services. According to the World Health Organization (WHO), infants are particularly

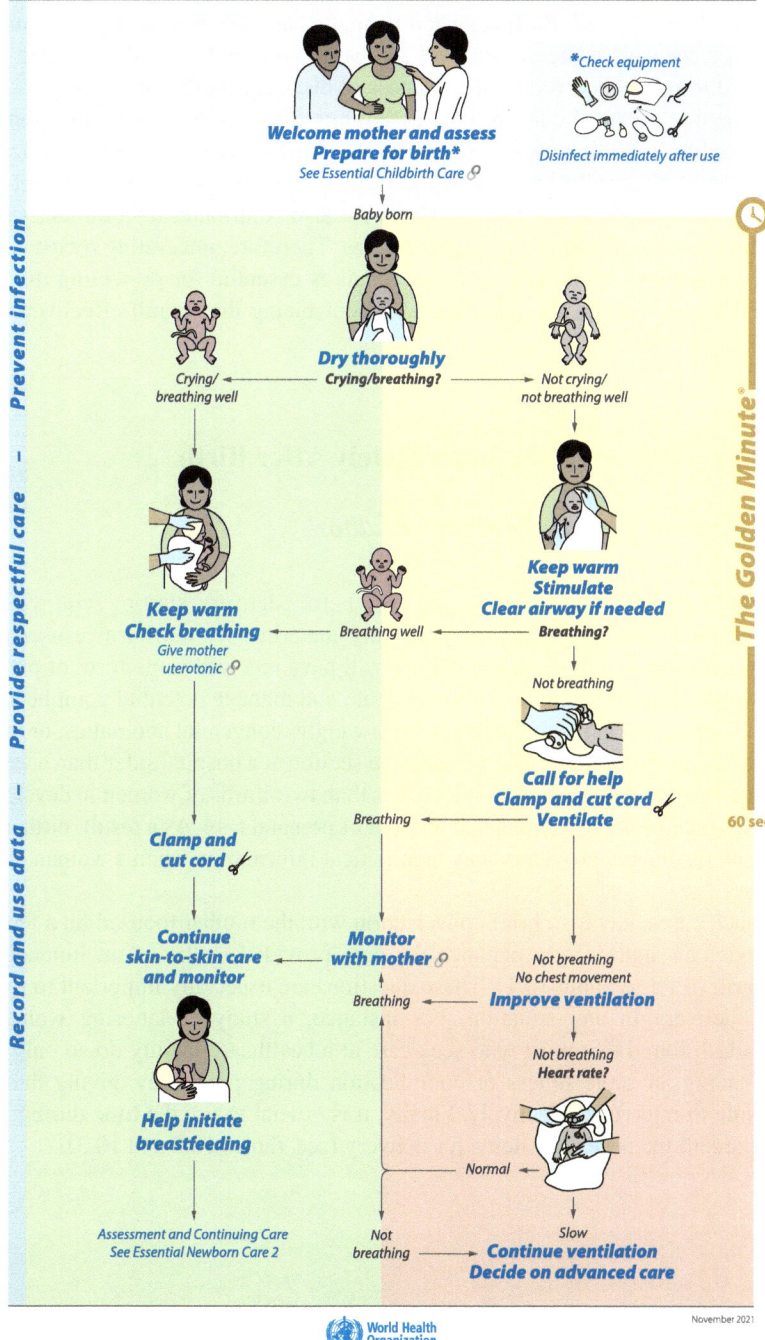

Fig. 10.1 Immediate care and helping babies breathe at birth

susceptible to conditions like hypothermia, respiratory distress, and infections, which can worsen in the chaotic and resource-limited conditions typical of disasters. The WHO highlights the critical need for tailored disaster preparedness and response plans that include specialized neonatal care. By addressing these unique challenges, we can ensure the survival and well-being of the most vulnerable newborns and improve the overall effectiveness of disaster relief efforts.

Addressing neonatal care in disaster settings also has broader implications for public health. Providing appropriate resuscitation and early care can significantly reduce long-term health impacts and prevent severe complications. This not only supports the immediate survival of infants but also contributes to community resilience by fostering healthier future generations. Therefore, integrating robust neonatal care practices into disaster response plans is essential for protecting the most vulnerable members of the population and enhancing the overall effectiveness of disaster relief efforts.

Routine Newborn Care Immediately After Birth

First Contact with the Mother in Labor

Providing care for the newborn begins even before delivery, starting with welcoming the mother and preparing the necessary materials for newborn resuscitation. Ideally, every woman presenting in labor will have received some form of prenatal care, which helps the medical team anticipate and manage potential complications. These complications may include low birth weight, congenital anomalies, or maternal conditions that would make a Caesarean section at a hospital safer than a vaginal delivery. However, according to WHO, less than two-thirds of women in developing countries receive the recommended amount of prenatal care. As a result, birth attendants and healthcare providers may lack critical information when a woman arrives in labor.

In such cases, having a brief conversation with the mother focused on a few key questions can significantly enhance the care provided to the infant immediately after birth (refer to Table 10.1). These questions are especially important to review before delivery in any situation. For instance, a study of laboring women in Bangladesh found that most who seek care at a healthcare facility do so only after experiencing an acute illness or complication during pregnancy, giving the staff little time to intervene effectively. Finally, it is crucial to use the time during labor to prepare all the necessary items for delivery (see Tables 10.2 and 10.3).

Table 10.1 Questions to ask mothers when they arrive for a delivery

How many times have you seen a doctor or nurse before today? When is the last time you saw them?
When is your due date? How many weeks along are you?
What problems have you had with this pregnancy?
Has your baby been growing well? Have they had any problems that your doctor has told you about?
Have you ever had a baby before? How is that child doing? Did you or they have any problems during delivery?
Do you have any medical conditions? Do you take any medications? Are you allergic to anything?
Have you been feeling the baby move like normal? Have you noticed any blood from your vagina or bad smelling discharge? Have you been sick recently?
If used in the healthcare system, request if mother has a government issued mother and child health booklet

Table 10.2 List of items needed for delivery

Hand sanitizer or water and soap for washing hands
Flat firm surface for resuscitation
Sterile gloves
Gowns and drapes if available
Clean clamps, cord ties, or strings
Sterile scissors
Suction device (penguin sucker or suction machine)
Ventilation bag (250–300 ml size) and mask (preemie (0) size or neonate (1) size)
Stethoscope
Warm hat for an infant
Blankets (at least 2 pieces of towel/linen for baby and extra blanket to cover mom and baby after delivery)
Room heater

Table 10.3 Preparing for birth

Ensure privacy
Ensure that the delivery suite/room is warm, between 25 and 28 °C
Ensure the delivery area is draft-free, turn off fans, and/or air conditioning units, close windows
Introduce yourself to the mother and her companion of choice or support person if present
Review with the mother what care to expect for herself and her baby in the immediate postpartum period
Wash hands with clean water and soap
Gown in readiness for delivery
Place a dry cloth on her abdomen and ensure all resuscitation equipment is within easy reach

Immediately Following Delivery

The first place the newborn should be placed after delivery is directly onto the mother's abdomen. This immediate skin-to-skin contact allows the mother to see and connect with her baby, helps regulate the infant's temperature, and gives the healthcare provider the opportunity to assess the baby's condition. It is crucial to begin drying the baby right away, as they will be covered in fluids. Drying the infant not only stimulates their first breaths but also helps prevent hypothermia.

As the neonate is stimulated through drying and rubbing, the provider or birth attendant should conduct the initial assessment of the child:

- Are they crying? Breathing independently? Responding to vigorous touch?

  - Check for any danger signs that might indicate the need for ongoing or more advanced care. These signs include apnea (lack of breathing), poor muscle tone, blue discoloration, labored breathing with retractions or gasping, pulselessness, and others (refer to Table 10.4).
  - Keep in mind that a newborn who seems stable initially may deteriorate quickly. Continuous monitoring and assessment, especially in the period shortly after birth, is crucial.

- If the baby is doing well, focus on keeping them warm.

  - If there are no concerns about the baby's condition, continue skin-to-skin contact on the mother's abdomen, which is essential for thermoregulation. Ensure the baby is kept warm by placing a hat on their head and covering them with blankets in a way that does not interfere with skin contact with the mother.
  - Neonatal hypothermia can occur even in warm climates and is closely associated with increased mortality rates and brain injury.

- For healthy newborns, the umbilical cord should be cut after one minute of life.

  - Research has shown that waiting one minute before clamping the cord leads to better outcomes for all infants and can reduce morbidity and mortality in preterm infants by 17% at two years, with a 30% overall mortality reduction

Table 10.4 *Danger* signs that the baby needs emergency intervention	
	Lack of breathing
	Gasping for air, retractions, sucking, audible breathing noises
	Blue coloring of the tongue, lips, other mucous membranes and extremities
	No pulse / no heart sounds with stethoscope
	Poor tone, no crying, will not respond to stimulation

in this vulnerable group. After performing delayed cord clamping, proceed with the following steps to cut the cord:

> Place the first clamp or tightly tie with string about 4 cm from the infant's belly button.
> Without pulling too hard on the cord, push the blood in the cord away from the baby's abdomen starting at the first clamp, then place the second clamp or tie 2 cm away.
> Ensure there is enough space between the two clamps to cut cleanly with sterile scissors.

Managing Problems

Immediately following delivery, the essential steps of newborn care involve placing the infant on the mother's abdomen, vigorously rubbing and drying the infant with a towel, keeping them warm with a hat and blanket, and cutting the umbilical cord after the first minute of life. However, if at any point the neonate begins to decompensate, such as by stopping breathing, experiencing a heart rate drop below 100 bpm, or displaying any of the danger signs mentioned in Table 10.4, immediate intervention is required. In such situations, the cord can be cut right away to allow the healthcare team to move the infant to a more accessible work surface. Alternatively, cord clamping can be delayed until additional help is available.

- If the infant is not breathing despite vigorous rubbing and stimulation, examine their mouth and nose.

  - If you observe fluid or if the amniotic fluid is stained with meconium—even if nothing is immediately visible in the oral cavity—gently suction the mouth first, followed by the nose. Suctioning is not necessary for all neonates and should be avoided if it is not indicated.

- Call for additional help.

  - Even if the infant begins to breathe independently, they might still need more advanced care than can be provided at the delivery location.

- Begin ventilation. It is crucial that every newborn starts breathing, either spontaneously or with assistance, within their first minute of life.

  - To administer breaths, gently extend the infant's head with one hand.
  - Form a 'C shape' with the other hand to hold the mask.
  - Place the edge of the mask on the chin first, then over the nose, ensuring a seal over both the mouth and nostrils (Fig. 10.2).
  - Firmly compress the bag. If the mask is correctly sealed and appropriately sized, the newborn's chest should rise and fall visibly with each squeeze of the bag.

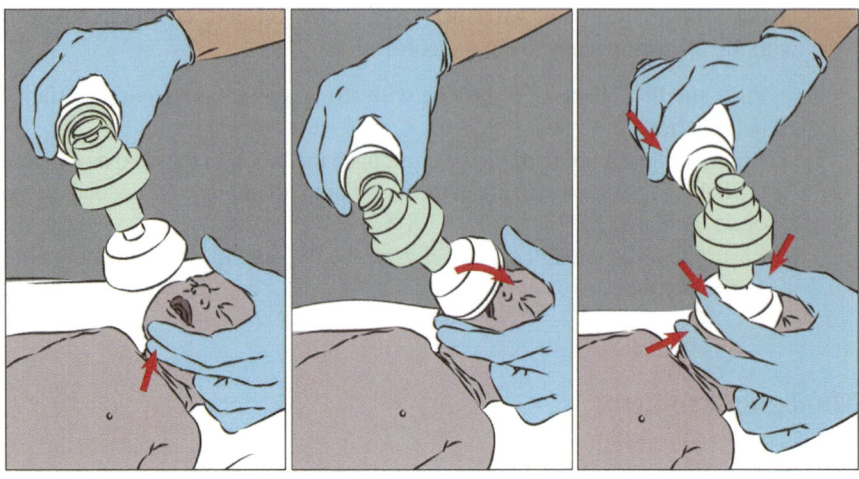

Fig. 10.2 Mask positioning (Source: Laerdal Global Health, Helping Mothers and Babies Survive. https://hmbs.org/training-program/enc1/#learning-materials)

- – Aim for a rate of 40 respirations per minute.
- – Continue rescue breaths until the baby breathes regularly without pauses, gasping, or retractions.
- • During ventilation of an infant:
  - – Verify the effectiveness of bag-mask ventilation by checking the equipment and seal.
  - – If secretions are visible, consider additional suctioning of the nose and mouth.
  - – Monitor the infant's pulse every 3–5 minutes.
  - – It is crucial to identify the newborn with an I.D. band and footprints before transporting them for more intensive medical care.
- • After several minutes, reassess the situation and consider transferring the infant if needed.

When to Halt Resuscitation Efforts

If the newborn has never had a pulse and has received 10 minutes of effective oxygen delivery, or if the pulse has been lost and resuscitation efforts have continued for 20 minutes, it may be appropriate to discuss discontinuing interventions with the team. In such cases, it is crucial to swaddle the baby and allow the mother to see and hold them.

The First Hour of Life

Once the newborn has been stabilized and the umbilical cord has been cut, continue skin-to-skin contact with the mother for at least the first hour of life. This practice helps keep the newborn warm, promotes bonding, and has been shown to reduce the risk of early postpartum depression. It also improves interactions and stress levels for both the mother and the child, with benefits extending into the months following delivery. During this hour, the healthcare team should monitor the newborn's breathing, heart rate, temperature, and any concerning signs without disrupting the skin-to-skin contact.

Breastfeeding should be initiated within the first hour, if possible, to encourage milk letdown, nourish the infant, enhance bonding, and provide the mother with her first chance to learn how to recognize and respond to her baby's hunger cues. Breast milk consistently offers the best nutritional support for the newborn, with the only absolute contraindications being certain medications. Other potential concerns should be evaluated by a provider. Absence of skin-to-skin contact and separation of mother and infant are linked to lower breastfeeding rates within this crucial timeframe.

To help new mothers breastfeed:

- Recognize when the baby is hungry. When the infant starts moving their tongue, "rooting" around, and crying more often, encourage the mother to initiate breastfeeding by first tickling her baby's nose with her nipple.
- Wait for the infant to open their mouth; when they do the nipple should be inserted directly inside their mouth.
- The signs of a good attachment include:
  - More areola above the infant's mouth than below
  - The baby's chin is directly in contact with the breast, and their nose is free
  - Their mouth is wide open with the lower lip not visible.
  - The mother experiences no pinching or pain.

A proper attachment is essential for ensuring good milk production, adequate feeding for the neonate, and a comfortable experience for the mother.

Referral Considerations for Neonates During Disasters

Limited referral options for neonatal patients in disaster or humanitarian settings present a major challenge to effective newborn care. The destruction of healthcare infrastructure, including specialized neonatal units and referral centers, leads to a severe shortage of resources and facilities capable of managing complex neonatal cases. This scarcity is compounded by logistical difficulties, such as damaged infrastructure and disrupted supply chains, which hinder the transport of critically ill neonates to appropriate care facilities. When healthcare facilities are overwhelmed or non-functional, the delays in receiving specialized care can significantly increase mortality and morbidity rates among newborns.

The International Committee of the Red Cross (ICRC) highlights that inadequate transportation options and unsafe conditions further exacerbate the difficulties of referring neonates to appropriate facilities. Many disaster-affected regions have limited access to functioning hospitals, and the lack of trained healthcare personnel to provide emergency care during transit intensifies these challenges. These issues make it difficult for neonates to receive timely and adequate treatment, thereby increasing their risk of adverse outcomes.

Médecins Sans Frontières (MSF) / Doctors Without Borders underscores the critical need for well-coordinated referral systems and the enhancement of local healthcare capacities to address these challenges effectively. MSF's experience in humanitarian settings shows that strengthening referral networks and improving the capabilities of local health facilities are crucial for managing severe neonatal conditions. By addressing these gaps, humanitarian organizations can better support neonates and improve survival rates, even in the most challenging environments.

Conclusion

Immediate newborn care at delivery is a crucial and cost-effective intervention that significantly improves neonatal survival, reduces long-term morbidity, and fosters mother-baby bonding. By following the outlined steps and strategies, complications during the immediate postpartum period can be minimized. Consistent, focused training for healthcare providers is essential to ensure effective resuscitation of distressed neonates at delivery.

For additional information, refer to "Essential Newborn Care 2," which covers the comprehensive care of infants from after their first hour of life through to their discharge.

Bibliography

1. Abiramalatha T, Ramaswamy VV, Bandyopadhyay T, et al. Delivery room interventions for hypothermia in preterm neonates: a systematic review and network meta-analysis. JAMA Pediatr. 2021;175(9):e210775. https://doi.org/10.1001/jamapediatrics.2021.0775.
2. Bollipo S, Pagali D, Korrapolu HB, Rahman MA. The first golden hour of breastfeeding: where do we stand? Int J Contemp Pediatr. 2018;6:27–32.
3. International Committee of the Red Cross (ICRC), ICRC Health Care in Danger (created September 19, 2014), accessed Sept 2024.
4. Kampalath V, MacLean S, AlAbdulhadi A, Congdon M. The delivery of essential newborn care in conflict settings: a systematic review. Front Pediatr. 2022;10:937751. https://doi.org/10.3389/fped.2022.937751.

5. Kreutz IM, Santos IS. Contextual, maternal, and infant factors in preventable infant deaths: a statewide ecological and cross-sectional study in Rio Grande do SUL, Brazil. BMC Public Health. 2023;23:87. https://doi.org/10.1186/s12889-022-14913-z.

6. Lama TP, Munos MK, Katz J, Khatry SK, LeClerq SC, Mullany LC. Assessment of facility health and health worker readiness to provide quality antenatal, intrapartum and postpartum care in rural Southern Nephal. BMC Health Serv Res. 2020;20:16. https://doi.org/10.1186/s12913-019-4871-x.

7. Médecins Sans Frontières (MSF), MSF Emergency Care (created June 22, 2016), accessed Sept 2024.

8. Mehler K, Hucklenbruch-Rother E, Trautmann-Villalba P, Becker I, Roth B, Kribs A. Delivery room skin-to-skin contact for preterm infants—A randomized clinical trial. Acta Paediatr. 2020;109:518–26. https://doi-org.proxy.hsl.ucdenver.edu/10.1111/apa.14975.

9. Perin J, Mulick A, Yeung D, Villavicencio F, Lopez G, Strong KL, Prieto-Merino D, Cousens S, Black RE, Liu L. Global, regional, and national causes of under-5 mortality in 2000-19: an updated systematic analysis with implications for the sustainable development goals. Lancet Child Adolesc Health. 2022;6(2):106–15. https://doi.org/10.1016/S2352-4642(21)00311-4.

10. Rasheda K, Baqui AH, Ibne Moin SM, Harrison M, Nazma B, et al. Can facility delivery reduce the risk of intrapartum complications-related perinatal mortality? Findings from a cohort study. J Glob Health. 2018;8:1. https://doi.org/10.7189/jogh.08.010408.

11. Robledo KP, Tarnow-Mordi WO, Rieger I, Suresh P, Martin A, Yeung C, et al. Effects of delayed versus immediate umbilical cord clamping in reducing death or major disability at 2 years corrected age among very preterm infants (APTS): a multicentre, randomized clinical trial. Lancet Child Adolesc Health. 2022;6(3):150–7.

12. Sharrow D, Hug L, You D, Alkema L, Black R, Cousens S, Croft T, Gaigbe-Tagbe V, et al. Global regional and national trends in under 5 mortality between 1990 and 2019 with scenario-based projections until 2030: a systematic analysis by the UN Inter-agency Group for Child Mortality Estimation. Lancet Global Health. 2022;10:e195–206.

13. Stanescu AMA, Totan A, Mircescu D, Grajdeanu IV, Serban B, Bratu OG, Diaconu CC. Contraindications to breastfeeding – current issues at the border between myth and reality. Mod Med. 2019;26(3):105–10.

14. United Nations Inter-agency Group for Child Mortality Estimation (UN IGME). Levels & Trends in Child Mortality: Report 2022, Estimates developed by the United Nations Inter-agency Group for Child Mortality Estimation, 2023. https://childmortality.org/wp-content/uploads/2023/01/UN-IGME-Child-Mortality-Report-2022.pdf.

15. World Health Organization. WHO recommendations on antenatal care for a positive pregnancy experience. Guideline WHO/RHR/16.12. 2016. https://www.who.int/publications/i/item/9789241549912.

16. World Health Organization. 14th March 2024. Newborn mortality. https://www.who.int/news-room/fact-sheets/detail/newborn-mortality. Accessed 9th May 2024.

17. World Health Organization (WHO), WHO Emergencies (created April 7, 2003), accessed Sept 2024.

Chapter 11
Understanding and Addressing the Emotional Impact of Disasters on Children and Families

Gwen V. Mitchell, Rosco Kasujja, Veehangi Singh, Kathryn Ahearne, Emilee Flynn, Audrey Norton, and David Schonfeld

Introduction and Objectives

The past two decades have seen a notable rise in both the frequency and intensity of major disaster events globally [33]. These events include natural disasters like earthquakes and hurricanes, as well as human-made crises such as industrial accidents and conflicts, resulting in extensive repercussions. The staggering loss of life, displacement, and economic damages from these disasters is estimated at about US$2.97 trillion. This increase in the scale and severity of disasters highlights the pressing need for effective response and mitigation strategies.

While the tangible and economic effects of disasters are clear, it's equally important to acknowledge the deep emotional and psychological toll they take on

G. V. Mitchell (✉) · V. Singh · K. Ahearne · A. Norton
University of Denver | International Disaster Psychology: Trauma & Global Mental Health Program, Denver, CO, USA
e-mail: gwen.mitchell@du.edu; Veehangi.singh@du.edu; veehangi.singh@healthonecares.com; Kathryn.ahearne@du.edu; Kahearne@readykidscville.org

R. Kasujja
Makerere University-School of Psychology, Department of Mental Health & Community Psychology, Kampala, Uganda
e-mail: rosco.kasujja@mak.ac.ug

E. Flynn
Emory University School of Medicine and Children's Healthcare of Atlanta, Atlanta, GA, USA
e-mail: Emilee.Flynn@choa.org

D. Schonfeld
National Center for School Crisis and Bereavement at Children's Hospital Los Angeles, Los Angeles, CA, USA

USC Keck School of Medicine, Los Angeles, CA, USA

© The Author(s), under exclusive license to Springer Nature Switzerland AG 2025
L. Umphrey et al. (eds.), *Pediatric Considerations in Disaster Settings*, https://doi.org/10.1007/978-3-031-85501-6_11

individuals, especially children and families [11]. Billions have suffered social distress and emotional trauma due to these events. Addressing these emotional challenges necessitates collective action at various levels, including international collaboration, regional partnerships, and local community involvement [11].

This chapter seeks to equip global health clinicians with a thorough understanding of the emotional effects of disasters on children and families. We will explore the complexities involved in caring for pediatric patients in such challenging contexts and delve into the emotional experiences of children, adolescents, and families impacted by disasters. By examining case studies from Africa, Southeast Asia, and North America, we aim to humanize the statistics and terminology related to disasters, providing insights into the varied challenges survivors face. It is crucial to approach these narratives carefully, ensuring cultural sensitivity and avoiding the reinforcement of stereotypes or the marginalization of historically vulnerable groups.

The chapter is grounded in the principle of "nothing about us without us," highlighting the importance of involving children and families directly affected by disasters in decision-making processes. This phrase was coined by Tshililo Michael Masutha, a South African advocate for disability rights, who emphasized that individuals with disabilities know what is best for themselves and should therefore have a role in shaping the programs and interventions that affect their lives [13]. By integrating the voices and perspectives of those with lived experience, we can better understand their unique needs, aspirations, and challenges.

We will start by examining the factors that affect vulnerability and resilience in children and adolescents in the aftermath of a disaster. Understanding the interplay of individual traits, family dynamics, community support, and environmental conditions is essential for developing effective strategies to support emotional well-being in these situations. Additionally, we will explore protective factors that can lessen the emotional effects of disasters and enhance resilience among individuals and communities. By recognizing and leveraging these factors, healthcare clinicians and caregivers can significantly contribute to positive outcomes for children and families impacted by disasters.

This chapter emphasizes the necessity of proactive, systemic interventions and preparedness initiatives to bolster resilience before, during, and after a disaster. By raising awareness and fostering capacity for protective factors, we can enhance individuals' abilities to cope with the emotional challenges that arise in disaster contexts. While protective factors are linked to improved outcomes, it's important to recognize that they do not ensure complete immunity from emotional distress. Each individual's experience and reaction to a disaster are distinct, and personal needs must be considered. Nevertheless, by integrating the insights and practices presented in this chapter, global health clinicians can help create a supportive environment that promotes emotional well-being and resilience in the wake of a disaster.

Objectives

1. Explain the emotional effects of disasters on children, adolescents, and families.
2. Identify the factors that affect vulnerability and resilience in children and adolescents after a disaster.
3. Explore protective factors that can reduce the emotional impact of disasters and foster resilience.
4. Analyze case studies to understand the varied challenges encountered by children and families in disaster situations.
5. Discuss strategies and interventions that global health clinicians can use to support the emotional well-being of pediatric patients in disaster contexts.
6. Highlight the significance of proactive and systemic interventions, along with preparedness efforts, in building resilience before, during, and after a disaster.

Emotional Vulnerability, Influences, and Risk Factors in Children and Adolescents in Disaster Situations

Children and adolescents in disaster situations are affected by a variety of factors that influence their emotional vulnerability and resilience. Recognizing these factors is essential for developing effective strategies to support their well-being. Individual characteristics, such as developmental stage, past experiences, the level of disruption caused by the disaster, the relationship between maternal and child well-being, family dynamics, social connections, and interactions with the broader community, significantly affect vulnerability. Additionally, the nature and severity of exposure to the disaster, the availability of support systems, children's perceptions of the events, the extent of disruption to daily life, and the resources present in their environment and community all contribute to the emotional health of young survivors.

Developmental Stages

Understanding the emotional responses of children and adolescents to disasters necessitates a thorough exploration of their age and developmental stages. Younger children may struggle to comprehend and process the event, while adolescents might face challenges related to identity formation and existential issues. Jean Piaget, a Swiss psychologist, developed a theory of cognitive development that outlines how a child's understanding of the world evolves from birth to adulthood [52].

The first stage, known as the sensorimotor stage, spans from birth to about 2 years old, during which children explore their environment through sensory and motor interactions. Key concepts such as object permanence and separation anxiety begin to form in this stage. The second stage, the preoperational stage, occurs from ages two to seven, where children can engage in imaginative play and use symbols to represent objects, though they remain egocentric. The third stage, the concrete operational stage, lasts from ages seven to twelve, during which children can think logically and connect concepts to tangible situations. Finally, the formal operational stage, which encompasses adolescents from age twelve through adulthood, is characterized by the ability to reason abstractly and think hypothetically. It's essential to recognize that while specific ages are linked to each stage, children develop at their own pace, so their understanding of the world may progress either faster or slower than their chronological age (Table 11.1).

Experiencing disasters can significantly affect a child's development and may lead to developmental regression. Children may exhibit a wide range of psychological, emotional, and behavioral responses. These reactions can arise in response to specific situations or events after a disaster, but they may also be more general and linked to underlying personality changes without an obvious trigger. The duration of these reactions can vary and is strongly influenced by resilience factors, which will be discussed in more detail later. Much like cognitive development stages, a child's responses will be unique and not strictly tied to their chronological age (Table 11.2).

Individual Life Experiences

Age, gender, prior trauma exposure, and mental health history are critical factors affecting the emotional well-being of children and adolescents in disaster situations. The age at which young people experience a disaster is a significant variable in the level of distress they may face. Dependency on adults for care is a vital consideration; infants, toddlers, and preschoolers are highly reliant on caregivers, while school-age children are somewhat less dependent but still need adult support. Although adolescents are less reliant, they may lack the experience and cognitive

Table 11.1 Piaget's stages of cognitive development

Stage	Approximate age range	Developmental concepts
Sensorimotor	0–2 years	Explores the world through direct sensory and motor contact. Object permanence and separation anxiety develop
Preoperational	2–7 years	Uses symbols (words and images) to represent objects and has the ability to pretend. Is not able to reason logically and maintains an egocentric perspective
Concrete operational	7–12 years	Can think logically about concrete objects and situations. Can add, subtract, and understand the conversation
Operational	12 year-adulthood	Can reason abstractly and think about hypothetical situations. Can strategize and plan for future events. Can apply concepts learned in one area to other contexts

Table 11.2 Common negative reactions to disasters

Age ranges	Common regressive reactions	Common psychological reactions	Common emotional and behavioral reactions
Infants	Crying, clinginess	Disorientation, irritability	Fear, distress, increased need for comfort
Toddlers	Thumb-sucking, bedwetting	Separation anxiety, sleep issues	Tantrums, clinginess, regression in behavior
Preschoolers	Regression in speech, toileting	Nightmares, phobias	Anxiety, fear, withdrawal, aggressive behavior
School-age	Regression in academic skills	Concentration difficulties	Irritability, mood swings, social withdrawal
Adolescents	Risk-taking behavior	Identity confusion, decreased self-esteem	Anger, rebellion, depression, substance use

abilities to fully understand the consequences of a disaster. The emotional availability and support from caregivers greatly influence a child's ability to adapt, especially for younger children who might feel abandoned when separated from their caregivers. Adolescents are particularly susceptible to developing major depressive episodes and are at a higher risk for substance use after a disaster [56]. Recognizing age-specific vulnerabilities helps inform targeted interventions and support.

Gender identity can also be a risk factor in post-disaster contexts, with female-identifying individuals facing a higher likelihood of additional distress. Internalizing symptoms refer to psychological distress that manifests without obvious external behaviors, while externalizing symptoms involve visible behaviors that tend to be directed outward, such as substance use disorders. Research from SAMHSA [56] indicates that female-identifying individuals, including transgender women, may be more likely to experience internalizing symptoms, such as major depressive episodes, and meet criteria for conditions like post-traumatic stress disorder (PTSD) and substance use disorders. Gender-based violence is also more prevalent in post-disaster settings.

Research has emphasized the unique risks faced by those who identify as lesbian, gay, bisexual, transgender, queer (or questioning), intersex, asexual, or non-binary (LGBTQIA+) in disaster scenarios [27]. Studies indicate that these populations disproportionately encounter disaster-related mental health challenges, often exacerbated by factors like discrimination, stigma, and insufficient support systems. The risk of gender-based violence in post-disaster environments further heightens vulnerabilities for LGBTQIA+ and non-binary individuals, underscoring the need for targeted interventions.

Individuals with pre-existing physical and mental health conditions are particularly susceptible to the emotional fallout of disasters. Those with chronic health issues—such as diabetes, epilepsy, or asthma—may encounter additional difficulties if their medication supplies are disrupted [41]. The mental state and cognitive development of children before a disaster also influence their ability to adapt [41]. Additionally, children and adolescents with neurodivergent conditions, like autism spectrum disorder (ASD), require specialized care and support during and after disasters due to challenges in sensory processing, executive functioning, and emotional regulation. These children face a heightened risk of experiencing familial abuse, neglect, and stress, which can worsen in disaster situations. Prioritizing their care and providing tailored support to meet their unique needs is essential.

Familial Connections and Interactions

In discussing the emotional effects of disasters on children and families, it's vital to highlight how parental well-being affects infants and young children. This is especially relevant for paternal mental health, including perinatal or postpartum mood and anxiety disorders (PMAD), which refer to the distressing emotions experienced during pregnancy and the first year after childbirth. These disorders can affect both women and men, regardless of age or background. Symptoms can vary in intensity and duration, significantly impacting the daily lives of both parents and their children. PMAD includes mood disorders, anxiety disorders, psychosis, and obsessive-compulsive disorders. Factors such as hormonal changes, social support, personal or family history of mental health issues, and childbirth-related stressors contribute to the onset of PMAD. Prognostic variability is considerable; some individuals may recover within weeks, while others might experience symptoms for months or even years. Experiencing a disaster during this period introduces additional risk factors, heightening the vulnerability of both parents and their children.

Research has linked PMAD during pregnancy to negative outcomes for infants, such as premature birth and low birth weight. Children of depressed mothers may show deficits in social, cognitive, and emotional development. Untreated PMAD can lead to serious consequences for families, as depressed and anxious parents may interact less with their infants, resulting in developmental challenges. Babies might face colic, feeding issues, and sleep disturbances, while older children may struggle with learning, attention, or behavioral problems. Furthermore, untreated PMAD can strain partner relationships and family dynamics. Resilience is associated with supportive adults in children's lives, including fathers, grandparents, or teachers [17]. Therefore, addressing the mental health of mothers, fathers, and primary caregivers is essential for effective interventions, as involvement from fathers and grandparents can mitigate the impact of maternal depression on children's outcomes [17, 42].

Understanding PMAD and its effects on children and families during and after disasters is crucial for providing appropriate support and interventions. Recognizing symptoms, seeking professional help, and addressing both maternal and paternal mental health are vital for lessening the effects of PMAD on family dynamics and child development. Additionally, acknowledging the complex connections between child mental health and parental mental health, along with the health outcomes related to parental depression and acute stress following a disaster, highlights the need for a holistic approach to disaster recovery.

Community Interactions

The extent of disruption and social cohesion within a community plays a crucial role in the emotional well-being of children and adolescents in disaster situations. When fundamental physiological needs—such as food, water, shelter, and clothing—are unmet, a child's sense of security is severely compromised. Damage to infrastructure, displacement from homes, and the loss of loved ones can heighten distress and lead to post-traumatic stress symptoms. Additionally, a lack of healthcare facilities, the loss of individual and family employment, and the destruction of personal property further diminish a person's sense of safety and security, exacerbating emotional distress and hindering recovery.

Specific Community Factors Influencing the Emotional Impact of Disasters on Children

- *Injured Survivors and Bereaved Family Members*: Individuals who have suffered injuries or lost loved ones in a disaster are at risk of heightened emotional responses [67, 68]. Physical injuries and grief can lead to intense feelings of guilt, anger, emptiness, and despair. The emotional trauma these individuals experience can be long-lasting, necessitating specialized support and interventions for healing and resilience.
- *Survivors with High Exposure or Evacuated from Disaster Zones*: Those directly exposed to the traumatic event or evacuated from disaster areas may face significant emotional challenges. They may have witnessed traumatic scenes, felt fear for their lives, or been displaced from their homes and communities. These experiences can hinder their ability to adjust to future situations and may lead to anxiety, depression, or post-traumatic stress disorder (PTSD). Providing immediate and ongoing support is crucial for their emotional recovery.

  - *Levels of Exposure*: Research on the Population Exposure Model highlights how varying levels of exposure to a disaster affect the risk of developing PTSD symptoms. This model acknowledges that while some community members may experience direct exposure, all individuals are impacted to some degree and must navigate their own experiences.
  - *The Dose-Related Model*: Studies show a dose-dependent relationship, indicating that children and adolescents facing greater threats or multiple disaster experiences often exhibit more trauma reactions and reduced adaptive functioning afterward. The type, extent, and duration of a disaster significantly affect children's psychological well-being [69] [16]. Generally, acute, short-lived disasters result in less psychological damage compared to prolonged ones that severely disrupt the social environment. Those exposed to successive disasters are at a higher risk for anxiety disorders, major depressive disorder, PTSD, and physical health issues. Therefore, screening for previous trauma exposure in children after a disaster is essential.

- *Separation from Caregivers*: Immediate separation from parents or primary caregivers can lead to lasting emotional consequences for children. Disasters often disrupt family stability, resulting in temporary or permanent separations. Such separations may occur during evacuation, displacement, or in the disaster's aftermath, where parents and children might be taken to different facilities for care. The absence of familiar, nurturing caregivers can heighten children's distress and increase the risk of negative emotional outcomes.

- *Loss of Homes, Jobs, Possessions and Schools*: Disasters frequently result in the loss of homes, jobs, and possessions, creating significant emotional and psychological stress. Forced relocation is a critical consideration when supporting children and families in crisis. Stressors related to evacuation often correlate with greater psychological distress and somatic complaints in youth affected by natural disasters [37]. Inability to meet basic needs, such as food, water, and shelter, can drain an individual's physical and emotional energy, making it challenging to address higher-level concerns. The upheaval, financial strain, and uncertainty about the future can lead to anxiety, depression, and a sense of loss. The age at which children relocate and its impact on their education can also influence their emotional responses [30]. Younger children may show fewer initial symptoms but may experience increased distress upon returning to their original communities. Providing school- and community-based resources is essential in post-disaster contexts.

- *Affected Individuals from the Larger Community*: The emotional impact of a disaster extends beyond those directly affected, influencing the larger community as well. Witnessing devastation, experiencing fear and uncertainty, and dealing with collective grief can adversely affect community members' mental and emotional well-being. Community-wide mental health support, fostering solidarity, and promoting resilience are vital for mitigating long-term emotional impacts on the affected population.

- *Additional Considerations for First Responders*: First responders who encounter traumatic scenes and support individuals during disasters may also experience emotional distress, known as "compassion fatigue" or "secondary trauma" [29]. This group includes law enforcement, firefighters, healthcare workers, mental health clinicians, and victim assistance professionals. Their roles expose them to personal physical harm while they assist survivors. Witnessing the suffering of others and hearing accounts of traumatic experiences can lead to high distress levels. The demands of their work often leave little time for emotional processing, and cumulative exposure can worsen symptoms. Recognizing and addressing the emotional needs of first responders, along with providing mental health support, is essential for effective disaster response and recovery efforts.

The Impact of Adverse Childhood Experiences

Adverse Childhood Experiences (ACEs) encompass various traumatic events or negative circumstances that a child may endure, such as physical and emotional abuse, neglect, domestic violence, the incarceration of a family member, divorce or parental abandonment, substance abuse within the family, and socioeconomic hardships [18]. These experiences can profoundly affect a person's long-term health outcomes and are associated with a heightened risk of stress responses following acute disaster events (Table 11.3).

ACEs and Autism Spectrum Disorder

Moreover, research by Kerns et al. [35] has emphasized the connection between Autism Spectrum Disorder (ASD) and Adverse Childhood Experiences (ACEs). Their study found that children diagnosed with ASD experience higher rates of ACEs compared to those without the diagnosis. Furthermore, the rates of ACEs are even greater among children with ASD from low-income families. This indicates that children with ASD, especially those in disadvantaged circumstances, may already face a heavier load of adverse experiences prior to a disaster. These children, along with others with disabilities, may need more comprehensive and specialized treatment and care both during and after disasters, as the physical demands of evacuation and sheltering can present additional challenges. Sensory sensitivities, difficulties with transitions, and communication barriers often linked to ASD can intensify their reactions to disasters and heighten their vulnerability [35].

By acknowledging these various factors influencing the emotional impact of a disaster, interventions and support services can be customized to meet the specific needs of different groups. Adopting a holistic approach to emotional well-being and recovery will enhance the overall resilience and healing of individuals and communities affected by the disaster.

Table 11.3 Common ACEs and associated poor health outcomes captured in the literature [20, 39, 53, 55]

Adverse childhood experiences (ACEs)	Poor health outcomes
Physical Abuse	Increased risk of diabetes
Emotional Abuse	Higher likelihood of smoking
Sexual Abuse	Increased risk of disability
Neglect	Higher rates of mental health disorders
Household Dysfunction	Elevated risk of chronic diseases (e.g., heart disease, obesity)
Parental Incarceration	Increased likelihood of engaging in risky behaviors
Socioeconomic Disadvantage	Reduced access to healthcare and higher rates of chronic illnesses

The Impact of Climate Change on Children in the Setting of Natural Disasters

In addition to the previously mentioned risk factors that heighten the effects of disasters on children, a 2017 survey by the American Psychological Association revealed that climate anxiety affects the mental health of over two-thirds of Americans. This form of anxiety, often referred to as eco-anxiety, arises from worries about the impacts of climate change [70], solastalgia (the yearning for a home environment that has changed) [71], or ecoangst [72]. Eco-anxiety specifically relates to the stress or distress triggered by environmental changes and the knowledge of these shifts. It is fueled by uncertainties about the future and highlights the risks associated with a changing climate. With the increasing frequency of natural disasters linked to climate change—such as severe weather events, hurricanes, tornadoes, floods, blizzards, and droughts—the prevalence of eco-anxiety among adults, adolescents, and children is also growing. Self-reported symptoms can include panic attacks, insomnia, obsessive thoughts, and changes in appetite due to environmental concerns [10].

Climate change poses significant threats to the health and futures of children and young people, who often lack the power to mitigate its effects, making them especially vulnerable to climate anxiety. A Lancet study (2021) found that 84% of individuals aged 16 to 25 express at least moderate concern about climate change, with 59% experiencing extreme worry. This concern is justified, given the disproportionate effects of environmental changes on younger generations. UNICEF (2021) reports that climate anxiety particularly affects children and youth, with projections indicating that around one billion children will face an "extremely high risk" of mental distress that impacts their overall functioning due to climate change. Children and young adults, already susceptible to chronic stress, face heightened risks of developing conditions such as depression, anxiety, and substance use disorders as a result of climate anxiety. For mental health clinicians, it is vital to consider culturally relevant factors in the context of specific disasters and climate change that may influence mental health outcomes and recovery.

Case Studies

In the following sections of this chapter, we will explore the intricate emotional experiences of individuals impacted by disasters through various case studies. These real-life stories bring to life the statistics and terminology associated with disasters, offering a deeper insight into the challenges faced by children, adolescents, and families. From a mother striving to stabilize her family after an earthquake in Nepal to assisting an adolescent trauma survivor in a refugee settlement in Uganda, and supporting a neurodiverse child coping with the aftermath of a climate-related disaster in Louisiana, these narratives provide valuable perspectives on the diverse reactions, resilience, and pressures encountered by survivors. By examining these cases, we aim to deepen understanding and inform strategies for delivering culturally sensitive and responsive support to disaster survivors, particularly children. Throughout this chapter, we will revisit these case studies as we delve into specific concepts.

Case 1: Nepal: A Mother's Effort to Restabilize Her Family After an Earthquake in Nepal

Ms. Puklong, a 35-year-old woman, lived with her husband and two young children, aged 4 and 7 years old. Her eldest daughter had a mild-mannered disposition, while her youngest child was prone to frustration and dysregulation. Ms. Puklong's husband had a history of depression related to complex childhood trauma and struggled with alcohol abuse for a decade before achieving sobriety, which he had maintained for the past 5 years. Although he had an aggressive attitude towards family and community members, his sobriety helped him control his temper. However, Ms. Puklong's family disapproved of her marriage due to differences in caste, resulting in her being completely disconnected from her kin relationships and not participating in local temple activities. Despite this, the family's economic condition was relatively stable. They owned a buffalo and goats and could afford their children's school fees.

An earthquake in 2015 brought significant changes to Ms. Puklong's life. Her home collapsed in the earthquake and subsequent aftershocks, leaving the family homeless. Her husband sustained a severe leg injury, preventing him from working and leading to a relapse in his alcohol consumption. Though estranged, she received word that her brother had been injured during the earthquake and subsequently died. Despite these losses, Ms. Puklong found purpose and energy in caring for her daughters and was determined to get them back in school. However, her youngest daughter experienced regression, exhibiting bedwetting, night terrors, and frequent conflicts with neighborhood children. Meanwhile, her eldest child was helpful and assisted with gathering firewood but stopped talking, often entering a dazed state or falling asleep.

MHPSS Interventions in a Complex Setting

To support Ms. Puklong and her family effectively, mental health and psychosocial support (MHPSS) interventions should be tailored to their immediate and long-term needs:

1. *Immediate Crisis Support:* It is crucial to provide a safe and private environment where Ms. Puklong and her children can receive psychological first aid. This can help them regain a sense of stability and process their immediate emotional distress.
2. *Routine and Structure:* Establishing a predictable daily schedule for the children, including designated times for meals, activities, and relaxation, can help reduce anxiety related to the loss of routine.
3. *Parenting Support and Education:* Providing Ms. Puklong with parenting support, including strategies for managing her youngest daughter's behavioral

issues and fostering open communication with her eldest child, can empower her in her caregiving role.

4. *Trauma-Informed Care:* Ensuring the children receive trauma-informed care from trained mental health professionals can help them process their experiences and develop healthier coping mechanisms.

5. *Family and Community Engagement:* Engaging supportive community members or extended family), even those initially estranged, can provide Ms. Puklong with additional resources and reduce her sense of isolation.

6. *Economic Assistance:* Providing economic assistance or linking the family to resources like temporary shelter, food, and school fees can help alleviate some of the financial burdens and allow Ms. Puklong to focus on her family's well-being.

7. *Alcohol Use Intervention:* Offering her husband access to alcohol use interventions and support groups can help him regain sobriety and become a more stable presence for the family.

Case 2: Uganda: Supporting an Adolescent Following a Traumatic Incident in a Refugee Settlement

In the Bidibidi Refugee Settlement in Northwestern Uganda, which hosts over 270,000 South Sudanese refugees, a 12-year-old girl named Abdo seeks medical assistance at the health post due to severe abdominal pain. During the examination, she discloses that she has been sexually abused by her maternal cousin, who is 10 years older than her and resides in the same area of the settlement.

Although there is an obligation to report such cases to child protective services, Abdo strongly emphasizes her unwillingness to involve her family or the police. She explains that her grandfather is a police officer, and notifying the authorities could lead to her immediate family being alerted. She worries that if her family is made aware of what has happened, they will force her into marriage with her cousin. Overwhelmed by distress, Abdo begins crying and shaking uncontrollably.

Legal Mechanisms and Cultural Considerations

There is a need to clarify the legal mechanisms that will consider the minor's cultural wishes while ensuring that decisions made are commensurate with the law. In Uganda, the National Child Act mandates reporting of child abuse cases to protect the victim. However, it also provides guidelines for ensuring the child's best interests are considered. In this context, it's essential to balance adherence to the law with the cultural sensitivities surrounding Abdo's wishes. The health post workers must navigate the complexities of mandatory reporting while addressing Abdo's fears of familial pressure and forced marriage.

Diverse Contexts of Laws and Medical Procedures

It is crucial to recognize that the legal and medical frameworks will differ significantly across various refugee settlements and regions. In Bidibidi, the legal requirement to report cases to child protective services remains clear. However, health workers should be prepared for diverse cultural norms and legal interpretations, particularly regarding child protection and support for vulnerable individuals.

MHPSS Interventions in a Complex Setting

To support Abdo effectively, mental health and psychosocial support (MHPSS) interventions should be tailored to her immediate and long-term needs:

1. *Immediate Crisis Support:* Providing a safe and private environment for Abdo to express her fears and emotions is crucial. Immediate psychological first aid can help her regain some sense of control over her situation.
2. *Legal and Medical Guidance:* Educating Abdo about her legal rights and the medical processes available to her can empower her to make informed decisions. However, care should be taken to respect her cultural background and concerns.
3. *Family Engagement:* Where appropriate, involving a trusted family member or community leader who can advocate for Abdo's safety and well-being may help in finding a solution that aligns with both legal and cultural norms.
4. *Community Support Networks:* Linking Abdo to community-based support networks can offer her additional protection and resources. Such networks can help her navigate complex cultural expectations while ensuring her safety.

Case 3: Neurodivergent Child Coping Following a Disaster Event

Aiden is a 12-year-old neurodivergent child living with autism spectrum disorder (ASD). Neurodivergence is a term used to describe individuals whose cognitive and sensory processing differs from the general population. Aiden's unique presentation of cognitive and social functioning due to his ASD diagnosis contributes to his neurodivergence.

Aiden lives with his family in Louisiana when a category 5 hurricane strikes the area. The hurricane brings significant wind and rain, resulting in widespread flooding, power outages, and destruction of buildings and roads. Although Aiden's family home is not destroyed, it has suffered flooding and requires repairs that will take several weeks to complete. In the interim, the family is staying in a shelter established for families with children temporarily displaced from their homes.

As you begin your volunteer shift in the shelter, you observe Aiden experiencing an emotional outburst with yelling and screaming as a result of the overstimulation he has encountered within the context of the disaster and need to reside in the shelter. The disruption of routine, compounded by unfamiliar surroundings and increased stress levels, has significantly affected Aiden's well-being.

Aiden faces specific challenges related to his condition, including:

1. *Sensory Sensitivities:* Aiden experiences heightened sensitivities to loud noises, bright lights, strong smells, and tactile sensations, leading to distress, anxiety, and sensory overload.
2. *Difficulty with Transitions:* Changes in routines, environments, and expectations pose significant challenges for Aiden, who struggles to adapt and experiences increased anxiety during transitions.
3. *Communication Barriers:* Aiden encounters difficulties with both verbal and nonverbal communication, making it challenging to express emotions, needs, and concerns, often resulting in frustration and behavioral outbursts.

4. *Emotional Regulation:* Aiden struggles with regulating emotions and managing stress and anxiety, which can manifest as emotional outbursts, withdrawal, self-injurious behaviors, or aggression toward others.

MHPSS Interventions in a Complex Setting

To support Aiden effectively, mental health and psychosocial support (MHPSS) interventions should be tailored to his immediate and long-term needs:

1. *Immediate Crisis Support:* It is crucial to provide a quiet, sensory-friendly environment within the shelter where Aiden can retreat to calm down and feel safe. Psychological first aid can help him manage immediate emotional distress.
2. *Routine and Structure:* Establishing a predictable daily schedule for Aiden within the shelter, including designated times for meals, activities, and relaxation, can help reduce his anxiety around transitions.
3. *Sensory Regulation Tools:* Providing sensory regulation tools like noise-canceling headphones, weighted blankets, or fidget toys can help Aiden manage sensory overload.
4. *Communication Support:* Using visual aids, social stories, or communication boards can help Aiden express his needs and emotions more effectively.
5. *Family Involvement:* Engaging Aiden's family in developing coping strategies and communication methods can reinforce a supportive environment and improve his ability to navigate the shelter setting.
6. *Access to Specialized Care:* Ensuring Aiden has access to specialized mental health professionals with expertise in neurodivergent care is essential for more comprehensive support.

Factors Promoting Children's Emotional Well-Being and Resilience in Disaster Situations

Individual Trauma vs. Collective Trauma: Understanding the Emotional Impact on Children in Disaster Situations

In disaster scenarios, both individual and collective trauma significantly influence the emotional effects on children. Individual trauma refers to the direct experiences and responses of individuals to traumatic events, while collective trauma involves the shared experiences of grief, loss, and disruption that affect a community following a disaster. This can manifest through the death of loved ones and community leaders, a breakdown in community cohesion, and a loss of security. Additionally, communities experiencing high levels of violence are at greater risk for collective trauma, which can severely disrupt social relationships and norms. Structural violence pertains to the harm experienced by individuals, families, and communities due to socioeconomic conditions, social institutions, and systemic inequalities that hinder access to basic needs [24, 64].

The community environment encompasses the social-cultural context (the people), the physical or built environment (the place), and the economic and educational landscape (equitable opportunities). In communities affected by trauma, these aspects are often compromised, perpetuating challenges instead of fostering resilience. Social-cultural issues may include weakened intergenerational relationships, fractured social networks, harmful social norms, and a diminished sense of collective efficacy in political and social matters. These issues reflect the long-term consequences of economic and social isolation, lack of investment, reduced social capital, concentrated poverty, and exposure to violence.

While traumatic experiences during childhood rarely result in post-traumatic stress disorder (PTSD), over 20% of children exposed to traumatic events exhibit emotional or behavioral difficulties. Moreover, 50% of those who have faced multiple traumas confront additional issues, including health problems, a higher likelihood of substance misuse, early pregnancy, and lasting negative psychosocial effects [31, 56]. Earlier research primarily focused on trauma from singular distressing events such as rape, war, or natural disasters, analyzing children's symptoms following these experiences. However, recent studies have expanded to include poly-victimization, which refers to exposure to multiple forms of violence simultaneously or cumulatively over a lifetime. The National Survey of Children's Exposure to Violence [48] indicated that children experiencing one type of violence are more likely to encounter other forms. Poly-victimization can lead to complex trauma, characterized by exposure to various traumatic events—often interpersonal in nature—with profound and pervasive effects, including distress, anxiety, aggression, hyperarousal, and mental health disorders. Factors that contribute to multiple traumas include communities with high rates of community and domestic violence, substance misuse in the home, child abuse, and prevalent mental health issues, all of which affect a child and their family's response to disaster situations.

Trauma-informed care practices have been developed and widely implemented as standard care for individuals with trauma and PTSD, primarily focusing on individual-level interventions. However, there is increasing awareness of the impact of collective trauma on larger communities, which can reach epidemic levels [7, 40]. While many strategies still prioritize individual treatment, it is essential to address the broader implications of collective trauma. On a population level, trauma can hinder efforts to promote health, safety, and well-being in communities, affecting decision-making, goal-setting, problem-solving, and interactions among community members. Communities grappling with trauma often exhibit damaged social relationships, disrupted networks, dislocated social norms that may promote violence, and diminished collective efficacy. It is crucial to move beyond an individual focus and adopt a comprehensive approach that considers the social, communal, and environmental factors that shape trauma and resilience in communities affected by violence [59].

Protective Factors

In the aftermath of a disaster, the emotional well-being of individuals, especially children, becomes a critical concern. While disasters can significantly impact psychological and emotional health, not everyone experiences distress in the same way. Resilience and coping mechanisms are influenced by various factors. Protective factors are characteristics, conditions, or processes that serve as buffers against the negative effects of adversity, help maintain emotional health, and facilitate recovery for both individuals and communities following disasters. By recognizing and leveraging these factors, healthcare providers, caregivers, and communities can profoundly impact those affected by disasters. These factors include aspects at the individual, family, and community levels that enhance resilience and well-being [6, 57]. Examples of protective factors include fostering social support networks, ensuring access to resources, utilizing effective coping strategies, and promoting a sense of empowerment [14, 65]. Individual protective factors encompass self-esteem, optimism, and strong problem-solving skills [54].

It is crucial to incorporate proactive interventions and preparedness measures to enhance resilience before, during, and after a disaster. By raising awareness and building capacity for protective factors, we can improve individuals' ability to cope with and recover from the emotional challenges associated with disaster scenarios. It is also essential to recognize that while protective factors are linked to more favorable outcomes, they do not guarantee freedom from emotional distress. Each person's experience and reaction to a disaster is unique, and individual needs must be taken into account. Nevertheless, by applying the knowledge and practices outlined in this chapter, healthcare providers, caregivers, and communities can help create an environment that supports emotional well-being and resilience in the wake of a disaster.

Resilience

Resilience is a vital concept in understanding how children cope with and adapt to adversity. It is defined as the ability to withstand challenges and recover quickly from difficulties. Resilience involves adapting to tough life experiences through mental, emotional, and behavioral flexibility, enabling individuals to bounce back and maintain positive mental health. Related concepts include grit, which refers to perseverance and passion for long-term goals; hardiness, which is the ability to thrive in challenging circumstances; and psychocentric focus, highlighting an individual's capacity to maintain control and prioritize their well-being during adversity. Together, resilience, grit, hardiness, and psychocentric focus represent individual factors that help children manage and recover from trauma.

Various elements contribute to personal resilience, such as an individual's worldview, engagement with their surroundings, access to quality social resources, and effective coping strategies during stressful times. Traits like optimism, a positive attitude, emotional regulation, and viewing challenges as growth opportunities can significantly bolster resilience. At the individual level, resilience focuses on enhancing psychological strengths, coping mechanisms, and emotional control. At the family level, it emphasizes fostering communication, cohesion, and support networks that can buffer against adversity. At the community level, it involves developing resources, social connections, and collaborations that promote cohesion and a shared vision.

Community support, resources, and infrastructure can provide protective buffers that enhance adaptive coping. Access to mental health services, community programs, and social networks can help children build resilience and navigate the emotional challenges of recovery after a disaster. Evaluating a child's social environment for resources and support is crucial for understanding their emotional distress and crafting effective interventions. By recognizing vulnerability factors and supporting children and families accordingly, we can improve their ability to cope with and recover from the emotional impact of disasters. Tailoring interventions to address specific needs can enhance the emotional well-being and recovery of children and adolescents affected by disasters, emphasizing a comprehensive approach that includes individual support, strengthening support systems, promoting social cohesion, and mobilizing resources.

Promoting resilience also involves minimizing situations where children take on parental roles that conflict with their developmental and emotional needs. Younger children should engage in age-appropriate activities, while older children may benefit from structured activities that provide stability when their routines are disrupted, along with opportunities to participate in recovery efforts. By identifying vulnerability factors and providing suitable support, we can help children and families better navigate challenges and recover emotionally from disasters.

Resilience after a disaster can manifest in various ways, all of which should inform behavioral health interventions in post-disaster contexts [43]. The primary objective of post-disaster behavioral health is to enhance adaptive functioning at individual, family, and community levels. Multiple frameworks, such as multisystem resilience and the Resilience Activation Framework, offer valuable insights into resilience and coping following disasters [1].

The Resilience Activation Framework highlights the significance of strengthening adaptive capacities across multiple levels. This holistic perspective acknowledges that resilient outcomes arise from the interactions between these different levels of influence. By addressing individual, family, and community dynamics, this framework helps establish a more solid foundation for recovery and growth after disasters. It underscores the need for integrated interventions that cater to the unique needs and strengths of individuals within their broader contexts, fostering adaptive functioning and overall well-being.

The goal of post-disaster behavioral health should be to enhance adaptive functioning. The Resilience Activation Framework views resilience not merely as a personal trait but as a dynamic interplay among individuals, families, communities, and larger societal factors. Multisystem resilience combines individual-focused and family-focused theories, emphasizing the importance of external factors that support mental health, such as social networks, healthcare access, and stable housing conditions. According to this theory, the ability of individuals or communities to respond to disasters depends on various components, including resource activation and depletion. The specific challenges faced by individuals, families, or communities also influence their capacity to respond effectively [43].

Thus, assessing children's emotional distress after disasters should also involve evaluating their social environment's capacity to provide resources that can mitigate the effects of exposure. These protective resources may exist at family, peer, school, and community levels. Resilient children can focus their energy on developmentally appropriate activities, such as play, building friendships, and learning.

Post-traumatic Growth

Post-traumatic growth (PTG) can emerge after grappling with the challenges of a disaster and its aftermath, resulting in positive transformations for individuals and communities. Research indicates that children as young as six can experience PTG [73]. While exposure to trauma is a significant factor, other elements also contribute to PTG, including intrusive and deliberate rumination. Deliberate rumination involves constructive cognitive processing of the trauma, whereas intrusive rumination consists of unwanted, repetitive thoughts that can exacerbate issues like anxiety and depression. Transitioning from intrusive to deliberate rumination is essential for promoting PTG. Studies have shown that when intrusive rumination lasts more than 12 months after a disaster, individuals are more likely to experience prolonged Post-Traumatic Stress Syndrome (PTSS) and are less likely to achieve states of PTG [4, 5, 8].

Social and Emotional Support

Evaluating the availability of social and emotional support for children and families is crucial in post-disaster contexts. Research indicates that emotional support serves as a protective factor, helping to moderate perceived stress and shaping social behavior in youth [44]. Interventions that encourage social engagement can reduce the emergence of emotional symptoms in children, especially in situations where families must migrate or relocate. Providing opportunities for youth to join clubs, participate in activities, and engage in community programs can help establish social networks and foster a sense of belonging, enhancing their emotional well-being.

The capacity of youth and families to adapt to a disaster is influenced by various dynamics and systems present in their lives before, during, and after the event. These include factors such as family functioning, community cohesion, resource access, and cultural context. Acknowledging and addressing these elements can enhance support and interventions for children and families affected by disasters. By adopting a holistic approach that considers the interconnectedness of these factors, we can offer comprehensive care and promote resilience in the face of adversity.

Cultural Considerations

Understanding the specific needs, cultural traditions, and capacity for behavioral health initiatives within a community after a disaster is essential. Tailoring interventions to fit the community's strengths and requirements enhances their effectiveness and ensures cultural sensitivity. Healthcare providers should be mindful of cultural nuances and offer care that respects and supports the community's unique perspectives and practices. Cultural diversity plays a vital role in disaster response, as different cultures have distinct ways of understanding and addressing trauma. By honoring these cultural differences, healthcare clinicians can build trust and deliver more effective support.

To comprehend a community's needs, it's important to consider factors such as language preferences, religious beliefs, and social structures. Collaborating with local leaders and community members can provide valuable insights into existing support systems and culturally appropriate interventions. Healthcare providers should actively listen to and value the lived experiences of the communities they serve. Utilizing language interpreters, providing translated materials, and incorporating cultural rituals can enhance the effectiveness of interventions. Regular feedback from community members is crucial for assessing intervention effectiveness and making necessary adjustments. Cultural considerations should be applied thoughtfully, acknowledging the diversity within a community. By prioritizing cultural sensitivity, healthcare clinicians can promote cultural safety, increase community engagement, and improve behavioral health interventions in post-disaster contexts.

When Should Professional Help Be Sought?

Knowing when to seek professional help is essential for ensuring the well-being of individuals and families affected by disasters. While community support is invaluable, there are situations where professional assistance may be necessary. Some indicators that suggest the need for professional help include:

• *Severe or Persistent Emotional Distress*: If an individual experiences intense or prolonged emotional distress, such as severe anxiety, depression, or post-traumatic stress symptoms, which significantly impact their daily functioning and overall quality of life.

- *Significant Impairment in Functioning*: If the individual's ability to perform daily activities, such as self-care, work, or school, is notably affected by emotional or psychological difficulties, including trouble concentrating, maintaining relationships, or fulfilling responsibilities.

- *Safety Concerns*: If there are worries about self-harm, harm to others, or the presence of immediate danger. In such cases, contacting emergency services or crisis hotlines is necessary to provide immediate assistance.

- *Lack of Improvement with Community Support*: If community support and self-help strategies have not led to meaningful improvements in the individual's well-being.

- *Co-occurring Physical Health Concerns*: If the individual is facing physical health issues related to or worsened by their emotional distress, mental health professionals can work alongside medical clinicians to ensure comprehensive care and address the interconnectedness of physical and mental health.

In situations where professional help is needed, it is crucial to connect individuals with qualified mental health professionals who specialize in trauma-informed care and have experience working with disaster-affected populations. These professionals can provide evidence-based interventions, such as cognitive-behavioral therapy (CBT), eye movement desensitization and reprocessing (EMDR), or medication management when appropriate. Unfortunately, in acute disaster scenarios, specialized mental health services often rank lower on the priority list for interventions. Clinicians in any disaster setting involving children must rise to this challenge by advocating for the unique emotional needs of children and actively seeking support and referral options whenever and wherever they are available.

Case Example of Recovery Process

In the aftermath of Hurricane Katrina in 2005, sociologists Lori Peek and Alice Fothergill initiated a 7-year research project to explore the disaster's effects on children. Their findings, presented in the book "Children of Katrina," offer valuable insights into the experiences of around 700 children aged 3 to 18 who were impacted by the hurricane [21]. They encouraged children to articulate their thoughts and feelings about the hurricane, uncovering three distinct trajectories in their post-disaster experiences: "declining," "finding equilibrium," and "fluctuating." Those in the "declining" group faced a downward spiral of increasing disadvantages, while children categorized as "finding equilibrium" encountered initial challenges but had access to resources and support that helped them regain stability. The "fluctuating" group experienced a mix of ups and downs, often lacking stability in some areas of their lives while enjoying a stabilizing influence in others.

The study emphasized the resilience and active involvement of children in the recovery process. Despite their challenges, many children engaged in supportive actions within their communities, organizing activities and helping others. Peek and Fothergill also highlighted the critical role of friendships in children's lives, especially after a disaster [22]. The disruption of social connections and separation from friends were significant challenges for many children, as they were frequently relocated to new schools where they lacked familiar faces. This research stresses the importance of considering children's perspectives when examining the impacts of disasters. Directly interviewing children reveals unique insights that might be overlooked if only parents were consulted. The authors found that children often shielded adults from their own difficulties by minimizing or concealing their troubles.

By recognizing the experiences and voices of children, we can gain a deeper understanding of their resilience and the support systems they need during emergency response and recovery. The study by Peek and Fothergill [74] serves as a crucial resource for policymakers, educators, and professionals working with children in disaster-affected areas, emphasizing the importance of providing tailored assistance and acknowledging the multifaceted impacts of disasters on children's lives.

Revisiting Our Case Studies

Each of the case studies presented highlights the complex emotional challenges faced by children in the aftermath of a disaster. Intervention consideration should include the following:

- *Case 1: Nepal*—Ms. Puklong and her family experienced significant disruptions due to the earthquake. Her children exhibit various trauma reactions, which can be influenced by individual characteristics, exposure levels, and social support. The Population Exposure Model suggests that while Ms. Puklong's family may have experienced direct exposure to the disaster, the entire community was impacted to some degree. Ms. Puklong's youngest child's regression and emotional distress align with common regressive reactions observed in preschoolers after a disaster. The loss of their home and support networks, combined with the disruption of daily life, can exacerbate their emotional distress. The dose-related model indicates that the extent and duration of the disaster have contributed to their trauma reactions. Providing comprehensive support, including trauma-informed care, access to mental health services, and community resources for housing and economic stability, is essential for their emotional recovery and resilience. Providing effective support to Ms. Puklong requires a sensitive and tailored approach that recognizes the unique challenges of her family dynamics. By offering trauma-informed care, economic assistance, and parenting support, MHPSS interventions can help her rebuild her family's stability and well-being amid the challenges following the earthquake.

- *Case 2: Uganda*—Abdo, a teenager, disclosed abuse and faces a difficult decision regarding involving authorities. The emotional impact on Abdo can be influenced by individual characteristics, exposure levels, and available support systems. Abdo's reluctance to involve authorities may be related to her fear of forced marriage and the potential consequences of reporting her cousin. The Dose-Related Model suggests that the intensity of the trauma experienced by Abdo can lead to post-traumatic stress symptoms and adjustment difficulties. Addressing gender-based violence and providing a safe and confidential support network is crucial in supporting vulnerable populations who may face increased risks in disaster settings. Trauma-informed therapy and legal assistance should be accessible to Abdo in order to promote her emotional well-being and recovery. Supporting Abdo requires a careful and sensitive approach that respects her wishes while ensuring that decisions are made in accordance with both the law and her best interests. Cultural considerations, legal obligations, and the unique challenges of refugee settlements must all be balanced to provide effective MHPSS interventions in this complex setting.

- *Case 3: Louisiana, USA*—Aiden, a neurodiverse child with ASD, requires tailored support to address sensory sensitivities, communication barriers, and emotional regulation. The emotional impact on Aiden can be influenced by individual characteristics, including his neurodevelopmental disorder and direct and indirect exposure to the disaster. Aiden's heightened sensitivities and difficulties with transitions align with the challenges commonly observed in neurodivergent children coping with disasters. The Population Exposure Model recognizes that all members of the community are impacted to some degree, but Aiden's unique needs require specialized interventions. Strategies should focus on establishing a routine, creating quiet spaces with low or gentle stimulation, providing specialized communication supports, and offering interventions to enhance emotional regulation and stress management, in line with the guidelines for addressing children's emotional well-being in disaster situations. Providing effective support to Aiden requires a sensitive and tailored approach that respects his neurodivergent needs. By creating a structured, sensory-friendly environment and equipping his family and caregivers with appropriate tools, MHPSS interventions can help Aiden regain a sense of stability and well-being amid the challenges of the disaster setting.

By considering the diverse factors that influence the emotional impact of a disaster and the unique needs of each child, interventions and support services can be tailored to promote emotional recovery and resilience. Taking a comprehensive approach that accounts for age, developmental stage, exposure levels, and the impact of the disaster on children and adolescents will contribute to their overall well-being and facilitate their recovery process. Healthcare clinicians and caregivers play a vital role in addressing the emotional needs of young survivors, and equipping them with the knowledge and tools to understand, intervene, and prevent mental health problems in children is essential for building a more resilient future for them.

Strategies to Support Coping and Accommodation Following Disasters

It is essential for healthcare clinicians and caregivers to acknowledge the various factors that can influence a child's experience and response during a disaster. By understanding the importance of these factors, they can provide appropriate interventions and support to help children manage their emotional reactions and reduce the long-term psychological impact. To reassure children about their safety, it is important to implement strategies that foster a sense of security. This can be achieved by creating safe spaces, connecting children with empathetic caregivers, and utilizing the Engage, Calm, Distract approach discussed below.

Considering each child's individual experiences and perspectives is crucial for gaining a deeper understanding of their emotional well-being after a disaster. Recognizing the subjective nature of their perceptions, as well as the challenges posed by separation from caregivers, loss of possessions, displacement, and the death of loved ones or community members, allows for more targeted and effective support. By addressing these factors in disaster response and recovery efforts, healthcare clinicians and caregivers can play a vital role in promoting children's emotional well-being and helping them navigate the challenges they encounter in the aftermath of a disaster.

Engage, Calm, Distract Approach

The Engage, Calm, Distract approach is a technique aimed at helping healthcare clinicians and caregivers effectively support children and families in the aftermath of a disaster [15]. This approach emphasizes the importance of connecting with children on an individual level and providing them with the time and space needed to process their emotions and redirect their energies into constructive activities.

Engage Engaging with children involves building a connection and establishing rapport. Creating a safe and supportive environment is crucial for children to feel comfortable expressing their emotions and concerns. This can be achieved through active listening, validating their experiences, and demonstrating empathy. Clinicians and caregivers can use open-ended questions to encourage children to share their thoughts and feelings, and they can involve them in decision-making processes by offering choices about what they want to share and what activities they would like to pursue next. This engagement fosters trust and collaboration, enhancing the effectiveness of the support provided.

Calm Promoting calmness is vital for helping children regulate their emotions and alleviate anxiety or distress. Clinicians and caregivers can model calmness through their demeanor and behavior by speaking in soothing tones, maintaining relaxed postures, and practicing patience. Techniques such as deep breathing exercises, muscle relaxation, guided imagery, and sensory awareness—encouraging children to name what they can see, hear, smell, and feel—can help them manage their emotional responses. Creating a calm and predictable environment contributes to a sense of stability and security for children.

Distract Distracting children from distressing thoughts or overwhelming emotions is a helpful strategy for redirecting their focus and providing temporary relief. Caregivers can introduce engaging activities that capture children's attention and allow them to channel their energy into positive pursuits. Activities may include art therapy, music, storytelling, play therapy, or engaging in hobbies that the child enjoys. By offering distractions, clinicians and caregivers help children shift their focus away from distress and encourage participation in more constructive experiences.

The Engage, Calm, Distract approach recognizes that each child is unique, and different strategies may be more effective for different individuals. It is essential for clinicians and caregivers to remain flexible and adaptable, considering each child's specific needs and preferences. By implementing this approach, healthcare professionals and caregivers can aid children in their emotional recovery, promote resilience, and support their overall well-being in the challenging aftermath of a disaster.

Enhancing Family Dynamics and Resilience in Post-disaster Response

Promoting strong family relationships and respectful communication within the family can enhance positive and adaptive responses in children. Tense and conflictual family dynamics can lead to disorganized and nonadaptive responses during interactions, negatively impacting children's sense of security.

- *Collaborative Engagement*: In the aftermath of disasters, children should receive age-appropriate information and have opportunities to ask questions. Involving them in decision-making processes and providing reasonable options for what they would or would not like to do is essential. By fostering open communication, healthcare clinicians and disaster responders can empower families and support effective coping strategies. Encouraging collaboration and active participation in family tasks and recovery activities strengthens support and fosters a sense of unity.
- *Limiting Exposure to Mass Media:* Continuous exposure to distressing images on television or social media can heighten emotional distress and anxiety in children. Many children may not realize that repetitive media coverage refers to the same event, leading them to believe that traumatic incidents are occurring repeatedly. Therefore, monitoring and limiting children's exposure to graphic images

is vital for their well-being. Media outlets can be encouraged to provide warnings about potentially disturbing content, allowing families to make informed choices about viewing. Caregivers can help by offering age-appropriate explanations and engaging in discussions about media coverage to alleviate fears and anxieties.

- *Attending to Cultural and Contextual Differences:* Children and families who have experienced prior trauma or chronic adversity may have heightened emotional reactions to disasters. Understanding cultural expressions of distress, along with traditional healing practices and rituals, can aid in delivering culturally relevant disaster response. Healthcare clinicians should approach children and families with cultural humility, respect, and sensitivity to ensure that their unique needs are met.

- *Acknowledge Lack of Trust Due to Historical Trauma*: The level of trust between a community and its institutions is crucial for successful disaster recovery. Addressing systems of oppression and marginalization is essential for healthcare clinicians to build trust and effectively engage with the community. Acknowledging historical trauma and promoting culturally responsive approaches can foster trust and facilitate meaningful connections within the community.

Promoting Community-Level Response

In times of disaster, community-level response and recovery efforts are vital for creating a supportive environment for children and families. Effective and coordinated community response plans significantly contribute to the resilience and well-being of children. Here are some key considerations for community-level responses.

- *Schools as Disaster Preparedness Hubs:* Schools can serve as essential centers for disaster preparedness by integrating drills and simulations into their regular activities. They can facilitate discussions about the roles individuals can play during disasters and assist families in creating personalized emergency preparedness kits and contingency plans. These exercises familiarize children with emergency procedures, enhancing their resilience. Additionally, schools can promote resilience-building activities and provide a safe, nurturing environment during and after disasters. Collaborating with local emergency management agencies and community organizations can further strengthen preparedness efforts.

- *Comprehensive Pre-Disaster Planning*: Prevention initiatives should begin well before a disaster strikes. Community stakeholders, including healthcare clinicians, should engage in thorough pre-disaster planning. This planning should incorporate strategies to identify and address the emotional and mental health needs of children and adolescents. By integrating mental health considerations into disaster response plans, communities can better tackle emotional challenges when they arise.

- *Mental Health Awareness Promotion*: Raising mental health awareness is crucial, particularly following a disaster. Community-wide campaigns can educate residents, parents, educators, and other stakeholders about the signs and symptoms of mental health issues in children and adolescents. Enhancing mental health literacy can lead to earlier detection and intervention, resulting in better outcomes for young individuals impacted by disasters.

- *Training for Professionals and Caregivers*: Building the capacity of professionals and caregivers is essential for providing effective support to children and adolescents post-disaster. Training programs should emphasize trauma-informed care, psychological first aid, and other evidence-based practices tailored to the emotional needs of young people. This training can be extended to healthcare clinicians, educators, social workers, spiritual leaders, and other community members who interact with children and families.

By implementing proactive measures at the community level—such as comprehensive pre-disaster planning, mental health awareness promotion, and training for professionals and caregivers—communities can establish tools and practices to help minimize the emotional impact on children and adolescents during and after disasters. A well-coordinated community response fosters a supportive environment that enhances the resilience and overall well-being of young individuals during challenging times.

Implementing a Whole Community Approach

Addressing the emotional needs of children in disaster situations necessitates a comprehensive strategy that extends beyond individual-focused interventions. While personal factors like resilience, grit, hardiness, and psychocentric focus contribute to coping and recovery, systems-level influences and community support are equally important for children. Cultural considerations are vital for customizing interventions to align with the specific needs and traditions of the affected community. Understanding the dynamics and systems in a child's life before, during, and after a disaster is essential for delivering effective support and interventions.

A whole community approach acknowledges that the most successful disaster response and recovery efforts engage the entire community. This strategy involves collaboration, coordination, and active participation from various stakeholders, including community members, government agencies, nonprofits, healthcare providers, and local organizations [19]. It highlights the significance of community resilience and collective action. By fostering strong partnerships and communication channels, a comprehensive strategy can be developed to support children and families throughout the recovery process. Suggested methods for implementing a whole community approach include:

- *Strengthen Community-Level Strategies:* Health clinicians should focus on strategies that build on existing community infrastructure and create safe community spaces to address symptoms of community trauma while fostering healing and connections among individuals. Reclaiming public spaces and enhancing the physical environment can enhance community cohesion and promote recovery. This approach is especially effective in collectivistic cultures, where community membership is vital for trauma recovery. Examples of community-level strategies include creating child-friendly areas for families, utilizing vacant lots for community gatherings, and identifying trusted community leaders to facilitate communication.
- *Establish Community Resilience Committees:* Forming committees or task forces that include representatives from various sectors can help plan, coordinate, and implement disaster response and recovery initiatives. It is crucial that these committees incorporate individuals from diverse backgrounds to ensure inclusive decision-making.
- *Improve Economic Opportunities:* Enhance economic prospects for youth and adults in heavily impacted neighborhoods through multi-sector strategies. These should involve increasing access to education, providing job training, and facilitating job placement to strengthen community networks and help individuals achieve a livable wage.
- *Foster Cultural Humility:* Interventions should be tailored to meet the specific needs and cultural traditions of the community to maximize their effectiveness and promote cultural sensitivity. Acknowledge and respect diverse cultural practices and beliefs, and incorporate indigenous knowledge and leadership to develop culturally relevant strategies.
- *Enhance Social and Emotional Support:* Evaluate and strengthen the social and emotional support available to children and families. Implement programs that encourage social engagement and build networks to reduce the risk of emotional symptoms, particularly for families who have been displaced.
- *Engage Community Leaders:* Community leaders, including religious figures, elders, and officials, can play a vital role in mobilizing communities and sharing important information. Leveraging their knowledge and networks can enhance community-wide support and participation.
- *Address Trauma at the Population Level:* Acknowledge that trauma resulting from disasters affects communities as a whole, not just individuals. Implement comprehensive strategies that bolster resilience, provide acute responses to community trauma, and promote healing in the aftermath of disasters.
- *Recognize the Fluidity of Gender:* Incorporate research and practices that highlight the significance of recognizing diverse gender identities and expressions. Emphasize the need for inclusive and equitable support for all individuals, regardless of their gender identity.

- *Special Considerations for Children with Disabilities:* Provide targeted guidance and resources for supporting children with disabilities in disaster contexts. Address their unique challenges, such as sensory, cognitive, and mobility issues, ensuring that interventions and support systems are accessible and inclusive.
- *Differentiate Individual and Collective Trauma:* Discuss the distinctions between individual trauma and collective trauma in the wake of disasters. Highlight the relationship between personal trauma experiences and their broader impact on communities, recognizing the importance of addressing both individual and collective trauma in healing efforts.

Revisiting the Case Studies: Understanding the Human Resilience in the Face of Disaster

Let us return to the case studies one final time. We have witnessed how a whole-community approach, the engagement of caring professionals, and tailored interventions can pave the path to healing and recovery. These case studies shed light on the importance of understanding the diverse factors that influence emotional well-being and resilience in children and adolescents after a disaster.

- *Ms. Puklong—Nepal Earthquake* Ms. Puklong and her family experienced significant disruptions due to the Nepal earthquake. The impact of the disaster on her children's emotional well-being can be influenced by individual characteristics, exposure levels, and social support. Recognizing the importance of engaging with Ms. Puklong and her family, a healthcare clinician from a local community organization reaches out to offer support. Through active listening and empathy, the clinician gains insight into the family's subjective perceptions of the disaster. They learn that Ms. Puklong's youngest child fears aftershocks and is worried about their father's relapse into alcoholism, which has worsened due to the stress from the earthquake. The clinician acknowledges the child's fears and reassures them that safety measures are in place. They provide Ms. Puklong with additional tools and strategies to continue to explore her child's fears and worries and offer continued reassurance of their safety and security where appropriate. Understanding the significant impact of the earthquake on the community, the clinician collaborates with community leaders and organizations to create support groups and coordinate counseling services. These resources provide Ms. Puklong and her family an outlet to express their emotions and concerns, fostering resilience and a sense of togetherness. Additionally, through community collaboration, the family gains access to housing and economic stability resources, reducing the acute stress and uncertainty they face.

- *Abdo—Uganda Flooding*—Abdo faces a challenging decision regarding involving authorities following her sexual assault. The healthcare clinician recognizes the importance of engaging with Abdo to understand her feelings and fears.

Through open communication, Abdo expresses her concerns about reporting her cousin, fearing potential consequences within her community. The clinician respects Abdo's wishes while ensuring her safety by establishing a confidential support network involving Abdo's identified trusted individuals within the community. Recognizing that post-disaster situations can increase vulnerability; the clinician may further choose to collaborate with local child protection services to ensure Abdo's well-being. Abdo is also offered trauma-informed therapy to help her process the trauma and to promote healthy coping strategies. Additionally, Abdo is encouraged to engage in community activities to promote access to social support systems. By addressing gender-based violence that may occur in post-disaster settings, the community works towards supporting vulnerable populations like Abdo.

- *Aiden—Louisiana Hurricane*—Aiden requires tailored support to address his sensory sensitivities and difficulties with emotional regulation. The healthcare clinician recognizes the importance of calmness and stability in helping Aiden manage his emotional responses. They create a sensory-friendly environment in the shelter by providing quiet spaces, visual supports, and structured routines. Engaging volunteers with knowledge of ASD, the clinician ensures that Aiden's unique needs are understood and met. Working in collaboration with other professionals, the clinician offers specialized interventions focused on emotional regulation and stress management. These interventions help Aiden cope with the overwhelming emotions and uncertainties of the disaster. By fostering a supportive and inclusive environment, the community facilitates Aiden's emotional recovery and resilience in the aftermath of the hurricane.

By implementing a whole community approach and seeking professional help when needed, disaster responders can effectively support individuals and families, address their unique challenges, and promote their well-being in the face of adversity. Engaging community members, leaders, and professionals creates a supportive and resilient environment that fosters emotional recovery and overall well-being.

Conclusions

The case studies featured in this chapter highlight the crucial need to incorporate cultural considerations, community-level strategies, and individualized approaches when supporting children, families, and communities after disasters. The varied experiences of Ms. Puklong, Abdo, and Aiden illustrate the complex emotional challenges faced by young survivors.

Integrating cultural factors, community strategies, and personalized care empowers clinicians and disaster responders to deliver more inclusive, culturally sensitive, and resilience-enhancing support. By advocating for and addressing each child's unique needs, clinicians in disaster contexts can cultivate a sense of safety, community support, and emotional recovery, contributing to the overall healing and well-being of those impacted by disasters. Cultural sensitivity is essential in tailoring interventions to align with the specific needs, traditions, and strengths of the affected community. Community-level strategies can create equitable job opportunities, enhance social networks, foster trust, and encourage collective action for the common good. Individual approaches, such as trauma-informed care and mental health services, support healing on a personal level.

The Engage, Calm, Distract approach fosters a supportive environment that provides age-appropriate information and engages children in decision-making. The whole community approach emphasizes collaboration, coordination, and widespread mental health awareness to ensure the well-being of children and adolescents post-disaster. Implementing population-level strategies and preventive measures can further mitigate trauma and enhance community resilience. Last, recognizing when professional help is necessary is vital; by adopting a comprehensive approach that encompasses all these aspects, we can work toward building a more resilient and compassionate society that can thrive despite challenges.

Acknowledgments Acknowledgement for contribution in this chapter: David Schonfeld.

References

1. Abramson DM, Grattan LM, Mayer B, Colten CE, Arosemena FA, Bedimo-Rung A, Lichtveld M. The resilience activation framework: a conceptual model of how access to social resources promotes adaptation and rapid recovery in post-disaster settings. J Behav Health Serv Res. 2015;42(1):42–57. https://doi.org/10.1007/s11414-014-9410-2.
2. Advocacy pcackage: IASC guidelines on mental health and psychosocial support in emergency settings. Inter-Agency Standing Commitee Reference Group. 2009. Accessed 12 September 2024. https://interagencystandingcommittee.org/sites/default/files/migrated/2018-10/1304936629-UNICEF-Advocacy-april29-Enghlish.pdf.
3. Anda RF, Brown D, Dube SR, Bremner JD, Felitti VJ, Giles WH. Adverse childhood experiences and chronic obstructive pulmonary disease in adults. Am J Prev Med. 2008;34(5):396–403. https://doi.org/10.1016/j.amepre.2008.02.002.
4. Andrades M, García F, Calonge I, Martínez-Arias R. Posttraumatic growth in children and adolescents exposed to the 2010 earthquake in Chile and its relationship with rumination and posttraumatic stress symptoms. J Happiness Stud. 2018;19(5):1505–151.
5. Andrades M, García FE, Kilmer RP. Post-traumatic stress symptoms and posttraumatic growth in children and adolescents 12 months and 24 months after the earthquake and tsunamis in Chile in 2010: a longitudinal study. Int J Psychol. 2021;56(1):48–55.
6. Beatriz E, Kaufman A, Salhi C, Kohrt BA. Integrating mental health into global development: Psychosocial programming in humanitarian settings. Global Mental Health. 2022;9:e32. https://doi.org/10.1017/gmh.2022.30.
7. Benjet C, Bromet EJ, Karam EG, Kessler RC, McLaughlin KA, Ruscio AM, Shahly V, Stein DJ, Petukhova M, Hill E, Alonso J, Atwoli L, Bunting B, Bruffaerts R, Caldas-De-Almeida JM, De Girolamo G, Florescu S, Gureje O, Huang Y, et al. The epidemiology of traumatic event exposure worldwide: results from the World Mental Health Survey Consortium. Psychol Med. 2015;46(2):327–43. https://doi.org/10.1017/s0033291715001981.

8. Bonanno G, Brewin C, Kaniasty K, La Greca A. Weighing the costs of disaster: consequences, risks, and resilience in individuals, families, and communities. Psychol Sci Public Interest. 2010;11(1):1–49.

9. Bürgin D, Anagnostopoulos D, Vitiello B, Sukale T, Schmid M, Fegert JM. Impact of war and forced displacement on children's mental health-multilevel, needs-oriented, and trauma-informed approaches. Eur Child Adolesc Psychiatry. 2022;31(6):845–53. https://doi.org/10.1007/s00787-022-01974-z.

10. Castelloe M. Collective trauma and the social healing project. Community Healing Initiative. 2018. Retrieved from https://www.martha@castelloe.com.

11. Centers for Disease Control and Prevention (CDC), Office of Readiness and Response. Caring for Children after a Disaster. Centers for Disease Control and Prevention. 2020, December 18. Retrieved September 11, 2023, from https://www.cdc.gov/childrenindisasters/features/disasters-mental-health.html#:~:text=After%20a%20disaster%2C%20children%20may,can%20cause%20stress%20for%20families.

12. Ćerimović E. At risk and overlooked: children with disabilities and armed conflict. International Review of the Red Cross. 2022. Accessed 19 June 2024. https://international-review.icrc.org/articles/at-risk-and-overlooked-children-with-disabilities-and-armed-conflict-922#footnote6_f2p06on.

13. Charlton JI. Nothing about us without us: disability oppression and empowerment. Univ of California Press; 1998.

14. Cherewick M, Dahl RE, Bertomen S, Hipp E, Shreedar P, Njau PF, Leiferman JA. Risk and protective factors for mental health and wellbeing among adolescent orphans. Health Psychol Behav Med. 2023;11(1):2219299. https://doi.org/10.1080/21642850.2023.2219299.

15. Colorado Department of Public Health & Environment (CDPHE). Engage – Calm – Distract: Understanding and responding to Children in crisis a toolkit for EMS and emergency department providers. 2020. Cdphe.colorado.gov. https://cdphe.colorado.gov/engage-calm-distract.

16. Dohrenwend BS, Dohrenwend BP. Stressful life events: their nature and effects. John Wiley & Sons; 1974.

17. Duan Z, Wang Y, Jiang P, Wilson A, Guo Y, Lv Y, Yang X, Yu R, Wang S, Wu Z, Xia M, Wang G, Tao Y, Xiao-Hong L, Ma L, Shen H, Sun J, Deng W, Yong Y, Chen R. Postpartum depression in mothers and fathers: a structural equation model. BMC Pregnancy Childbirth. 2020;20(1):537. https://doi.org/10.1186/s12884-020-03228-9.

18. Felitti VJ, Anda RF, Nordenberg D, Williamson DF, Spitz AM, Edwards V, Koss MP, Marks JS. Relationship of childhood abuse and household dysfunction to many of the leading causes of death in adults. The Adverse Childhood Experiences (ACE) Study. Am J Prev Med. 1998;14(4):245–58. https://doi.org/10.1016/s0749-3797(98)00017-8.

19. FEMA. A whole community approach to emergency management: principles, themes, and pathways for action. Federal Emergency Management Agency; 2008. Retrieved August 31, 2023, from https://www.fema.gov/sites/default/files/2020-07/whole_community_dec2011__2.pdf.

20. Fergusson DM, Horwood LJ, Lynskey MT. Childhood sexual abuse and psychiatric disorder in young adulthood: II. Psychiatric outcomes of childhood sexual abuse. J Am Acad Child Adolesc Psychiatry. 1996;35(10):1365–74. https://doi.org/10.1097/00004583-199610000-00024.

21. Fothergill A, Peek L. Children of Katrina. University of Texas Press eBooks; 2015. https://doi.org/10.7560/303894.

22. Fothergill A, Peek L. Kids, creativity, and Katrina. Contexts. 2017;16(2):65–7. https://doi.org/10.1177/1536504217714263.

23. Frounfelker R, Nargis I, Joseph F, et al. Living through war: mental health of children and youth in conflict-affected areas. International Review of the Red Cross; 2019. Accessed 16 June 2024. https://international-review.icrc.org/articles/living-through-war-mental-health-children-and-youth-conflict-affected-areas.

24. Galtung J. Violence, peace, and peace research on JSTOR. JSTOR. 1969; https://www.jstor.org/stable/422690.

25. Girls Associated with Armed Forces and Armed Groups. UNICEF. Accessed 12 September 2024. https://alliancecpha.org/sites/default/files/technical/attachments/tn_gaafag_eng.pdf.

26. Global multisectoral operational framework for mental health and psychosocial support of children. Adolescents and Caregivers Across Settings. 2022;2024:1–134. https://www.unicef.org/media/109086/file/Global%20multisectorial%20operational%20framework.pdf.

27. Gorman-Murray A, McKinnon SJ, Dominey-Howes D. Queer domicide. Home Cult. 2014;11(2):237–61. https://doi.org/10.2752/175174214x13891916944751.

28. Greeson JK, Briggs EC, Layne CM, Belcher HME, Ostrowski SA, Kim S, Lee RJ, Vivrette RL, Pynoos RS, Fairbank JK. Traumatic childhood experiences in the 21st century. J Interpers Violence. 2013;29(3):536–56. https://doi.org/10.1177/0886260513505217.

29. Greinacher A, Derezza-Greeven C, Herzog W, Nikendei C. Secondary traumatization in first responders: a systematic review. Eur J Psychotraumatol. 2019;10(1):1562840. https://doi.org/10.1080/20008198.2018.1562840. PMID: 30719236; PMCID: PMC6346705.

30. Hansel TC, Osofsky JD, Osofsky HJ, Friedrich PF. The effect of long-term relocation on child and adolescent survivors of Hurricane Katrina. J Trauma Stress. 2013;26(5):613–20. https://doi.org/10.1002/jts.21837.

31. Hillis SD, Anda RF, Dube SR, Felitti VJ, Marchbanks PA, Marks JS. The association between adverse childhood experiences and adolescent pregnancy, long-term psychosocial consequences, and fetal death. Pediatrics. 2004;113(2):320–7. https://doi.org/10.1542/peds.113.2.320.

32. Information Note: Disability and Inclusion in MHPSS. IASC reference group on mental health and psychosocial support in emergency settings. 2024. Accessed 12 September 2024. https://interagencystandingcommittee.org/sites/default/files/2024-01/IASC%20Information%20Note%20on%20Disability%20and%20Inclusion%20in%20MHPSS.pdf.

33. International Federation of Red Cross and Red Crescent Societies, IFRC. World disasters report 2020. Come heat or high water: tackling the humanitarian impacts of the climate crisis together. 2020. https://www.ifrc.org/document/world-disasters-report-2020.

34. Jordans MJD, Tol WA. Mental health and psychosocial support for children in areas of armed conflict: call for a systems approach. BJPsych Int. 2015;12(3):72–5. https://doi.org/10.1192/s2056474000000490.

35. Kerns CM, Newschaffer CJ, Berkowitz S, et al. Brief report: examining the Association of Autism and Adverse Childhood Experiences in the National Survey of Children's Health: the important role of income and co-occurring mental health conditions. J Autism Dev Disord. 2017;47:2275–81. https://doi.org/10.1007/s10803-017-3111-7.

36. Kiss L, Quinlan-Davidson M, Pasquero L, et al. Male and LGBT survivors of sexual violence in conflict situations: a realist review of health interventions in low-and middle-income countries. Confl Heal. 2020;14:11. https://doi.org/10.1186/s13031-020-0254-5.

37. La Greca AM, Burdette ET, Brodar KE. Climate change and extreme weather disasters: evacuation stress is associated with youths' somatic complaints. Front Psychol. 2023;14:1196419. https://doi.org/10.3389/fpsyg.2023.1196419.

38. LGBTQ lives and conflict and crisis: a queer agenda for peace, security, and accountability. Outright International. 2023. Accessed 19 June 2024. https://outrightinternational.org/sites/default/files/2023-02/LGBTQLivesConflictCrisis_0.pdf.

39. Lown EA, Lui CK, Karriker-Jaffe K, Mulia N, Williams E, Ye Y, Li L, Greenfield TK, Kerr WR. Adverse childhood events and risk of diabetes onset in the 1979 national longitudinal survey of youth cohort. BMC Public Health. 2019;19(1):1–13. https://doi.org/10.1186/s12889-019-7337-5.

40. Magruder KM, McLaughlin KA, Elmore Borbon DL. Trauma is a public health issue. Eur J Psychotraumatol. 2017;8(1):1375338. https://doi.org/10.1080/20008198.2017.1375338.

41. Mann M, McMillan JA, Silver EJ, Stein RE. Children and adolescents with disabilities and exposure to disasters, terrorism, and the COVID-19 pandemic: a scoping review. Curr Psychiatry Rep. 2021;23(12). https://doi.org/10.1007/s11920-021-01295-z.

42. Maselko J, Hagaman A, Bates LM, Bhalotra S, Biroli P, Gallis JA, O'Donnell K, Sikander S, Turner EL, Rahman A. Father involvement in the first year of life: associations with maternal mental health and child development outcomes in rural Pakistan. Soc Sci Med. 2019;237:112421. https://doi.org/10.1016/j.socscimed.2019.112421.
43. Masten AS, Motti-Stefanidi F. Multisystem resilience for children and youth in disaster: reflections in the context of COVID-19. Advers Resil Sci. 2020;1(2):95–106. https://doi.org/10.1007/s42844-020-00010-w.
44. McDonald-Harker C, Drolet J, Sehgal A, Brown M, Silverstone PH, Brett-MacLean P, Agyapong VIO. Social-ecological factors associated with higher levels of resilience in children and youth after disaster: the importance of caregiver and peer support. Front Public Health. 2021;9:682634. https://doi.org/10.3389/fpubh.2021.682634.
45. MHPSS key message bank for children and families in emergencies â the MHPSS network. UNICEF; 2022. Accessed 12 September 2024. https://app.mhpss.net/resource/cf-mhpss-message-bank.
46. Moore MW, Barner JR. Sexual minorities in conflict zones: a review of the literature. Aggress Violent Behav. 2017;35:33–7. https://doi.org/10.1016/j.avb.2017.06.006.
47. Morina N, von Lersner U, Prigerson HG. War and bereavement: consequences for mental and physical distress. PLoS One. 2011;6(7):e22140. https://doi.org/10.1371/journal.pone.0022140.
48. N A T I O N A L S U R V E Y O F, N., Slowikowski, J., & Administrator, A. Children's Exposure to Violence Children's Exposure to Violence Access OJJDP publications online at ojjdp.ncjrs.org A Message From OJJDP. 2009. https://www.ojp.gov/pdffiles1/ojjdp/227744.pdf.
49. Nctsnadmin. Understanding child traumatic stress: a guide for parents. The National Child Traumatic Stress Network. 2018, October 3. https://www.nctsn.org/resources/understanding-child-traumatic-stress-guide-parents.
50. Oliveros B, Agulló-Tomás E, Márquez-Álvarez LJ. Risk and protective factors of mental health conditions: impact of employment, deprivation and social relationships. Int J Environ Res Public Health. 2022;19(11):6781. https://doi.org/10.3390/ijerph19116781.
51. Peterson S. Interventions. The National Child Traumatic Stress Network. 2018, August 14. https://www.nctsn.org/treatments-and-practices/trauma-treatments/interventions.
52. Piaget J. The theory of stages in cognitive development. In: Green DR, Ford MP, Flamer GB, editors. Measurement and Piaget. McGraw-Hill; 1971.
53. Rich-Edwards JW, Spiegelman D, Hibert EN, Jun HJ, Todd TJ, Kawachi I, Wright RJ. Abuse in childhood and adolescence as a predictor of type 2 diabetes in adult women. Am J Prev Med. 2010;39(6):529–36. https://doi.org/10.1016/j.amepre.2010.09.007.
54. Rincón Uribe FA, Espejo CAN, Pedroso JDS. Role of optimism in adolescent mental health: a protocol for a systematic review. BMJ Open. 2020;10(7):e036177. https://doi.org/10.1136/bmjopen-2019-036177.
55. Salokangas RKR, Schultze-Lutter F, Schmidt SJ, Pesonen H, Luutonen S, Patterson PH, Von Reventlow HG, Heinimaa M, From T, Hietala J. Childhood physical abuse and emotional neglect are specifically associated with adult mental disorders. J Ment Health. 2019;29(4):376–84. https://doi.org/10.1080/09638237.2018.1521940.
56. SAMHSA. 2018. https://www.samhsa.gov/sites/default/files/srb-childrenyouth-8-22-18.pdf.
57. SAMHSA. Risk and protective factors. Substance Abuse and Mental Health Services Administration. 2019. https://www.samhsa.gov/sites/default/files/20190718-samhsa-risk-protective-factors.pdf.
58. Sarwer DB, Siminoff LA, Gardiner HM, Spitzer JC. The psychosocial burden of visible disfigurement following traumatic injury. Front Psychol. 2022;13:979574. https://doi.org/10.3389/fpsyg.2022.979574.
59. Saul J. Collective trauma, collective healing: promoting community resilience in the aftermath of disaster. Routledge; 2022.
60. Schonfeld DJ, Demaria T, Nasir A, Kumar S. Supporting the grieving child and family: clinical report. Pediatrics. 2024; https://doi.org/10.1542/peds.2024-067212.

61. Schonfeld DJ, Demaria T. Providing psychosocial support to children and families in the aftermath of disasters and crises. Pediatrics. 2015;136(4):e1120–30. https://doi.org/10.1542/peds.2015-2861.

62. The Human Cost of Disasters – An overview of the last 20 years 2000-2019 – World. 2020, October 12. ReliefWeb. https://reliefweb.int/report/world/human-cost-disasters-overview-last-20-years-2000-2019.

63. The impact of conflict on women and girls: a UNFPA strategy for gender mainstreaming in areas of conflict. United Nations Population Fund; 2002. Accessed 12 September 2024. https://www.unfpa.org/sites/default/files/pub-pdf/impact_conflict_women.pdf.

64. Weigert KM. Structural violence. In: Elsevier eBooks; 2008. p. 2004–11. https://doi.org/10.1016/b978-012373985-8.00169-0.

65. Wille N, Bettge S, Ravens-Sieberer U. Risk and protective factors for children's and adolescents' mental health: results of the BELLA study. Eur Child Adolesc Psychiatry. 2008;17(S1):133–47. https://doi.org/10.1007/s00787-008-1015-y.

66. 5 ways that conflict impacts children's mental health. Save the Children. 2024. Accessed 12 September 2024. https://www.savethechildren.org/us/what-we-do/protection/mental-health/ways-conflict-impacts-childrens-mental-health.

67. Keyes CLM, Dhingra SS, Simoes, EJ. (2012). Change in level of positive mental health as a predictor of future risk of mental illness. American Journal of Public Health, 100(12):2366–2371. https://doi.org/10.2105/AJPH.2010.192245.

68. Makwana, N. (2019). Disaster and its impact on mental health: A narrative review. Journal of Family Medicine and Primary Care, 8(10), 3090-3095. https://doi.org/10.4103/jfmpc.jfmpc_893_19.

69. Wyler AR., Masuda M, Holmes TH. (1971). Seriousness of illness rating scale. Journal of Psychosomatic Research, 11(4), 363–374. https://doi.org/10.1016/0022-3999(71)90020-2.

70. Clayton S, Manning CM, Krygsman K, Speiser M. (2017). Mental health and our changing climate: Impacts, implications, and guidance. American Psychological Association and ecoAmerica. https://www.apa.org/news/press/releases/2017/03/mental-healthclimate.pdf.

71. Albrecht, G. (2005). 'Solastalgia': A new concept in health and identity. PAN: Philosophy Activism Nature, 3, 41–55.

72. Goleman, D. (2009). Ecological intelligence: How knowing the hidden impacts of what we buy can change everything. Broadway Books.

73. Cryder CH, Kilmer RP, Tedeschi RG, & Calhoun, LG. (2006). An exploratory study of posttraumatic growth in children following a natural disaster. American Journal of Orthopsychiatry, 76(1), 65-69. https://doi.org/10.1037/0002-9432.76.1.65.

74. Peek L, Fothergill A. (2009). Parenting in the wake of disaster: Extraordinary stories of hope and healing. International Journal of Mass Emergencies and Disasters, 27(1), 41–53.

Further Reading

Peck SC, Dutta M, Patel R, Ramaswamy S. Community-based healing in the aftermath of mass trauma: A participatory action research approach. International Journal of Social Psychiatry. 2022;68(7):1258–1271. https://doi.org/10.1177/00207640221098654.

Index